THE 150 MOST EFFECTIVE WAYS TO

BOOST YOUR ENERGY

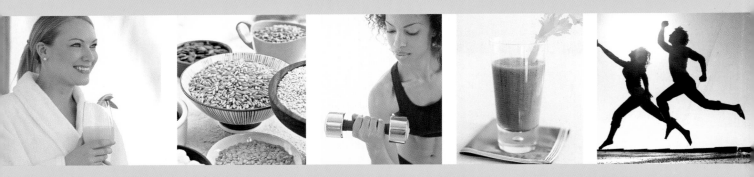

THE 150 MOST EFFECTIVE WAYS TO

BOOST YOUR ENERGY

The Surprising, Unbiased Truth about Using Nutrition, Exercise, Supplements, Stress Relief, and Personal Empowerment to Stay Energized All Day

JONNY BOWDEN, PH.D., C.N.S.

Best-selling author of *The Most Effective Natural Cures on Earth*

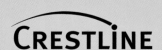

CRESTLINE

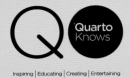

Inspiring | Educating | Creating | Entertaining

Brimming with creative inspiration, how-to projects, and useful information to enrich your everyday life, Quarto Knows is a favorite destination for those pursuing their interests and passions. Visit our site and dig deeper with our books into your area of interest: Quarto Creates, Quarto Cooks, Quarto Homes, Quarto Lives, Quarto Drives, Quarto Explores, Quarto Gifts, or Quarto Kids.

Text © 2009 Jonny Bowden

This edition published in 2018 by Crestline,
an imprint of The Quarto Group
142 West 36th Street, 4th Floor
New York, NY 10018 USA
T (212) 779-4972 F (212) 779-6058
www.QuartoKnows.com

10 9 8 7 6 5 4 3 2 1

Crestline titles are also available at discount for retail, wholesale, promotional, and bulk purchase. For details, contact the Special Sales Manager by email at specialsales@quarto.com or by mail at The Quarto Group, Attn: Special Sales Manager, 401 Second Avenue North, Suite 310, Minneapolis, MN 55401, USA.

ISBN-13: 978-0-7858-3593-6

Printed and bound in China

The information in this book is for educational purposes only. It is not intended to replace the advice of a physician or medical practitioner. Please see your health-care provider before beginning any new health program.

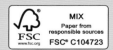

MIX
Paper from
responsible sources
FSC® C104723
FSC
www.fsc.org

To Anja

who makes me see what's possible . . .
and then helps make it happen

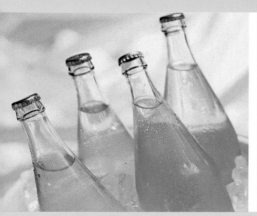
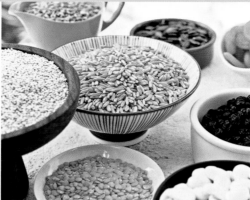
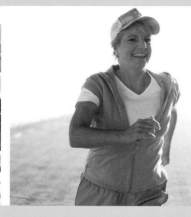

CONTENTS

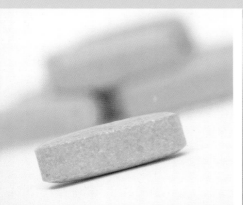
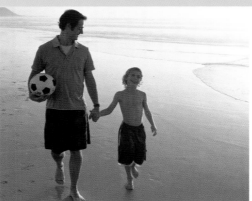
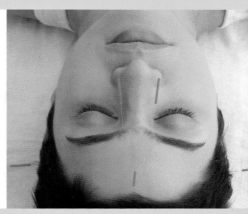

Chapter 10: Make Personal Changes for Inner Energy 232

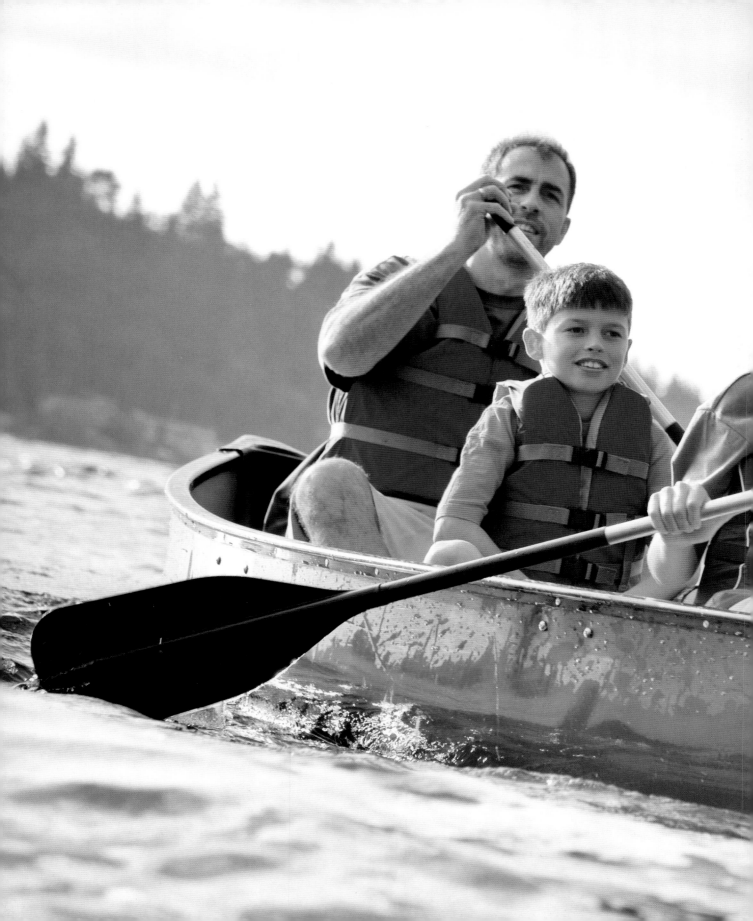

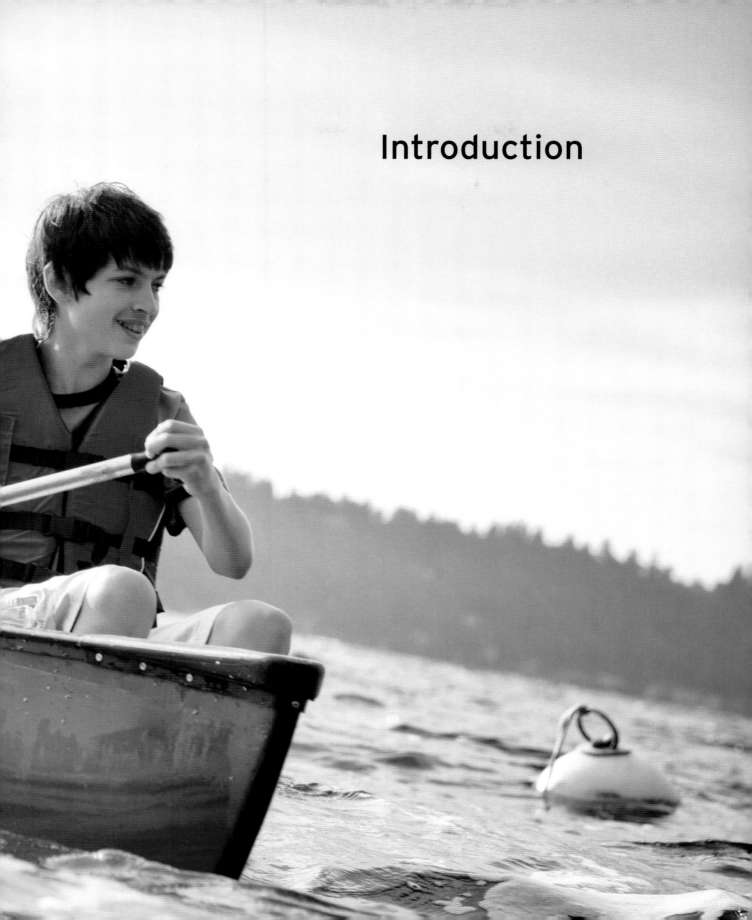

Introduction

"I'm tired all the time."

"I can't seem to get going."

Do these refrains sound familiar? They sure do to me. It seems hardly a day goes by when I don't hear from people asking about the best *food* they can eat for energy, the best *supplements* they can take for energy, and the best *exercise* they can do for energy. People all over are genuinely searching for anything to improve their rapidly diminishing stores of energy.

We all want that get-up-and-go we remember having—or seem to remember having—at one time in our lives. That motivation. That drive. That mental alertness and aliveness. That sense of excitement and power and optimism.

Where did it go? How did we lose it? And more important, how do we get it back?

In more ways than one we're in an energy crisis in this country. We're burned out, fatigued, overstressed, not sleeping, overstimulated, and just plain tired. And I'm talking about otherwise healthy people, or at least people who don't have any real pressing medical conditions. I'm talking soccer moms, NASCAR dads, executives of both sexes. I'm talking teenagers falling asleep at their desks. I'm talking average folks nodding off in front of the 6:00 p.m. news because they don't have the energy to stay awake. Not only are we tired, but we're also tired of *being* tired!

If energy is a concern to you—and I suspect you wouldn't have picked up this book if you didn't want more of it—you've come to the right place. This book is about energy. About that feeling of being alive, being awake, ready to take on the world.

Throughout these pages, you'll find strategies to promote optimal energy and particulars on how to fuel your body, nourish your mind, and power your spirit. I'll help you recognize the situations,

relationships, thoughts, and habits that deplete your energy. I'll also help you incorporate the energizing power of the sun, and discover how to use simple organizational tips to free up energy that gets wasted and depleted when you're multitasking. And I'll help you remove (or at least reduce) one of the biggest energy depleters on the planet: stress.

Once you let go of the negative blocks, you'll be open to accept positive energy.

FINDING LOST ENERGY

I'm known as a high-energy kind of person. I'm sixty-two years old as of this writing (2008), I wake up every morning without an alarm clock at around 6:00 a.m., and I can't wait to get started with my day. I take no medications or drugs, am in virtually perfect health, and approach the vast majority of my days with optimism and spirit and enthusiasm. Not *all* the time, of course, but *most* of the time, and I've been that way for quite a while.

But it wasn't always that way for me. I know what it's like to have energy, to lose energy, and to get it back. And I understand this both as a health professional *and* as a person struggling with the same issues that everyone else struggles with, issues that sap energy for everyone. And the first thing I know is this: We all want to find a quick fix to the problem of energy.

Let's face it. It's deep within our national character to want solutions, and to want them fast—doubly so if we happen to be male. We look at a problem, figure it out quickly, find a fast and easy solution, and move on. Late night infomercials make a fortune selling programs that promise a quick fix to your financial problems. ("Make a fortune in real estate—here's how!") They don't do so badly in the diet industry, either. All across the country, garages are packed with rusting gym equipment that promised "instant abs" in just minutes a week.

So is there an easy and quick solution to our energy crisis?

Well, yes and no.

Yes, in that there are *absolutely* certain strategies that you can put into effect right now that are relatively easy and that will make a huge difference to your well-being and overall sense of energy and vitality. You'll find many of them in the course of this book. *The 150 Most Effective Ways to Boost Your Energy* offers powerful approaches that you can start using today. But it also offers some long-term strategies that can really add to the quality of your life and ultimately add up to a huge difference in your well-being and overall sense of energy. You'll find those in every chapter.

But there is a "but." Energy is not something you get from a pill or a food alone. Sure, the right foods can help—and they do!—and so can the right supplements and the right exercise. (We'll talk about all of these in great detail in the coming chapters.) Remember, though, the causes of energy loss can be a lot more complicated than just the absence of a single nutrient or the presence of a single bad habit.

I'm hoping you'll be so excited about the changes that can be produced in your life with some of the easy, "right now" strategies we're going to talk about that you'll want to continue on the journey that will ultimately result in your removing all the barriers to the fabulous energy and glowing good health that can be yours on a daily basis for the rest of your (hopefully long) life.

So, to start, let's talk about removing those energy-blocking barriers!

Conducting Your Own Energy

Years ago, the world-famous conductor Herbert von Karajan allowed himself to be studied by the neurologist Antonio Damasio. In an ingenious demonstration that he later discussed in his book, *Descartes' Error*, Damasio hooked von Karajan up to all sorts of fancy instruments and measured what was going on in his body at different times of the day and during different activities (such as conducting or studying a score).

Damasio found that von Karajan's heart beat just as wildly and quickly when he was *listening* to music as when he was *conducting* it! Just hearing a piece of music—imagining himself conducting it, feeling the emotions and passions that stirred in him—changed von Karajan's heart rate, his blood pressure, and his entire physiology.

In short, what we *think about* has the power to create—or take away—energy.

Make sense?

THE TRUTH ABOUT ENERGY

As I worked on this book over the past six months, it became increasingly clear to me that trying to get more energy was like trying to grab a fistful of water. The way to hold water in your hand is to *create the conditions where water can be held*. You empty your hand of whatever it's holding, you cup your hand and make a little bed in your palm, and guess what—water will stay there! But if you try to grab it, it disappears.

Energy will flow right into your life and stay there like water in your cupped palm if you simply create the proper conditions for it, which means removing all the obstacles to it (we'll talk about them in this book) and creating a lifestyle in which energy is the natural outgrowth of your habits (we'll talk about that as well)!

How do you do this? Read on!

Achieving a high-energy lifestyle and being able to happily zip through your day with cheer and pizzazz require an exquisitely balanced and fine-tuned system. That's hard to achieve without enough sleep, a nourishing diet, regular exercise, stress management, and nurturing relationships.

High energy means a healthy body, which in turn supports a healthy mind and a healthy spirit. All the parts that make you the unique individual that you are have to work well. Otherwise, trying to increase your energy will be like trying to increase the performance of your car when the wheels are out of alignment or the tires are bald.

Which, by the way, is what many people do.

Imagine a car with a flat tire and an owner who's frantic to get somewhere, consequences be damned. If he puts pedal to the metal, the car *will* actually go, and if he ignores the crunching sound of the deflated tire and eventually the cracking metal of the axle, he may even make it to his destination.

But he will have done irreparable damage to the structure of the car, and he'll have to pay for it later.

How many of us do exactly the same thing to our bodies, refusing to slow down (until we reach utter and complete exhaustion or until disease forces us to)? Metaphorically, we're putting the pedal to the metal in a car that isn't functioning properly. By tuning it up first, making sure the oil is changed, the parts are lubricated, and the tires are aligned, we can be sure that the car will perform as good as new.

Let's stay with the car analogy just a little longer. David Kruger, M.D., an executive coach and the head of curriculum at Coach Training Alliance in Boulder, Colorado, poses this question to his students: If you were going to buy a car and knew—*absolutely knew*—that this car would be the one you'd be driving for the rest of your life, that you would never be able to trade it in, that you could never replace it, and that you'd have it forever, wouldn't you'd be a lot more careful about how you took *care* of that car? If you knew that this particular automobile would have to last a lifetime—*your* lifetime—you'd be much more likely to have regular tune-ups, right?

Well, that's the case with our bodies. We're issued one at birth, and one only. What we do with it (or neglect to do with it) affects what will happen to us down the road, including—*especially*—whether we have the energy needed to make the journey a blast.

HOW YOUR BODY FIGHTS BACK

My good friend Mark Houston, M.D., who lectures on medicine, hypertension, and metabolic syndrome around the country, is fond of saying, "The body has a *finite* number of ways to respond to an *infinite* number of insults."

Here's what he means: There are absolutely countless ways you can insult, injure, destroy, damage, harm, and wear down (or wear *out*) your body. You can assault it with junk food, pent-up anger, environmental pollutants, a sedentary lifestyle, too little sleep, too much alcohol, and not enough interpersonal connection. The list of things—and *combination* of things (including a particular *genetic* vulnerability to some of the stressors on this list)—is really, no kidding, endless.

But the body *doesn't* have an endless number of ways of responding to this long laundry list of things that can go wrong. Pain is one response. The breakdown of an organ system is another. A weakened heart or immune system is a third. There's an eruption or outbreak on the skin. Asthma or allergies. Heartburn and indigestion. Lower back pain. Headaches. Cancer. Depression. No matter how long the list is, it's *not* infinite, and it *certainly* isn't as long as the list of things that can conspire to create those effects.

Energy at Every Age

A few years ago, I attended a seminar where a silver-haired gentleman inspired the audience with stories about his life. He talked about all the projects he was involved in, including a new solar energy company that he was very excited about. He had written another book that was about to be released (I think it was book number twenty-two). His various businesses were thriving, as was his family life. He spoke glowingly about Lois, his wife of more than sixty-five years, and about his grandkids. Although his work and travels kept his schedule full, he still found time for regular walks in the mountains. And he ate well!

The speaker was Art Linkletter. At the time, he was ninety-one.

The audience responded with a standing ovation. As he left the stage, the crowd started buzzing—not about his rhetorical skills, but about his energy. Over and over I heard the same refrain, "Where does this guy get his energy?" (Where, indeed. If we could bottle that and sell it, we'd be set for life.)

Actually, his speech provided important clues about how to have a ton of energy. Clue number one: Be passionate about your work. Clue number two: Surround yourself with people you love. Clue number three: Keep your mind and body active. And clue number four: Eat the right food!

It's that simple—which doesn't mean it's easy.

But it *is* doable. This book is about helping you attain that kind of optimal energy. Now, I'm not saying that you'll become a multimillionaire, best-selling author who'll travel the world inspiring people at the age of ninety-one.

What I *am* saying is this: If you follow the strategies outlined in this book and make some positive lifestyle changes, then you *will* increase your energy, you *will* feel better, you *will* look better, and you *will* improve the quality of your life.

What Is Energy, Anyway?

In 1964, the state of Ohio convicted and fined the manager of the Heights Art Theater in Cleveland Heights, Ohio, $2,500 for showing a French art film called *The Lovers*, on the grounds that it was obscene. The case made it all the way to the Supreme Court, where Justice Potter Stewart, struggling to come up with a workable definition of "obscenity," finally threw up his proverbial hands and admitted, essentially, that while he couldn't define it, *"I know it when I see it."*

That's pretty much how most people feel about energy.

Tell some friends that you "just don't have any energy today" and absolutely everyone knows what you're talking about—this would not be a good day to bet on you winning a marathon.

That works, you think. Let's just think of energy as a feeling of "get up and go!"

Food manufacturers play on this commonly understood meaning of the word when they sell us "energy" bars and hope that you'll think that eating their product will make you want to do some wind sprints.

But nutritionists mean something entirely different when they talk about energy. To them, energy is another word for calories. In this sense, all food on the planet (except for water) has energy. But all food does not make you feel like going to the gym, or taking on a new project. Far from it. (We'll come back to this at length later on.)

Talk to a nuclear physicist about energy and you get a much different definition—energy, for that person, is some *measurable force* that is released from the nuclei of atoms—not exactly the same definition you'd use if you were talking about having enough energy to go to the movies tonight.

Even in general conversation, we frequently talk to each other about *physical* energy and *mental* energy, although, as we'll see, they're very hard to separate. In fact, the whole premise of this book is based on the fact that they're not just difficult to separate, they're *impossible* to separate, and that they influence each other in a continuous feedback loop, even at the cellular level.

But I digress.

For now, let's agree that even if we can't settle on a perfect definition of energy, virtually all of us can agree on one thing—that whatever energy is, it feels good.

Since we know that feeling good and feeling *energetic* tend to go together, understanding exactly why and how we feel good to begin with will go a long way toward helping us create that desirable feeling of energy more often. We also know that what we *think* about has a big effect on how we *feel* (as we'll see time and time again in the pages that follow). Therefore, it makes perfect sense that what we *think about* has a big effect on our energy levels.

However, one item that consistently finds its way onto the list of things that can go wrong—one of Houston's "finite ways" of responding to that "infinite number of insults"—is a *lowered energy level*. If you accept, as I do, that high energy and well-being is the *natural birthright* of every person alive, then any decrease in your energy, any increase in your fatigue, any diminishment of your *joie de vivre* is worth addressing.

When your body is overstressed—whether from an unhealthy lifestyle or relationship, a lack of sleep or a lack of purpose, too many obligations or too few connections—then all systems aren't go. Your body is screaming, "Houston, we have a problem."

This book is about checking in with mission control, making sure all parts are working properly, and all systems are go. Only then will you really have the kind of fantastic energy that it's possible to have every single day of your life!

RIDE THE FREEWAY OF ENERGY

Okay. Repeat after me: *Everything is connected to everything*. You might want to tattoo that under your eyelids, or at least imprint it in your brain. It's the guiding principle of this book, and we'll come back to it often.

Whether you're listening to music, reading a book, hiking a mountain, eating some protein, hanging with friends, taking a supplement, lifting weights, practicing yoga, getting a massage, meditating, chanting, smiling, dancing, laughing, or snuggling with your soul mate, each of these activities sets into motion a complicated string of messages and electric signals that start in the brain and produce powerful energy-creating messages.

You can think of those "energy circuits" as a giant freeway system. No matter which on-ramp you take, you can still find your way to the same destination. In these pages, we'll map out the various entry points to get you on the Autobahn of energy, where traffic flows freely, drivers are in control, and everyone's having fun.

It's gonna be a great ride.

Enjoy the journey!

—*Jonny Bowden*
Los Angeles, June 2008

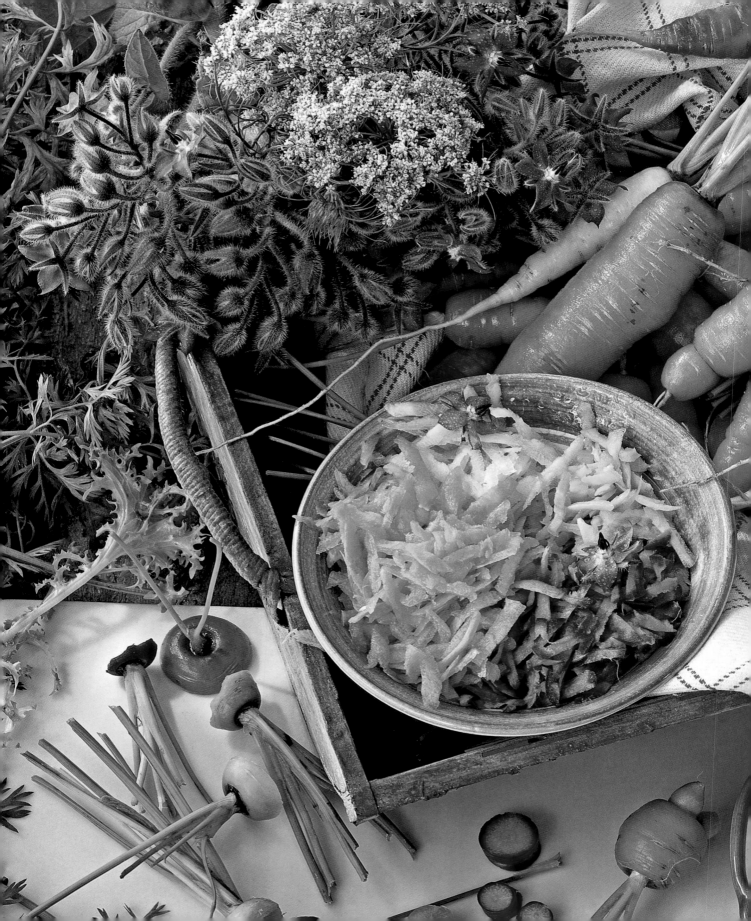

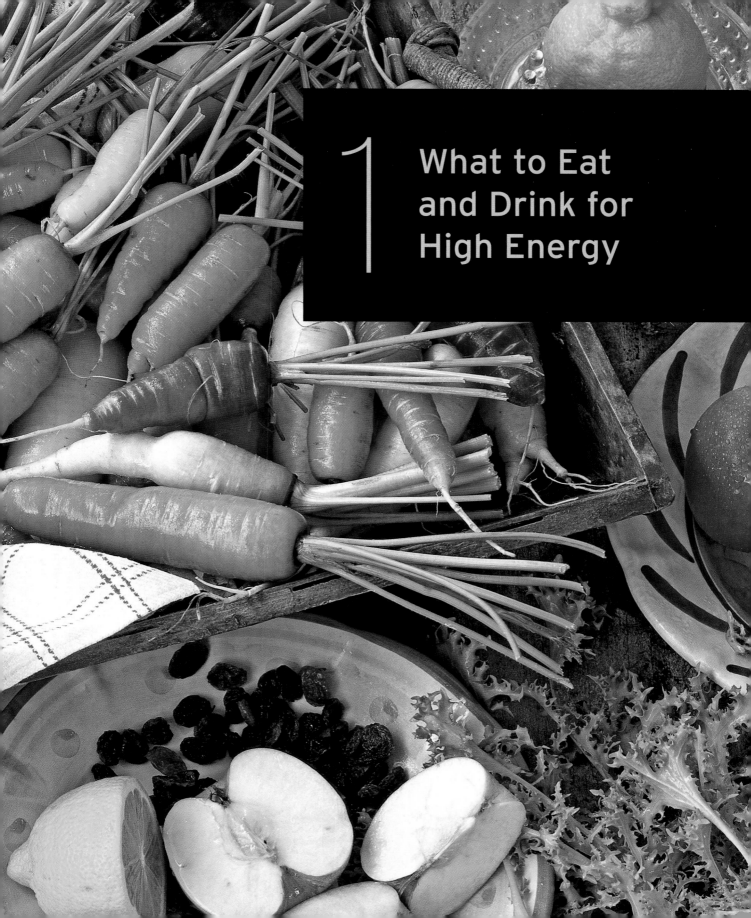

1 What to Eat and Drink for High Energy

Just in case you don't read any further than the first paragraph of this introduction, let me give you the take-home message right now: *Absolutely everything we do, feel, and think is influenced by the food we eat.*

Food is fuel. Our brains need it to think. Our muscles need it to move. The heart needs it to pump, the liver needs it to detoxify, and glands such as the thyroid and adrenals need it to make the very hormones that help drive your metabolism. Our organs, tissues, muscles, and bloodstream all need fuel (nutrients) to function, nutrients that we get from—guess where?—food!

But here's the key: If that food doesn't provide the right combination of nutrients and macronutrients (protein, fat, and carbohydrate), then eating can be like putting sugar into a gas tank. It will fill up the tank, but your car won't run very well. Too many of us use food merely as a way of staving off inconvenient hunger, rather than as a valuable asset in the quest for optimal health and energy.

When you give the body what it needs, it can—and *will*—do miraculous things. Remember, depression is not a Prozac deficiency and heart disease doesn't happen because you don't have enough Lipitor in your diet. Hippocrates, the father of modern medicine, had it exactly right when he said, "Let food be thy medicine and medicine thy food." The right food is truly the secret to high energy!

Would you ever sit down for a final exam when your blood sugar is plummeting? Would you go to an important meeting or interview when you're lightheaded from hunger? Do you feel like playing a competitive round of golf or tennis or running a race immediately after finishing a holiday dinner? Of course not, and that's precisely because food is fuel, and not having enough, or, just as bad, having the wrong kind, sets you up for guaranteed failure in any task you undertake.

Bottom line: If you want to perform like a high-energy person, you're going to have to eat like one. You should select your food the way Formula One drivers select their gasoline. Those Ferrari teams racing in Monaco don't just stop at any local gas station when they need fuel—they're driving highly tuned, multimillion dollar machines that require the highest quality gasoline on the planet. You can be sure they're not making pit stops at the local Al's Stop and Gas. Your body is at least as complicated and intricate and potentially as high performance a machine as a Formula One racing car, and it deserves the same quality of care.

It all starts with food. Rich, nutrient-dense, whole food carefully selected to give you the maximum nutritional bang for your buck, which means food that:

- keeps you *off* the blood sugar roller coaster.
- provides you with sustained energy throughout the day.
- gives your body *all* the nutrients—vitamins, minerals, and phytochemicals—it needs for every metabolic, energy-producing process.
- provides adequate protein for growth, repair, and performance.
- provides adequate fat for energy and health.

This section contains some of the most effective ways you can boost—and even more important, *sustain*—your energy using food and drink. Remember, when all is said and done, what you put in your mouth is the number one source of energy in the world.

Enjoy!

#1

Eat Protein at Every Meal for All-Day Energy

In my early days as a personal trainer, I believed the myth that carbs give you energy. That's why I was always surprised that I didn't feel very energetic after eating a high-carb snack. In fact, quite the opposite.

I later learned why. The appetite control mechanisms that send messages from your *gut* to your *brain* signaling that you've had enough to eat work very well with protein and fat, which have been in the diet of the human genus for 2.4 million years. The "satiety" molecules in the gut are exquisitely tuned to respond to those macronutrients, which they recognize quite well.

But those appetite control mechanisms don't work nearly as well with carbohydrates. For one thing, we haven't had as much "practice" with them, because most of the carbohydrates we eat (from grains) are relatively new in the human diet, and the highly processed kind, which make up most of the American diet, are virtually unprecedented. (In case you were wondering, that explains why it's so easy to eat six bowls of cereal watching reruns of *Friends*. Not that I've ever done that, of course, but I've *heard* of it.)

Because protein (and fat) just naturally activate the body's innate satiety mechanisms, it's a lot less likely you'll overeat, and if you don't overeat, you're a lot less likely to fall into that post-meal slump. Plus, when your meal has a greater ratio of protein to carbohydrate, it stabilizes blood sugar and reduces insulin response. As an added bonus, new research suggests that *leucine*, an amino acid found in protein, helps you maintain muscle mass while losing body fat during weight loss.

For high-energy snack food, think nuts, cheese (string cheese is a great choice), hard-boiled eggs, jerky, or some leftover chicken, all of which, by the way, are extremely portable. (There goes the excuse "the snack machine was the only thing around." Sorry about that!)

You can add a piece of fruit to the mix or some veggie crudités, such as carrots, celery, broccoli, and cauliflower, but what you *can't* do is grab a bag of chips or pretzels or a chocolate chip cookie. Or at least not if you want to boost your energy!

Because protein (and fat) just naturally activate the body's innate satiety mechanisms, it's a lot less likely you'll overeat, and if you don't overeat, you're a lot less likely to fall into that post-meal slump.

ENERGY FROM THE SEA

Another snack, the one that gives me the most energy—literally changing my mood and vigor for the rest of the afternoon—is tuna fish.

For a while, this kind of mystified me, especially because I was still under the sway of the prevailing myths about carbohydrates. But I felt energized for hours when I ate it, sometimes alone, sometimes on a single slice of high-fiber bread.

I found out that tuna contains a lot of the amino acid *tyrosine,** which converts to *dopamine,* a neurotransmitter that helps keep you focused and alert. (Dopamine is also a big player in the rush that comes from falling in love.) To this day, a tuna sandwich on whole-grain bread with a glass of raw** organic milk will keep my energy tank full for hours. Fact is, protein is highly energizing for many people.

So here's my number one tip for higher energy: Every single meal should contain protein. (Ideally, so should every snack, but let's fight the big battles first.)

To recap, protein has less of an effect on insulin ("the hunger hormone") than carbs do, is more satisfying, and sustains energy without making you tired. The body recognizes protein (and fat) as physiological and dietary requirements, and it knows quite well what to do with them.

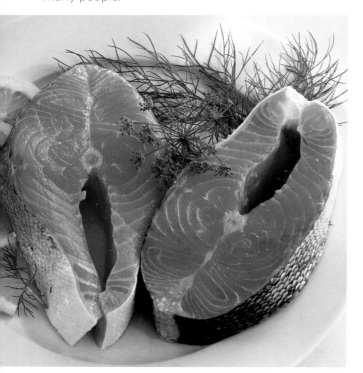

#2

Stop Ordering Egg White Omelets

Ordering egg white omelets is an idea whose time has come—and gone. (Long gone!) Mother Nature put the egg together the way she did for a reason.

Eggs—yolks and all—contain more than fifteen different vitamins and minerals, including double-digit percentages of the daily value for important energy vitamins such as riboflavin (vitamin B_2) and vitamin B_{12}, not to mention some of the highest quality protein on the planet. And that's a great recipe for energy.

The yolk is a rich source of an essential nutrient called *choline,* which is usually thought of as a member of the B-vitamin family. Choline is needed for the synthesis of *acetylcholine,* which is one of the major neurotransmitters in the body. That means it helps transmit information in the brain and is absolutely critical for memory and thought.

*Only protein contains amino acids such as tyrosine.
**To read why raw milk is one of the best foods on the planet, see my book The 150 Healthiest Foods on Earth.

Having adequate levels of acetylcholine also helps protect against dementia!

The choline in egg yolks also helps the body form a chemical called *betaine*, which in turn reduces another body chemical called *homocysteine*. Homocysteine can slow you down in a number of ways. It's a nasty little chemical compound that's made naturally in the body, but when it builds up, it can contribute to inflammation and increase the risk for heart disease and stroke, both of which are not exactly at the top of your must-have list. High levels of homocysteine are also linked to a greater risk of fractures, which isn't something that's likely to increase your get up and go either.

If all that weren't enough, the choline and phosphatidylcholine* in egg yolks help the liver get rid of the kinds of toxins that can drain your energy. Remember that the liver is ground zero for detoxification, and the more help you can give it, the better off you'll be.

With the number of energy-zapping toxins we're exposed to on a daily basis, your liver can use all the help it can get. Eggs—complete with the nutritious yolk—can help. Eggs are truly an energy superfood.

*A close relative of choline.

Confused About Protein?

Confused about protein? I don't blame you! For years we've been told that carbohydrates are the food we need for energy. However, carbohydrates (at least the processed variety, which is what most of us eat) do nothing but send you on a blood sugar roller coaster that is death to your energy levels. Protein comes from the Greek word meaning "primary." Protein is the real energy food.

Protein can make you feel satisfied without feeling stuffed, a surefire prescription for feeling energetic throughout your day. Eating protein is also a surefire way to stimulate your metabolism, especially when you combine it with weight training (see page 115). Weight training builds muscle, and muscle, in turn, burns both calories and fat. Protein has been shown in several studies to actually stimulate *thermogenesis* (the production of heat by burning calories). Together, they're a great formula boosting energy naturally.

When I see people with low energy, I'm almost always struck by how much better they do when they revamp their diet and increase their protein. Our Paleolithic ancestors, with whom we share a virtually identical digestive system, nourished themselves on a combination of protein and plant foods. If they could hunt, fish, gather, or pluck it, they ate it. And they weren't exactly low-energy folks—those protein-eating Paleolithic ancestors of ours had enough energy to typically travel twenty miles per day (on foot!).

Try Eating in the Zone

When my friend Barry Sears, Ph.D., first wrote his classic book *The Zone*, he intended it for cardiologists. Little did he suspect that his heart-healthy diet program of 40 percent carbohydrates, 30 percent protein, and 30 percent fat would soon catch on as one of the greatest high-energy eating programs on the planet. He called this diet "The Zone" because it kept blood sugar (and insulin levels) in the ideal "zone" for stable and sustained energy throughout the day.

Let's back up a second and you'll soon see why eating in the zone can be an easy prescription for higher energy. It all goes back to the founder of the Atkins Diet, Robert Atkins. Back in 1972, Atkins introduced the topic of insulin and its effects to the national conversation about diet. At the time, that conversation was limited to the profound effects of insulin on weight and weight loss.

As time went on, others—notably, Sears and Drs. Michael and Mary Dan Eades—expanded the discussion. They noticed the profound effects hormones such as insulin had not just on weight, but also on energy and well-being. The Eades' contribution to diet and energy is the foundation of what I've written here about protein (see page 24). Sears had a slightly different approach that many people have found to be the answer for increasing energy all day long.

Sears' book found a huge audience in the general public that identified with its fresh point of view about the effect food has on hormones and energy. These folks knew quite well that some meals made them tired and some gave them energy. They had correctly observed that some ways of eating seemed to make them fat and lethargic while others made them feel "lean and hungry" and energetic, and they intuited that the reason might have something to do with the *composition of the meals* rather than just the number of calories in them.

Borrowing a term well known to athletes and performers who understood intuitively what being "in the zone" meant, Sears argued that if you ate the right proportion of fats, carbs, and protein, you could get—and stay—in the zone, resulting in all sorts of benefits.

GET OFF THE ROLLER COASTER

Although many people didn't understand this, what Sears really meant was that there was an ideal *zone* for both blood sugar and the hormone insulin, a zone that would lead not only to weight maintenance but also to optimal energy and vitality.

Insulin is basically a storage hormone. High levels of insulin will eventually drive excess sugar into the fat cells and produce results that don't look very good in the dressing room mirrors of Macy's.

The high-carb diet so popular at the time had the unintended result of driving insulin through the roof, resulting in precisely the blood sugar roller coaster that zapped energy and made people fat, miserable, and ultimately unhealthy.

Sears argued for an ideal zone for both blood sugar and insulin levels, one that would produce sustained energy, good health, and, incidentally, natural weight loss. The ideal zone for both blood sugar and insulin is much like the porridge on Goldilocks' table—"not too hot, not too cold, but just right."

Sears also argued—absolutely correctly, as it turns out—that a diet high in carbohydrates and low in fat was likely to keep both blood sugar and insulin higher than ideal, ultimately leading to a form of blood sugar hell that looks exactly like the blood sugar roller coaster I described above. This is bad news from the standpoint of weight and health, but it's also bad news from the point of view of energy.

You see, insulin is basically a storage hormone. High levels of insulin will eventually drive excess sugar into the fat cells and produce results that don't look very good in the dressing room mirrors of Macy's.

In addition, high levels of blood sugar and insulin also lead to one of two scenarios, neither of them good. Eventually, either blood sugar responds to all that excess insulin and comes way, way down (basically decimating your energy levels) or both blood sugar and insulin stay elevated. The latter happens when the cells get so sick of insulin knocking on their doors that they basically shut down and start ignoring their pleas to let them in. The cells become what's known as *insulin resistant*.

This is the first step in a scenario that can and frequently does lead to either metabolic syndrome (a collection of symptoms that include high blood pressure and elevated triglycerides, increasing your risk for heart disease and stroke) or to full-blown diabetes.

One scenario it does *not* lead to is higher energy.

THE RIGHT BALANCE EQUALS GREAT ENERGY

Protein, fat, and carbohydrates are classes of food that are known as *macronutrients* (as opposed to the *micronutrients* that are vitamins, minerals, and the like). The balance of these three macronutrients is critical for controlling blood sugar and insulin, and ultimately for sustaining energy.

Too many carbs and you've bought yourself a ticket on the blood sugar roller coaster. Too few (of the good, natural, "slow-burning" carbs such as vegetables) and you've got too little fiber in your diet, not to mention too few of the important vitamins, minerals, and phytochemicals that stoke your metabolism and ultimately allow you to experience high energy.

Sears argued that a diet composed of about 40 percent carbohydrates, 30 percent fat, and 30 percent protein was the perfect balance, ideal for addressing all these concerns. His Zone program now seems so reasonable and conservative that it is hard to understand what all the fuss was about, but it caused nothing short of apoplexy in the moribund halls of the American Dietetic Association, a conservative (and often irrelevant) organization that pushed its high-carb diet on the world as the solution to all our nutritional woes.

No matter. It now appears that the only serious argument with Sears's prescription is that some people do well with (and may even need) far fewer carbohydrates than the 40 percent he recommends, an argument I suspect Sears himself would agree with if you asked him in private.

#4

Eat Low Glycemic for Enduring Energy

Your job as a high-energy person is to eat in such a way as to keep blood sugar and insulin levels at a nice even, sustained level, so that your energy stays that way.

Not so coincidentally, choosing foods that keep blood sugar even and energy up—what we call *low-glycemic* food—is a great weight-

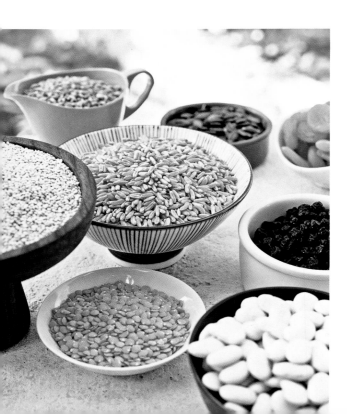

management strategy. Remember, foods that make you fat are highly unlikely to give you a feeling of boundless energy.

So you're going to want to eat low-glycemic foods, what some folks call "slow-burning carbs." Simply put, low-glycemic foods are those that raise your blood sugar slowly, and not too high. Too high, and your energy quickly spikes and then plummets.

So how do we know which foods are low glycemic?

Glad you asked.

FLAWED FOOD RATINGS

In the last few years, a scientific measure of just how high blood sugar is raised in response to food has become popular. It's called the *glycemic index*. Researchers at the University of Toronto developed the concept in 1981 by testing 50-gram portions of all sorts of carbohydrates and rating how they "performed" in the blood sugar department against a standard of pure glucose, the reference food to which they arbitrarily gave the rating "100."

Carbohydrates that were quickly broken down during digestion had the highest glycemic indexes, and those that had a lot of fiber and broke down slowly had lower indexes. Generally speaking, we consider foods with a rating of 70 or higher a high-glycemic-index food, foods rated less than 40 are low glycemic, and stuff in the middle is, well, in the middle.

It would seem as if this is the perfect way to figure out which foods to eat for energy. If a food has a high glycemic index, avoid it. If it has a low glycemic index, consume it. This makes a lot of sense, but the problem is, it's not completely true for three reasons.

Reason #1: The glycemic index is based on 50-gram portions of carbohydrate foods. But many foods we regularly consume have portion sizes way smaller or way larger than 50 grams, so the rating at 50 grams doesn't really tell us much about how our blood sugar is going to behave when we eat the food. Carrots, for example, have a very high glycemic index, but again, that's for a 50-gram portion of carbohydrate. There's only about 3 grams of carbohydrate in a carrot. You'd have to eat a ton of them to raise your blood sugar significantly.

Reason #2: The glycemic index only tells you what happens to your blood sugar if you eat that particular food by itself. Add some olive oil to your high-glycemic cornflakes and the mix is much lower on the glycemic index. (Okay, that's a stretch, but the same thing happens when you add cream or almonds. Fat lowers the total glycemic impact of a food, even one high on the scale such as cornflakes or white bread.)

Reason #3: There are certain situations when you actually *want* high-glycemic foods, though they don't necessarily apply to the average person. Athletes in training who practice twice a day actually do great replenishing with high-glycemic fruits and drinks; they burn the sugar right off in training. And there are plenty of high-glycemic foods that are extremely healthy (such as carrot juice) and plenty of low-glycemic foods (such as fried fish tacos) that aren't.

MORE FOR YOUR MOUTHFUL

So the glycemic index is not a perfect measure. But luckily, scientists figured this out and came up with a much better one. It's called the *glycemic load*. Glycemic load is a much more modern measure of the effect food has on your blood sugar because it's a measure that actually takes into account the real-life portion size of something you're likely to eat.

Think of it this way: Let's say you go into an exotic spice store and spot an unusual spice selling for $300 a pound. "Three hundred bucks a pound!" you exclaim. "That's expensive!" Well, that's true. But knowing the price per pound won't tell you how much you're actually going to pay at the cash register, which is what you *really* want to know. Who cares how much it costs per pound if you're only buying 1/2 teaspoon of the stuff? You're going to hit the checkout counter and find that the bill is only 55 cents!

Glycemic load is a much more modern measure of the effect food has on your blood sugar because it's a measure that actually takes into account the real-life portion size of something you're likely to eat.

High-Performance Foods Sit on the Low End of the Scale

The following is a much abbreviated list of some typical foods and where they stand on the glycemic load scale. (There are much more comprehensive charts of all foods that have been tested available on the Internet. One particularly good chart is at www.mendosa.com/gilists.htm.) There's nothing wrong with having the occasional high-glycemic fruit or grain, but you'll want to keep it to a minimum. Remember, too, that whenever you add fiber, protein, or fat to a meal or snack, you're lowering the overall glycemic impact on your blood sugar (and energy).

High-Glycemic-Load Foods (20 and above)

Cornflakes

Doughnuts

Linguini

Macaroni

Pancakes

Rice

Russet potatoes

Spaghetti

Medium-Glycemic-Load Foods (11–19)

Bananas

Navy beans

Pearled barley

Sweet potatoes

Low-Glycemic-Load Foods (10 or less)

Apples

Carrots

Cashews

Chickpeas

Grapes

Kidney beans

Lentils

Oranges

Pinto beans

Peanuts

Pears

Red lentils

Strawberries

Watermelon

Remember that most of the testing for glycemic values has been done on carbohydrate foods. Fat has almost no effect on insulin, and "mixed foods" (foods containing some combination of carb, protein, and/or fat) are rarely tested. That doesn't mean they don't affect your blood sugar, just that we know more about the effect of pure carbohydrate foods—from kidney beans (low) to jelly beans (high).

It's much the same way with glycemic index and glycemic load. Glycemic index is like knowing the "price per pound," but glycemic load is like knowing the price *you actually pay* based on the amount you actually consume. If you're consuming a 3-gram carbohydrate portion (one medium carrot), it's not that relevant what a 50-gram portion would do to your blood sugar. Glycemic load is calculated using a formula that takes the glycemic index *plus* the portion size into account. That's a lot more meaningful.

Let's use two foods as an example—carrots and pasta. Carrots have a glycemic index of 92, and because of that, many people will tell you not to eat carrots. But like much of conventional wisdom, that's dead wrong. Sure, a glycemic index of 92 seems "expensive," but remember, that's for the standard 50-gram carbohydrate portion. If you eat two carrots, you're consuming about 6 grams of carbohydrate, maybe 7. Plugging that into the formula for glycemic load (don't worry, the math is all done for you on the glycemic load charts) gives you a glycemic load of about 5, which is ridiculously low.

As my friend and colleague from the U.S. Department of Agriculture, C. Leigh Broadhurst, Ph.D., is fond of saying, "No one ever got fat or diabetic on peas and carrots."

Pasta, on the other hand, has a medium glycemic index of about 55, which pasta-apologists claim isn't so bad. True. But plug into the formula the typical portion of 200 grams—it's probably two or three times that in a typical restaurant portion—and you're looking at a glycemic load that's off the charts. You won't get fat on carrots, but you may well do so on pasta.

Try Bee Pollen and Bee Propolis

Bee pollen is one of the few nonmeat sources of the energy-essential vitamin B$_{12}$. But that's hardly the only reason to recommend it.

Bee pollen is also loaded with vitamins, enzymes, almost all known minerals, and tons of amino acids, which makes sense because bee pollen contains the essence of every plant from which the bees collect pollen. It also contains a number of bioflavonoids, a family of plant chemicals with multiple health and energy benefits.

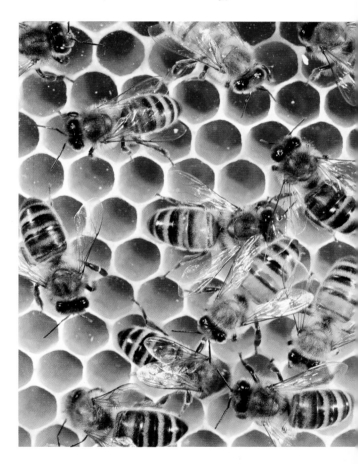

In one study, adolescent swimmers who took bee pollen experienced fewer missed training days due to colds and upper respiratory infections. I use bee pollen as an additive in my smoothies, especially in the afternoon, but many people eat it by the spoonful, straight from the jar. Try pollen or propolis (more on that below) and see what you think. One brand I really like is distributed by David Wolfe's Sunfood Nutrition (www.sunfood.com), but you can find others in your local health food supermarket.

Propolis is the stuff the bees create by mixing wax with a resinous sap from trees. The result is a substance that has documented antioxidative, antiulcer, antitumor, and antimicrobial properties. No wonder people find it energizing! At the very least, propolis protects against a host of microbes that can easily drain your energy in a number of subtle ways.

Although there isn't a ton of research on bee pollen, it's still a phenomenally nutritious and well-balanced food that's been a staple in folk medicine and healing traditions for more than two millennia. And many people swear by it as an energy food.

Add More Fiber to Your Diet

If your grandmother is still alive, she's probably chuckling over the number of things she turned out to be right about—especially when it comes to food.

One of those things she was right about—in spades, as it turns out—is fiber. Of course, in her day they called it roughage, but it's the same stuff. It was known then for "keeping you regular," and was probably not the sexiest part of her diet (or yours), nor the most discussed.

Nevertheless, whether you call it roughage or fiber, it's one of the single most important components of a high-energy diet.

#1 ENERGY DRAINER: THE BLOOD SUGAR ROLLER COASTER

Fiber does two major things in the body that can contribute directly and indirectly to energy. First and foremost, it helps control blood sugar. When your blood sugar is out of control, so is your energy. Low-fiber foods, especially processed carbohydrates that also don't contain much fat or protein, send your blood sugar rocketing, which, in short order, sets you up for a big fat crash in energy.

A candy bar may give you a rush of blood sugar, but half an hour later you'll be pinching yourself to keep your eyes open as your blood sugar plummets. On the other hand, eat some beans and your blood sugar will rise slowly and stay up there for a week. (I'm kidding, but you get the point.)

High-fiber foods, unlike that candy bar, slow the entrance of sugar into the bloodstream. Blood glucose levels rise and fall gradually and gently, like the waves in a lake on a nice summer day as opposed to the waves of the Atlantic Ocean during a hurricane. That's what you want. Slow and gentle. A sustained level of blood sugar means a sustained level of energy. A rollicking, out-of-control blood sugar roller coaster is an energy disaster, leading to cravings, hunger, foul moods, and fatigue, often at the same time.

The second way fiber helps increase your energy is indirectly, through its effect on weight. Although there are no magic weight-loss supplements, fiber probably comes the closest. Virtually every study shows that people who consume a high-fiber diet have an easier time controlling and losing weight, probably because fiber not only keeps you full and therefore less likely to overeat, but also because of its aforementioned positive effect on blood sugar.

It's hard to see why people don't make more of an effort to get fiber into their diet any way they can, including taking fiber supplements, when you consider fiber's other benefits, such as contributing to gastrointestinal and cardiovascular health, helping manage blood lipids, and potentially offering protection from certain cancers. (See www.jonnybowden.com for brand recommendations on fiber supplements, or visit your health food store.)

Energy Comes in Two Types of Fiber

Fiber is essentially indigestible carbohydrate. It comes in two "flavors" (or types)—insoluble and soluble. Both are important, but for different reasons.

Soluble fiber, like the name suggests, dissolves in water, and is made up of *polysaccharides* (carbohydrates that contain three or more molecules of simple carbohydrates). Insoluble fiber (which, obviously from the name, is *not* soluble in water) is actually made up of the plant cell walls.

Most fiber-containing foods have a combination of these two types, but they are usually known as sources of one or the other, depending on what's most predominant. A plum, for example, has insoluble fiber in the skin, but soluble fiber in the juicy meat of the fruit. (There's also a third kind of fiber called resistant starch, which has some of the benefits of both soluble and insoluble fibers.)

THE RIGHT AMOUNT
FOR THE RIGHT ENERGY

Our Paleolithic ancestors were thought to have consumed between 50 and 100 grams of fiber daily. The Institute of Medicine recommends 20 to 35 grams a day (but if you ask me, the higher number is way better). Are you ready for the amount the average American consumes? Between 4 and 11 grams daily.

If you want to correct that, and you start increasing your fiber intake (highly recommended) with food, supplements, or both, remember to drink plenty of water and add the extra fiber slowly. A big increase all at once can cause a lot of gas, and a big increase without enough water can cause constipation—neither of which are energy-friendly! Add the fiber gradually by eating more nuts, seeds, grains (if you tolerate them), bran, vegetables, and fruits. And if you need more reasons to increase your fiber, consider this: Fiber and the compounds produced by its fermentation in the gut stabilize insulin levels, help control LDL cholesterol and triglycerides, and may help protect the lining of the intestines from the formation of polyps. Those fiber by-products also help increase the absorption of dietary minerals and stimulate components of the immune system from cells to antibodies.

Insoluble fiber from plant cell walls includes substances such as lignins and lignans (both of which are found in flaxseeds) and cellulose. Top food sources include vegetables, unprocessed bran, nuts, seeds, certain vegetables, the skins of some fruits, wheat germ, and whole grains (but read the label for fiber content, because there are a lot of imposters out there).

Soluble fiber (pectins, gums, mucilages, etc.) is found in legumes, oats, some fresh and dried fruit (especially berries and prunes), vegetables (broccoli), and psyllium husks. Resistant starch— starch that resists digestion—can be found in legumes, under-ripe bananas, and whole grains.

According to the Linus Pauling Institute, the five top fiber-rich foods are:

1. Legumes (15 to 19 grams per cup)
2. Wheat bran (17 grams per cup)
3. Prunes (12 grams per cup)
4. Asian pears (10 grams each!)
5. Quinoa (9 grams per cup)

Raspberries and blackberries are both fiber heavyweights as well, weighing in at 8 grams and 7.4 grams, respectively, per serving.

A high-fiber diet is one of the dietary keys to high energy. Add that fiber and your body will thank you. I can almost hear your grandmother saying, "I told you so!"

Fiber helps control blood sugar. When your blood sugar is out of control, so is your energy.

Try These Three Carbs for Long-Lasting Energy

Fibrous—or slow-burning—carbs are energy foods.

I don't use the terms simple carbs and complex carbs anymore. The old idea that simple carbs raise blood sugar quickly while complex carbs do not is woefully out of date. Many simple carbs are high in fiber and raise blood sugar slowly (berries) while many complex carbs are treated by the body as one big bolus of sugar (pasta, rice, and most breads).

It's far better to use the distinction slow-burning carbs and fast-burning carbs. For sustained energy, you want the slow burn-ers, which are almost all vegetables and most low-sugar, high-fiber fruits.

Here are three of my favorite fibrous carbs for energy.

Kiwi—the Energy Promoter and Potassium Heavyweight

What fruit has the highest amount of vitamin C ounce for ounce? The orange? Not even close. The answer is kiwifruit, which contains twice as much vitamin C as an orange. It also outranks bananas on the potassium scale, and it's a good source of fiber and a decent source of magnesium. And kiwifruit made the Environmental Working Group's list of twelve foods least contaminated with pesticides. So you have your energy-promoting nutrients without a side of chemicals.

Eat Apples for All-Around Alertness

Apples are one of nature's great natural energy enhancers, and one of the best all-around fruits on the planet. In addition to their many health benefits (apple eaters have reduced risk of lung cancer, asthma, and diabetes), apples are a great source of an unsung hero of the mineral world—*boron*. My friend John Hernandez, M.D., director of the Center for Health and Inte-gration in San Antonio, Texas, tells of a study in which drowsy college sophomores were given supplements of 3 mg of boron—all of a sudden, no more falling asleep in class.

Pumpkins—the Secret Superfood

Most people are surprised to find that you can actually eat pumpkin when it's not autumn. But pumpkin is actually one of the best-kept secrets on the planet when it comes to superfoods for energy. First of all, it's loaded with potassium, which makes both your heart and your muscles work better, not to mention that it lowers blood pressure and reduces risk of stroke. Second, it's loaded with vitamin A, which helps your immune system fight off energy-draining viruses and other microbes. Third, it has fiber: $2\frac{1}{2}$ grams of it in one cup. Fourth, it's a low-glycemic food, which means it raises your blood sugar slowly, giving you sustained energy for very few calories. Bonus: It's one of the only canned vegetables that's actually good for you! Heat it up and season with butter, sea salt, cinnamon, and nutmeg and watch your energy skyrocket.

Enjoy a Green Drink Every Day

Recently, while promoting my book *The Most Effective Natural Cures on Earth*, I was lucky enough to be invited to spend a full hour with Mehmet Oz, M.D., who hosts an *Oprah and Friends* radio show on XM satellite radio. As I sat in his studio during the interview, I couldn't help but notice that he was sipping from a large container holding a liquid that looked suspiciously like the "green drink" I drink at the start of every single day.

That's because it was. Oz, along with many other high-energy health-minded people I know, is a big fan of green drinks.

So what are these things, anyway? No one knows how they got to be so big in the health food world, but I suspect their popularity came about when folks started noticing how great they'd feel after having a shot of wheatgrass juice, which is made from little plants that look like grass that you can find next to the big industrial-strength juicer at nearly any health food juice bar. Talk about energy!

PACKING A NUTRITIONAL WALLOP

Wheatgrass "shots" have been a staple of the high-energy health food crowd for decades, even before health food stores morphed into natural supermarkets and multiplied to the point where they can be found in every big city and mall in the United States. They've been a staple of that crowd for good reason. Wheatgrass is loaded with chlorophyll, a natural blood purifier and detoxifier that can contribute to a feeling of well-being and energy. It is bitter tasting and expensive, but thousands of people swear by it.

So now, thanks to high-tech manufacturing processes, you don't have to drink pure wheatgrass to benefit from the energy-enhancing effects of grasses. There have been an explosion of drinks and powdered drink mixes in the marketplace to fill the needs of consumers thirsty (forgive the pun) for the energizing, alkalizing, detoxifying, and immune-enhancing effects of wheatgrass and its relatives in the grass family.

I'm using the term *green drinks* to refer to the entire category of juices from barley, wheatgrass, magma, or any combination of whole green foods, including spinach, broccoli, parsley, and virtually any other healthy green thing that grows. Green drinks pack an incredible nutritional wallop and usually have amazing phytonutrients*.

A general name for the thousands of chemical compounds and nutrients (besides vitamins and minerals) that are found in plants, the majority of which have health benefits.

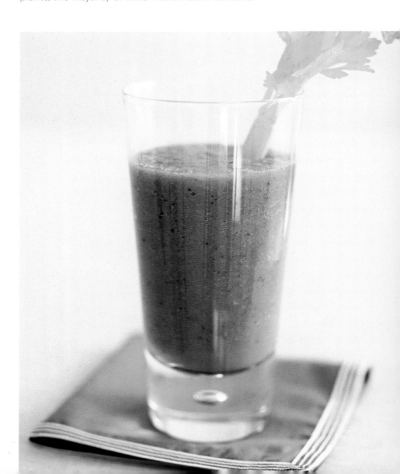

Green drinks are very alkalizing. You may recall from high school chemistry (or from gardening!) that many organic compounds have a pH value that can range from an extremely acid 1 (battery acid) to an extremely alkaline 14 (lye). The pH balance is very important for living things, and body fluids such as blood and saliva all have a very narrow range that is ideal for human health. However, a diet very high in meat and grains (and absent tons of vegetables) is likely to tip the balance more in the direction of acid, which is not a great thing for either energy or general health. Alkalizing green drinks help correct the balance and are a terrific counterpart to a higher meat diet.

On top of that, green drinks are usually made from organic sources, they're low in calories, and most have no more than 3 or 4 grams of (low-glycemic) carbohydrates. You can find them in most health food and whole food supermarkets, and you should definitely consider making them part of your energy-boosting program.

The best green drinks include all kinds of extracts from vegetables such as spinach and can be mixed with water for a low-calorie, low-glycemic, high-vitamin and -mineral snack, pick-me-up, or breakfast juice. I sometimes add in a couple of ounces of one of the newer, exotic "designer" juices, such as—my favorite—noni juice. Because they're so low in sugar, they don't give you the "spike and drop" in energy that commercial fruit juice would give you, so you get a nice sustained buzz, not to mention the gratification that comes from knowing you're doing something so good for yourself. They also do a nice job of taking the edge off your appetite, leaving you just "lean and hungry" enough to take on the world yet not so hungry that you can't concentrate on anything.

Use green drinks as a stand-alone energy boost, or in combination with solid foods. A green drink together with a high-protein snack such as tuna will keep you going for hours. My personal favorite is Barlean's Greens, available both on my website, www.jonnybowden.com, and at health food stores everywhere. For something so downright healthy, it tastes surprisingly good!

Because green drinks are so low in sugar, they don't give you the "spike and drop" in energy that commercial fruit juice would give you, so you get a nice sustained buzz.

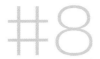

Don't Fear Fat!

Here's a pop quiz: What's the best source of energy in the human body?

If you answered carbohydrates, you're probably not alone. And, don't take this the wrong way, you're dead wrong.

Think about it. Your body stores roughly 1,800 calories of carbohydrates in the form of glucose and glycogen (the storage form of carbohydrates). It also stores, oh, I don't know, about eight gazillion calories of fat.

Doesn't it make sense that the most energetic people in the world are those that tap into that virtually unlimited source of biological energy?

Of course it does.

When a marathoner "hits the wall," it means he or she has run out of carbohydrates. However, experienced marathoners have trained their bodies to tap into their fat stores more effectively, because that source of fuel is virtually unlimited. They've literally become what's called "better butter burners." That's why they can run longer than mere mortals.

So for optimal energy, you need to eat fat. But that doesn't mean scarfing down fried potatoes from the fast food burger joint. To supercharge your energy batteries you also need to eat the right fat.

AVOID EATING UNDER OUTDATED STANDARDS

So if fat is so essential for our energy (not to mention for our health, but don't get me started), how did we ever come to fear this valuable macronutrient? To this day, when it comes to fats, most of us are still laboring under some of the most misguided and out-of-date information on the planet.

I'll give you a perfect example. The other day my tennis partner and I were playing a doubles match against two guys, one of whom also happens to be the other team's captain. After the first hour, the captain was running out of energy, not surprising because the match was brutal and we were playing in 98°F (37°C) heat in the California San Fernando Valley. On one of the breaks, the captain reached into his bag and brought out some cookies.

"I tell everyone to eat these to keep their energy up," he told me, "but I make sure to tell them to get the low-fat kind!"

How ironic. This is exactly the opposite of what you want to do if you want to keep your energy up.

It's time to set the record straight. Read on.

GET OVER THE FEAR OF FAT

Back in the 1970s and 80s, some well-meaning people came up with the theory that the reason Americans were getting too fat was that they were eating too much fat. Waistlines were expanding and heart disease was increasing. The good folks in charge of making health policy recommendations decided that eating fat *made* you fat. In short order, everyone got on board with what appeared to be the obvious solution: *Stop eating fat.*

Wrong.

I'll never forget when I first began to question this so-called conventional wisdom. I was working at Equinox Fitness Clubs in New York with the legendary ultra-marathoner and exercise physiologist Stu Mittleman. Ultramarathoners, by the way, are folks who run marathons as warm-ups. *USA Today* once called ultramarathoners "the ultimate road warriors," as their event is typically a six-day run of 100 miles. Stu held a number of records in the

UltraMarathon. We used to see him running every morning in Central Park, where he routinely did twenty miles a day. When asked why he ran twenty miles a day, he would answer, "'Cause that's all I have time for."

Which should give you some idea about Stu's energy.

Stu was big on eating butter and eggs. Especially in the morning.

At the time, that was nutritional heresy. But as Stu explained, fat is your best source of energy. If you want to effortlessly get through your day, you have to become one of those better butter burners. You have to train your body to use fat, not carbohydrates, as your primary energy source, because, as noted, you store a ton of it at any given time. So doesn't it make sense to train your body to use fat for energy?

To this day, Stu never eats more than about 40 percent of his calories from carbs, the rest coming from protein and fat.

So how did we ever go so wrong on our advice on fat? What were we thinking?

Well, look. It's not like the experts got together and said, "Hey, what can we do to really screw up everyone's health?" Experts are well-meaning people (at least they usually are). They sincerely wanted to help us get on the right track. Taking a page from recent historic events, we might say that their hearts were in the right place, but they had *bad intelligence*. Their information was just plain wrong. As professor Harlan Onsrud put it in *Science* magazine, "Most of us would have predicted that if we can get the population to change its fat intake . . . we would see a reduction in weight. Instead, we have seen the exact opposite."

And that's exactly what happened. Although the percentage of calories from fat in the American diet has actually gone down over the past couple of decades, obesity has gone up. And up. And up. And folks, it's not because we're eating fat. Fat is not the enemy, and cutting fat out of the diet is not the solution. Especially if you want to be at your energetic best.

So we, the experts, were wrong about cutting out fat. In fact, for many people, particularly those who have type 2 diabetes or are at risk for it, a low-fat diet can be the wrong approach. Fat helps make you feel satiated. Many fats—omega-3s from fish, for example—have anti-inflammatory properties. Some saturated fats, such as those found in coconut oil, have antiviral properties.

When you remove fat from the diet, you generally replace it with something else, usually carbs, which sends many people on a bumpy roller coaster ride of mood swings, blood sugar dips, insulin spikes, and increased fat storage. (Of course, this doesn't apply when the carbs you're eating are very, very high in fiber, but unfortunately that's not the case when you're eating most breads, pastas, and the majority of commercial cereals.)

The death knell to the idea that fat alone was the enemy of health, weight, and energy was sounded recently by professor Walt Willett of Harvard University, arguably the most prestigious nutrition researcher of our time and the lead researcher on both the Nurses Health Study and the Health Professionals Follow-Up Study. In these studies, Willett and his colleagues examined the eating habits of more than 100,000 people over three decades. Here's what he said: "We have found virtually no relationship between the percentage of calories from fat and any important health outcome."

In other words, fat doesn't make you fat. It doesn't make you sick. And it definitely doesn't rob you of your energy.

Quite the opposite.

What *does* seem to matter a lot, though, is the *type* of fat and the *type* of carbohydrate eaten (see "Good" Versus "Bad" Fats below).

Bottom line: Fat is the best source of sustained energy in the human body. It makes you feel satiated, helps manage your blood sugar, and keeps your energy tank full. But you want to make sure you're eating the right kinds. The best advice: Get a nice mixture in your diet of saturated fats (coconut oil, eggs), omega-3s (fish and flaxseed), and omega 9s (macadamia nut oil, extra-virgin olive oil), and some omega-6s (evening primrose oil, black currant oil, borage oil).

And if, like my tennis opponent, you're tempted to fall back into the anti-fat camp, remember this: If your calories are at the appropriate level for optimal energy (and for weight management), the percentage of calories from fat are of absolutely no importance.

"Good" Versus "Bad" Fats

Now if you've read even a minimum of information about nutrition and diet over the past few years, you're probably aware of the fact that there are "good fats" and "bad fats." You've also probably heard that the "bad fats" are saturated and the "good fats" are everything else.

Nope, again.

Bad fats are trans fats. It's now the law that trans fats have to be listed on the label of foods, but you have to be a detective to find them. Look on the label for "partially hydrogenated oil." (For arcane, bureaucratic, and political reasons, manufacturers can legally say "zero trans fats" if there is less than $1/2$ gram per serving, which has resulted in many foods having more than a few grams in a typical serving size. For the record, the amount of trans fats that a human should consume per day is zero.)

So if you see "partially hydrogenated oil" on the ingredients list, put the box back on the shelf and step away from the food, even if the label says "zero trans fats." (Trans fats, by definition, are partially hydrogenated oil. Period.) Trans fats are associated with every degenerative disease you can think of.

Another kind of "bad fat" is *damaged* fat. Fats can be damaged by high heat or chemical processing, or by being used for frying multiple times (fast food chains are notorious for this). And, contrary to popular opinion, too many omega-6 fats, which are a type of polyunsaturated fat found in vegetable oils that everyone used to think were always healthy, can be quite pro-inflammatory and have been linked to an increased risk of cancer, particularly when they are not balanced in the diet with the friendly omega-3s from fish, omega-9s from olive oil, and even some small amount of healthy, undamaged saturated fat, such as egg yolks.

Kick the Carbs, Kick-Start Your Energy

One of the biggest energy zappers on the planet is sugar. Although we've been taught that sugar gives you energy, it actually does nothing of the sort. In fact, it does quite the opposite.

The number one reason why sugar ultimately saps your energy and makes you feel like an extra from the cast of *Night of the Living Zombies* when 4:00 p.m. rolls around, has to do with dietary sugar's effect on blood sugar.

Here's how it works: Eating any food triggers a whole bunch of responses in the body, not the least of which is the release of certain hormones that have a profound effect on your energy (not to mention your weight). Those hormones lie in wait for the right signal for food, at which point they jump into the bloodstream like a sleeper cell given the "go" command, sending little messages to the important cells, tissues, and organs that they control. They're like a giant email system, each with a screaming headline in the subject line: *Build some muscle! Burn some fat! Store some fat! Burn some muscle!*

All those hormonal messages have a great deal to do with how you feel and with your energy levels.

FOR KILLER ENERGY, TAME THE HUNGER HORMONE

One of the big players in this little hormonal dance, a player that has a *profound effect* on your energy, is a hormone called *insulin*. When you eat almost any food (except pure fat), your blood sugar rises and your pancreas responds by saying, *"Uh-oh, blood sugar is going up; let's do something."* And what it does is secrete a powerful anabolic hormone called insulin, also known affectionately as "the Hunger Hormone" (for reasons which will soon be clear). Now insulin has a lot of jobs in the body, but one of its most important tasks is to get blood sugar back down to normal levels, which is a good thing indeed because over time, high blood sugar is extremely damaging to the body.

You may be shocked to learn that your body treats a bagel, most cereals, pastas, rice, and potatoes—all the low-fat staples of the high-carb diet so popular in the 1980s—*exactly* the same as it would a big, fat, incoming ball of sugar. Once you chew up that bread and swallow it, the body sees an incoming bolus of sugar, and treats it accordingly. From a hormonal, and an energy-related point of view, this is a complete disaster.

Here's why. Those "unsupervised" sugar molecules float around the bloodstream like teenagers after curfew, and much like those teenagers, they will eventually cause mischief. They glom on to protein molecules in the blood, resulting in sticky substances that clog up the works and eventually interfere with circulation, particularly in small capillaries such as those in the eyes and kidneys. They get shuttled into little packages called *triglycerides*, high levels of which are a definite risk factor for heart disease.

The point is, *your body doesn't want your blood sugar elevated*, thank you very much! Your body would *much* prefer to have sugar in the *cells*, where it can be burned for energy, rather than in the *bloodstream*, where it will eventually get you into trouble.

And that's where insulin comes in.

INSULIN RESISTANCE: THE ENEMY OF HIGH ENERGY

Insulin is a "sugar wrangler," whisking up the excess sugar from the bloodstream and attempting to deliver it to the muscle cells, where it can be burned for fuel. This makes perfect sense, and the system usually works pretty well when we're exercising or active all the time. When that's happening, the muscle cells actually put out the "welcome" sign for sugar.

Problem is, most of us aren't active. The only exercise we're getting—especially if we're low-energy folks to begin with—is moving the computer mouse around during the day and hitting the buttons on the remote control later at night. The muscle cells say to the insulin, *"No thanks, we gave at the office, go somewhere else, we don't need your sugar."* So insulin, quite rightly miffed, takes its business elsewhere—to the fat cells.

At first, the fat cells open their doors to the insulin and its payload of sugar, which accomplishes three things. Number one, it makes your jeans fit badly. Number two, it makes you feel horrible once you notice number one. And number three, because you've eaten so much sugar* in the first place, and because you've produced a lot of insulin to get rid of it, all that insulin eventually does its job so well that your blood sugar takes a nosedive as the fat cells scoop it all up. Your energy plummets. Now you'll kill someone if you don't get a bagel. You're tired, grumpy, low energy, and out of sorts. The office snack machine beckons, and the cycle starts again.

You want more energy? Cut out the white stuff. It's that simple. I'm not saying you can't occasionally have a slice of bread, but I am saying that by making processed carbs a once-in-a-while addition to your diet in tiny amounts, your energy will go through the roof.

Your Paleolithic ancestors had the energy to travel an average of twenty miles per day, often dragging along the carcass of a large animal they found on hunting trips. And they did it without ever eating a single slice of white bread. 'Nuff said.

Or anything that converts to sugar quickly, including the aforementioned bagel, or a bowl of pasta.

#10-17

Increase Your Energy by Eliminating Sugar with These Eight Ways

When it comes to energy, sugar is bad news. You may think it's giving you an energy boost, but the facts tell a different story. Although sugar in your diet might temporarily give you a short lift, it's invariably followed by a crash that leaves your energy in the dumpster.

Anyone wanting sustained energy, a clear and focused mind, and laser-sharp concentration and performance is well advised to do an exorcism as far as sugar in the diet goes.

I could go on. (And frequently do, especially when I'm giving talks about the effect of sugar on weight, hormones, cravings, fat storage, the immune system, athletic performance, and general health. The executive summary: Sugar does nothing good and plenty bad.) The bottom line is that if you want to be at the top of your game, energetically speaking, you'd be well off removing as much sugar as humanly possible from your everyday diet.

Several years ago, in my very first book (*Jonny Bowden's Shape Up! The Eight-Week Program to Transform Your Body, Your Health, and Your Life*), I wrote the following words: "To the extent that you can remove sugar from your diet, you will be doing a huge service to your body, your health, and your weight." Nothing has changed since I wrote those words in 2000, except that I'd add the following: You'll also be doing a huge service to your energy levels!

Is it easy to "get the sugar out"? Heck, no. It's in everything. But you can make a serious effort, and if you aim for the bulls-eye, you'll be close enough to make a big difference in your energy and well-being. Here are eight great tips to get you started on the path to a high-energy, sugar-free life!

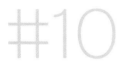

Don't Add Sugar or Salt to Your Food

First principles first. Don't add sugar to your food, and this includes coffee and tea. As someone who used to sweeten coffee with 3 teaspoons of sugar (granted, that was twenty-five years ago, but I still remember), I can assure you that you can learn to enjoy it without the added health hazard. Recent research indicates that added salt can, paradoxically, increase the consumption of sugar-sweetened beverages, and in addition, you don't need that additional sodium. Which leads to principle number two.

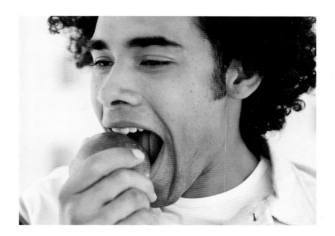

Learn What Real Food Tastes Like

You know, back in the day when my body was, shall we say, a bit more "polluted" than it is now (hey, that was back in the 60s and 70s, what do you expect?), I could have taken a horse tranquilizer and barely noticed any effect. After I got completely clean, I noticed an aspirin! That's what happens when you clear your body of toxins, and it's also what happens when you clear your palate of the taste of super-sweet and super-salty. Your senses become fine-tuned and you can actually start noticing real flavors.

It's true. Once we stop adding salt and sugar to everything, our taste buds quickly adapt and start to respond to subtle tastes that we never noticed before. Want proof? Try an heirloom tomato without anything but some pepper on it. But be forewarned—it may spoil you so you're never again satisfied with the run-of-the-mill, uniform, steroided-out giant red suckers that taste like wet cardboard. But you'll be developing a taste for real food.

#12

Experiment with Spices

Once you break the sugar and salt habit, there's a whole world waiting for you in delicious, nutritious spices that can not only add to your eating pleasure but also provide a cornucopia of medicinal benefits. Try turmeric on your eggs or vegetables. Give lemon pepper and Celtic sea salt a try while you're at it. And cinnamon and nutmeg aren't only for Thanksgiving—they're both healthy spices that can easily take the place of sugar with a lot more health benefit to boot. By the way, they taste great on mashed pumpkin with butter, an energy food if ever there was one!

#13

Beware of Fat-Free Food

Fat-free food is so yesterday. Forget it. If you're eating real, whole food, you don't need it. Fat will keep you full longer, making it less likely that you'll overeat. And remember, according to Walter Willett, M.D., Ph.D., lead researcher on the thirty-plus-year Nurses Health Study and the Health Professionals Follow-Up Study, there's no relationship between the percentage of fat in your diet and any major health outcome. Eat food the way it was intended to be eaten and you won't need all the added sugar. Virtually every fat-free fake food I've seen is manufactured with a ton of sugar, which food producers use to make up for the missing fat. From an energy (and a health) point of view, you're way better off with the real thing.

#14

Be a Smart Label Reader

Sugar comes in many disguises. High-fructose corn syrup is the nastiest and most prevalent, but beware of brown rice syrup, invert sugar, cane juice, evaporated cane juice, fruit juice concentrate, and anything ending in "ose," which includes fructose, lactose, glucose, maltose, and sucrose. Manufacturers frequently use a combination of these so they can hide the actual amount of sugar in any product. By law, ingredients have to be listed in order of weight, so by using just a little of five different sugars, sugar won't necessarily be the first ingredient on the label, even though the product in question may have more sugar in it than any other ingredient! These manufacturers can be sneaky devils!

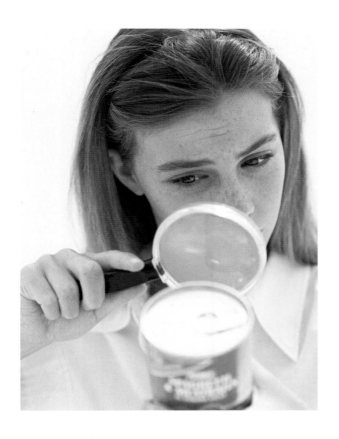

as well as in many health food stores.) If you're interested, it's also good for alcohol cravings, which are often sugar cravings in disguise.

Learn about Lo Han

No, not the bad-girl teen-queen actress, the sweetener. Lo Han sweetener is made from the Chinese fruit of the same name, is all natural, and offers a multitude of health benefits. It's a great alternative to sugar; it is a couple hundred times sweeter than the white stuff, has zero calories, and is safe for diabetics. Lo Han is available at many natural foods supermarkets and health food stores.

#15

Use This Natural Crave-Buster

If you experience sugar cravings, try glutamine. I wrote about L-glutamine in *The Most Effective Natural Cures on Earth* for the simple reason that it is a great natural crave-buster. An amino acid, glutamine is a natural energy fuel for the brain, and a spoonful of the powder in a glass of water will do wonders for knocking your sugar cravings right out of the park. (You can find powdered glutamine on my website, www.jonnybowden.com,

#17

Try Xylitol

This is one of my favorite sugar substitutes. It's actually a sugar *alcohol*, and although it has some (very few) calories it has a vanishingly small effect on blood sugar, helps prevent bacteria from adhering to surfaces (such as in the mouth, making it a key ingredient in "healthy" chewing gums), and looks, tastes, and cooks like the real thing. It's particularly great in energy smoothies. You can find xylitol on my website, www.jonnybowden.com, under shopping/supplements; more and more health food supermarkets are starting to carry it as well.

#18

Switch to Tea of Any Color

The Chinese have used green tea as a medicine for more than 4,000 years. Putting aside the fact that it's been shown to reduce the risk of at least one kind of cancer, improve immune function, and fight rheumatoid arthritis, cardiovascular disease, infection, and high cholesterol, it's also possibly the greatest energy drink around.

And although green tea gets a lot of attention in the media, truth be told, almost any high-quality tea is great for energy and health. All (except yerba maté, see page 49) are made from the same plant, *Camellia sinensis*, and differ only in the amount of processing and fermentation that the leaves get. So although green, white, black, and oolong tea may differ a little bit in their health profiles, all are superb when it comes to giving you an energy boost, especially mid-afternoon!

So what's so great about tea? Well, for me it has a terrific "brightening" effect without any of the jitters. Tea contains a substance called *the-anine*, an amino acid that is a natural relaxer with significant antianxiety properties. I believe that's why tea drinkers rarely get the jitters even though they enjoy the increased mental acuity and sharpness that the caffeine delivers.

In addition to the many benefits tea has for your health, it boosts your metabolism, which can be great for both energy and weight loss. In one study, published in the *American Journal of Clinical Nutrition*, one group of men was given some caffeine, and the other group the same amount of caffeine plus green tea. And guess what happened? The men who received green tea burned more calories than the men who were given the caffeine alone. So there's something specific to green tea (besides caffeine) that helps boost metabolism.

My friend, nutritionist Shari Lieberman, Ph.D., C.N.S.., points out that studies in humans have shown that green tea increases the rate at which you burn calories and fat over a 24-hour period! Lieberman calls it one of her favorite supplements for weight loss.

And by the way, if you're still worried about the caffeine, green tea has only one-third as much as coffee, and none of the toxins and acids that make cheap coffee a problem for many people. From a caffeine point of view, you could drink five cups of green tea a day for less than the caffeine load of one medium Starbucks! And that's really not a problem for most people.

Studies show great benefits from drinking between three and five (or more) cups a day. You can make a big pitcher of the stuff and just drink it like water, all day long. Or even start by substituting one cup of green tea for your regular coffee. It's soothing and calming, yet at the same time a fantastic energy booster. How great is that?

WORTH KNOWING

Herbal teas aren't really teas at all. They're actually herbal infusions made from fresh or dried flowers, seeds, or roots—anything but the Camellia sinesis plant. Although they're perfectly lovely and may have other benefits, you won't get the energy boost I'm talking about from using them.

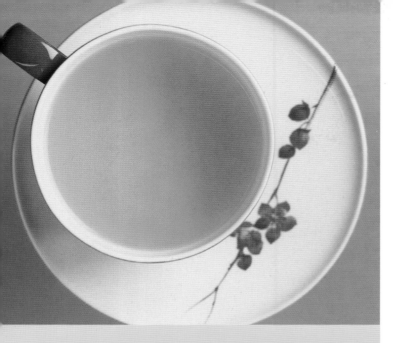

Try These Energy Snacks

The key to keeping energy up when you have to go a lot of hours without food is to pick the right snacks. Unfortunately, they can be hard to find.

Snack machines dispense nothing but sugar and processed carbs, such as pretzels, and fast food is no better. (Airports used to be the worst of all, but that's actually changing!) Running out to get a bagel, or grabbing a high-sugar low-fat muffin at the coffee emporium, is no solution and only adds to the problem of energy drain later in the day.

Fortunately, with just a little planning, you can create fantastic snacks that will keep your blood sugar stable, give you sustained energy for the afternoon (or evening), and keep your motor running smoothly and in high gear for hours.

Read on for three of my faves.

My Favorite Teas

A personal note: Although I love the buzz of my daily Starbucks, around midday I nearly always switch to tea.

I'm lucky enough to live close by to the famous Dr. Tea's Tea Garden and Herbal Emporium in West Hollywood (www.teagarden.com), so I never have to go without my fix of his amazing, delicious gourmet teas (which you can also get by mail, see resources).

But there are no shortages of superb brands to try. Four of my favorites are Choice Organic Teas (www.choiceorganic-teas.com), Numi Organic Tea (www.numi-tea.com), Tazo teas (www.tazo.com), which are carried by Starbucks, and the wonderful selection at The Coffee Bean & Tea Leaf (www.coffeebean.com). With a little poking around in the stores and coffee emporiums, you'll quickly discover your own personal favorites.

ENERGY SNACK #1: CELERY AND ALMOND BUTTER

Although I chose almond butter for this example, any one of the organic nut butters, such as walnut or cashew, for example, would work just as well. So would peanut butter (provided you don't buy the commercial kind that is loaded with sugar and trans fats). Even manufacturers are getting hip to how terrific peanut butter tastes on celery sticks; in Los Angeles, Trader Joe's now carries ready-made packs of celery sticks with a little tub of peanut butter for dipping.

Nut butters taste great smeared on some celery sticks or apple slices. The total calories are reasonable, and the nutrient density is terrific. It's energy in a pack, whether you buy it in the store or make it yourself and carry it with you!

ENERGY SNACK #2: WHEY PROTEIN SHAKE

Whey protein powder is one of the most absorbable sources of protein on the planet. In addition to providing all the goodness of high-quality protein, whey protein helps the body make more of the master antioxidant *glutathione*, which is critical for detoxification. It also helps protect the immune system. Both systems need to be working properly for your energy to be at its peak.

Whey contains all the amino acids a body needs in the best possible balance. It is easily my favorite form of protein powder. But not all whey protein is created equal. Although whey protein isolate is marginally higher in protein, it's frequently a distinction without a difference. Well-made concentrates, including my favorites, PaleoMeal and Whey Cool, both by Designs for Health (available on my website, www.jonnybowden.com) are excellent choices, the latter especially because it comes from grass-fed cows, is pesticide-free, contains no artificial sweeteners or flavors, and is fortified with a plethora of nutrients, including omega-3s.

The beauty of the whey protein shake as an energy pick-me-up is that you can make it a million different ways, from a low-calorie, bare-bones, midday energy booster to a full-out meal substitute. My favorite between-meals blood sugar stabilizer is to mix a scoop of PaleoMeal, Whey Cool, or other whey protein powder with water and a cup of frozen blueberries. The blueberries add flavor and creaminess, and the fact that they're frozen makes the result taste more like a shake. Bonus energy points: some high-quality cacao powder, such as Sunfood's cacao.

ENERGY SNACK #3: HUMMUS

Hummus makes a great energy snack and can be spread on celery just as easily as any nut butter. (You can also spread it on high-fiber whole-grain bread, but you might want to save the carbs and extra calories.)

Hummus travels surprisingly well in a small resealable container, and it's so easy even I can make it. There's a wealth of great recipes on www.about.com's guide to Middle Eastern food, but here's one of my favorites from about.com's own Saad Fayed:

Hummus

1 can (16 ounce, or 475 ml) chickpeas (garbanzo beans)
¼ cup (60 ml) liquid from canned chickpeas
3 to 5 tablespoons (45 to 75 ml) lemon juice
1 ½ tablespoons (30 g) tahini
2 cloves garlic, crushed
½ teaspoon salt
2 tablespoons (30 ml) olive oil

Drain the chickpeas and set aside the liquid from the can. Combine the chickpeas, lemon juice to taste, tahini, garlic, salt, and olive oil in a blender or food processor. Add the liquid from the chickpeas. Blend for 3 to 5 minutes on low until thoroughly combined and smooth.

#20

Try Yerba Maté Tea for a Caffeine Jolt without the Jitters

Although all teas make great energy drinks, one in particular—yerba maté—may be the biggest energy booster of all.

All of our more well-known teas—black, green, oolong, and white—are made from the leaves of *Camellia sinensis*, whereas yerba maté comes from an entirely different plant—*Ilex paraguariensis*. Yerba maté tea is grown mainly in four countries in South America—Brazil, Paraguay, Argentina, and Uruguay—and is the national drink in the latter two. And, yes, it deserves its growing reputation as a superfood and energy booster.

Yerba maté tea has antioxidant properties, contains important nutrients, and can you give the caffeinated jolt you need, all without adverse side effects. Pretty cool, right?

MORE CAFFEINE THAN COFFEE

Elvira de Mejia, Ph.D., of the University of Illinois, and her research team tested various forms of the tea using two sophisticated tests for the presence of antioxidants called the ORAC test and the DPBH test. In both, researchers expose dangerous free radicals (rogue oxygen molecules that damage your cells and DNA) to different amounts of a compound (in this case, yerba maté tea) and measure the ability of the compound to deactivate the free radicals. How well they do is a measure of their antioxident capacity.

"What we've seen in our research is that some types of maté tea are even higher in antioxidants than green tea," de Mejia told me.

But antioxidant power is only part of the story. "Maté tea in general contains high amounts of *chlorogenic acid*, a very powerful plant compound with antioxidant and possibly other healthy properties," she explained. "And it also contains substantial amounts of caffeine, sometimes higher than coffee."

Higher amounts of caffeine than coffee? Sure, that's great for giving you a boost, but can that be a good thing? "Actually, caffeine is an interesting molecule," de Mejia explained. "Caffeine has been shown in some studies to have a preventative effect on diabetes and Parkinson's."

Although she was careful to point out that high amounts of caffeine can be a problem for many people, she does not believe that the presence of caffeine in yerba maté tea is unhealthy—quite the opposite. "Sometimes there are synergistic effects between the caffeine and the antioxidants," she told me.

And it's not just the caffeine. Yerba maté tea contains *xanthines*, which are alkaloids in the same family as caffeine. It also contains *theo-phylline* and *theobromine*, the same well-known stimulants found in coffee and chocolate. (Bonus points: Maté also contains the minerals potassium, magnesium, and manganese.)

I've become a big fan of this tea. The physiological effects are similar to (yet distinct from) more widespread caffeinated beverages, such as coffee, tea, and guarana drinks. In my own admittedly unscientific survey of yerba maté fanatics, I heard many people mention a mental state of wakefulness, focus, and alertness that is reminiscent of most stimulants, but most enthusiasts remarked on maté's decided lack of the negative effects that sometimes accompany other such compounds (such as anxiety, diarrhea, jitteriness, and heart palpitations).

Some people find that maté has fewer negative effects (such as jitteriness) than do coffee and even strong tea from the *Camellia sinensis* plant. Researchers at Florida International University in Miami, for example, found that some people seem to tolerate a maté drink better than coffee or tea.

#21

Eat Nuts for Energy and for Your Heart

Nuts have fiber, protein, and minerals, and are a great energy food. So are nut butters. The protein and fat keep you full and stabilize your blood sugar, while the minerals help your energy and metabolism.

Nut eaters as a rule have significantly lower rates of heart disease than those who don't eat nuts. Because heart disease can really drain your energy—not to mention shorten or eliminate your life—it makes sense to make nuts and nut butters a part of your energy eating plan.

Truth be told, all nuts make a great snack and all are great energy foods. (I'm not necessarily including the salted peanuts you get at a bar, which are technically a legume anyway, not a nut, and are usually not the best snack for energy or health.) There's a reason that trail mix—the standard-issue snack food for hikers—contains a ton of nuts (as well as dried fruit such as cranberries). The mixture of the "good" carbs in the dried fruit together with the heart-healthy fat and moderate amount of protein in the nuts makes the perfect food for sustaining energy through a long day on the hiking trails.

I've written extensively about the other health benefits of nuts, especially almonds, walnuts, pecans, pistachios, and macadamia nuts, in *The 150 Healthiest Foods on Earth*. Suffice it to say here that 1 ounce (28 g) of almonds (or a smear of almond butter) together with a piece of fruit such as an apple make the perfect energy snack, and is hands-down one of my favorite preworkout snacks. (Come to think of it, it's pretty darn good *after* working out, too.)

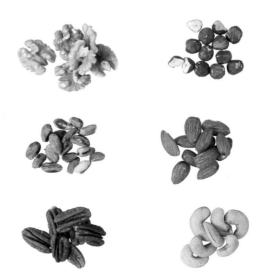

You can also try mixing 1 ounce of nuts (walnuts, pecans, or almonds) with an equal amount of one of the newer, more exotic berries now available in health food stores, such as goji berries or (my favorite) mungberries. Or even with good, old-fashioned raisins. Try sprinkling on some dried coconut flakes for even more of an energy boost.

#22

Reboot Your Brain with Breakfast

You can't be energetic if your brain is starving, which is what happens when you skip breakfast. Our brains need about 120 grams of glucose a day to function properly.

Unless you have a habit of sleepwalking to the refrigerator, I'm going to assume you're not eating during the night, so when you wake up in the morning, your levels of glucose are low and need to be replenished. That's where breakfast comes in.

If you don't start the day with a well-put-together breakfast, your brain will simply not generate enough energy to keep you on top of your game for the day. And I don't mean a bran muffin, a donut, or a bagel. I mean a moderate-calorie (300 to 500 or so), well-balanced meal with plenty of protein, some good fat, and maybe some high-fiber, slow-burning carbs such as those found in oatmeal.

When you skip breakfast—among the many other negative things that happen—more insulin (the "hunger" hormone) will be released after the next meal than it would have if you'd had your oatmeal. Blood sugar becomes destabilized. You're more likely to experience cravings. Next thing you know, you're running on empty, and it's probably going to get worse as the day wears on.

REPROGRAM YOUR BRAIN— AND YOUR STOMACH

If your excuse for not eating breakfast is that you have no appetite in the morning, get over it. (Sorry, but it's tough-love time.)

If you have no appetite in the morning, it's probably because you've conditioned yourself to morning fasting rather than morning breakfast. In that case, your appetite just needs to be reprogrammed, like rebooting a computer, and the way to do it is to start with a protein shake. Even people who aren't hungry in the morning can manage to down one of these babies.

Eventually, you should transition to a real-food breakfast (at least for most of the time), and make sure it contains protein and some good fats. (Note: You may be one of those people who does fine on a vitamin-rich green drink in the morning, but even so, at some point you should probably have some protein later on.)

Think about it: Studies show that teens who eat breakfast score higher on tests, are better able to concentrate, and exhibit greater overall mental performance than those who don't. Want your kids to nod off at their desks by 11:00 a.m.? Just make sure they go to school on an empty stomach. That holds true for you and me, too, though we sometimes mask that urge to doze with a few trips to the local coffee emporium.

And consider this if you need additional motivation: At least seven studies have found a correlation between being overweight and skipping breakfast. Since being overweight can sap your energy, any strategy that can help fend off unwanted pounds—while increasing your mental and physical performance—is going to be a welcome addition to your energy-boosting arsenal.

Three High-Energy Breakfasts That Fit Your Schedule

Try these recipes for high-energy breakfasts to start your day off right.

Fast Protein Shake

1 scoop high-quality whey protein powder (I like PaleoMeal or
Whey Cool, both available on my website, www.jonnybowden.com)
1 cup (235 ml) water
1 cup (155 g) frozen blueberries or strawberries
1 tablespoon (5 g) uncooked oats (optional)

*Combine all the ingredients in a blender and blend
until smooth.*

Easy Raw Foods Breakfast

1 cup (230 g) plain whole yogurt with live cultures
¼ cup (35 g) fresh blueberries
1 ounce (20 g) raw almonds or pecans
1 ounce (20 g) dried cranberries or raisins
1 to 2 tablespoons (7 to 14 g) Barlean's Forti-Flax or goji berries

*Stir together the yogurt, blueberries, almonds, and cranberries
in a small bowl until just combined. Sprinkle the Barlean's
Forti-Flax on top.*

Great Sit-Down Breakfast

1 tablespoon (14 g) butter or Barlean's extra-virgin 100 percent
organic coconut oil
1 apple, sliced
2 free-range eggs, whisked slightly with a fork
2 or 3 huge handfuls raw organic spinach
½ teaspoon turmeric
½ teaspoon lemon pepper

*Melt the butter in a skillet over medium heat. Add the apple
slices and stir-fry for a few seconds until they brown slightly.
Add the eggs and spinach and keep mixing. After a minute
or two, add the turmeric and lemon pepper. Mix until the
eggs are scrambled and the spinach is incorporated.*

(Optional: Serve with one slice whole-grain bread.)

Eat Some Hot Peppers!

While writing this book, I got an interesting phone call from Tara Parker-Pope of the *New York Times*, one of the best reporters in America covering science and health for national magazines and newspapers. Apparently, Hillary Clinton—who was then running for the Democratic presidential nomination—had told reporters that the secret to keeping her energy up on the campaign trail was eating plenty of capsaicin peppers. The *Times* wanted to know what I thought about that.

Truth be told, eating hot peppers for energy is a pretty interesting possibility. Hot peppers, such as cayenne, habanero, and jalapeño, have an active ingredient called *capsaicin*, which has a host of benefits and uses, one of which just might be increasing metabolism (and possibly energy).

Eating red hot chile peppers raises your levels of "feel-good" endorphins, according to my friend, Dharma Singh Khalsa, M.D. At the very least, hot peppers will definitely wake you up! Capsaicin is a vasodilator*, enhancing circulation and increasing body temperature. What's more, hot peppers may act as a metabolism booster. In one animal study, capsaicin promoted energy metabolism and suppressed the accumulation of body fat.

I think adding hot peppers to your diet makes a lot of sense. They're loaded with antioxidants, low in calories, and high on taste. They'll certainly wake you up and put a zing in your step!

Meaning it helps relax the muscles of the blood vessels, dilating them and allowing blood, nutrients, and oxygen to flow more freely.

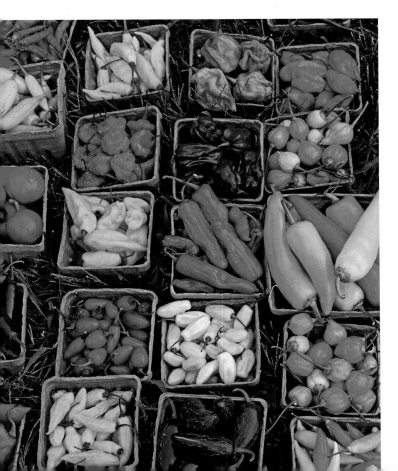

Prescription for Fatigue: Drink Water. Repeat

Years ago, I participated in a panel discussion about health at the *Los Angeles Times* annual festival of health and fitness. A couple of well-known Los Angeles health practitioners were also on the panel. I remember two things vividly about this experience. The first was a telling exchange between one of the docs and an audience member who asked for tips on working with patients.

"The single most important thing I do during the first session for almost everybody is to get them to double or triple the amount of water they're drinking," said the doc. "Then I tell them to come back in a week or two. In almost 80 percent of the cases, they report a huge improvement in energy levels and overall well-being."

The second thing I remember about that panel discussion is that *everyone else on the panel nodded affirmatively as the practitioner was speaking.*

Water is *that* important.

WATER: THE #1 ENERGY DRINK ON THE PLANET

I know water is probably not what you'd consider a high-energy drink, but maybe it should be. Studies have shown that athletes' performance can be significantly reduced if they're even 2 percent dehydrated. And that means it will have the same negative effect on your daily energy. You need water for virtually every metabolic process, including the production of cellular energy.

Water is essential for flushing out the waste products and toxins that can significantly contribute to fatigue. It's also essential for preventing constipation and optimizing kidney and liver function, all very important if you're going to operate at peak energy levels.

Your body is actually about 60 percent water, and to function efficiently—to maintain optimal health, vigor, and mental sharpness—you must keep the supply flowing. Eight glasses of water a day is the minimum you should drink (and even that may not be enough if you're overweight). Here's my personal formula for calculating how much water you should be drinking: Take your weight and divide it by two—that's the number of ounces a day to shoot for. So, if, for example, you're 200 pounds (91 kg), go for 100 ounces (3 L) of pure water a day.

Besides being quickly and easily absorbed, water has no calories and is almost always available. Much of what we perceive as hunger is actually thirst. (You can demonstrate this for yourself by simply drinking 8 to 12 ounces (235 to 355 ml) of water next time you feel hungry. Half the time the hunger will be gone in a few minutes.) For at least some of us, a drop in energy can be related to mild dehydration.

If you need more motivation to drink up, then consider this: Water is number one in the antiaging arsenal of Nicholas Perricone, M.D., F.A.C.N., formerly of Yale University and the chairman of the International Conference on Aging and Aging Skin. Perricone says, "If I could teach my patients and students three things that would keep them forever young, they would be 1. Drink water, 2. Drink water, and 3. Drink more water."

--------- **WORTH KNOWING** ---------

If you're tempted by the healthy-looking vitamin waters, don't be. They're overpriced nonsense. The amount of vitamins they contain is absolutely paltry, less than you'd get in the cheapest drugstore multiple. If the money is burning a hole in your pocket, get pricey artesian water and take a multiple vitamin.

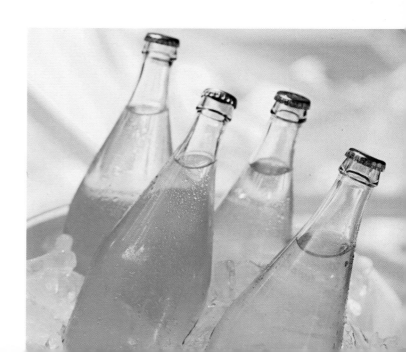

How Much Water Do We Actually Need?

Although practically everyone has heard the recommendation to drink eight glasses of water a day, this recommendation is based more on convention and tradition than on hard science.

We actually don't know that much about water intake and excretion patterns in what's called "free-living individuals" (i.e., us) because fluid intake, particularly from noncaloric, nonalcoholic, and noncaffeinated beverages, is very poorly documented. A growing number of scientists are asking "Where's the beef?" in the standard "eight glasses a day" recommendation. (Answer: There isn't any.)

The recommendation seems to have been originated in some anecdotal reports dating back to a 1796 German text by a physician named Christoph Wilhelm Hufeland. Hufeland wrote about the vibrant, eighty-year-old surgeon general to the King of Prussia who had "contracted the habit of drinking daily from seven to eight glasses" of cold water and "enjoyed much better health than in his youth."

Then in 1945, the U.S. government's food and nutrition board issued the statement that "a suitable allowance of water for adults is 2.5 liters daily in most instances," adding that most of this quantity is contained in prepared foods!

Many experts now think that you can get all the fluid you need from drinking when thirsty, and that there's generally enough fluid in food and beverages to more than provide the body with the water it needs. These experts say that if you had to actually drink those 2.5 liters the food and nutrition board recommended, you'd have to consume eight to ten glasses a day, but you don't, because there's plenty of water in the food you eat.

I don't buy it. I think it's like saying "you can get all the vitamins you need from food." You probably can if your purpose is to avoid deficiency diseases, but that's "minimum wage nutrition," and getting enough fluid to prevent clinical dehydration is "minimum wage hydration" and certainly won't do much for your energy.

Call me crazy, but I still think it makes sense to stay with the conventional wisdom. After all, you wouldn't wash your clothes in milk, would you? Water is noncaloric, cheap, and readily available. I'm sticking with the traditionalists on this one, even though I recognize that there really is no hard science to back up the value of actually drinking eight glasses a day.

And yes, flavored noncaloric sparkling waters count, but avoid the ones with artificial sweeteners, and be aware that the carbonation can make some people feel bloated.

#25

Step Away from the Diet Soda

If you think drinking diet soda has no effect on your health or energy, think again. For the past few years, mounting evidence has shown that diet soda will not only *not* help you lose weight, but it may also help you *gain* weight. It's a rare bird indeed who gets *increased* energy from unwanted weight gain!

Inconvenient fact: A 2005 study at the University of Texas Health Science Center found a 41 percent increase in the risk for being overweight for every single can of diet soda a person consumed daily.

There's more. Researchers studied the dietary information of more than 9,500 people over nine years to determine how diet might affect metabolic syndrome—the collection of risk factors for cardiovascular disease and diabetes that includes abdominal obesity, high cholesterol and blood glucose levels, and elevated blood pressure—a well-known energy drainer. Not surprisingly, they found those who ate a diet high in refined grains, fried foods, and red meat had a higher risk—18 percent higher—for metabolic syndrome. Those who ate

the most red meat increased their risk by 25 percent more than those who ate the least*.

But here's the kicker—people who drank one can of diet soda a day had a whopping 34 percent higher risk of developing metabolic syndrome than those who drank none. That's *one can* of diet soda per day. Sweetened beverages, such as juices and regular soda, carried no extra risk.

So, you might well ask, how can something with *no calories* increase the risk for obesity and heart disease?

*I think it's always worth mentioning an inherent limitation of these studies, which is that the meat they're talking about here is nearly always the commercial, factory-farmed meats, typically highly processed and filled with antibiotics, steroids, and hormones. The people eating the most meat in these studies also tend to eat the least amount of vegetables and fiber.

SUGAR CRAVINGS AND THE PAVLOVIAN RESPONSE

One theory, the one I hold dear, has to do with Pavlov's dogs. You may remember from high school that Pavlov fed his dogs steak at the same time as he rang a bell. Eventually, the mere ringing of the bell caused the dogs to salivate, exactly as they would if presented with an actual T-bone

One study found a 41 percent increase in the risk for being overweight for every single can of diet soda a person consumed daily. It's a rare bird indeed who gets *increased* energy from unwanted weight gain!

steak, even though there was no meat in sight. Pavlov named this a "conditioned response."

My long-held theory has been that the sweet taste of diet soda works in the brain to create a conditioned response, and the body responds as it usually does to normal sugar—with insulin, the fat-storing hormone. Those circuits in the brain are pretty primitive, and they don't immediately recognize chemical fakery; as far as your brain is concerned, sweet means sugar. It's entirely possible that physiologically, you would respond to aspartame—the artificial sweetener in most diet soda—in the same way as you would to table sugar.

Now Josephine M. Egan, M.D., and Robert F. Margolskee, M.D., Ph.D., of the National Institutes of Health and Mount Sinai School of Medicine, respectively, have published research that offers a variation on my explanation. They write, "Apparently, the gut 'tastes' sugars and sweeteners in much the same way as does the tongue and by using many of the same signaling elements. Taste receptors and other taste signaling elements in the gut may be contributors to obesity, diabetes, metabolic syndrome, and other diet-related disorders." Again, our body can't tell the difference between real and artificial sweeteners.

Another theory is that the taste of something sweet—even if it's fake—creates the same cascade of cravings in a carb addict that real sugar does. Cravings lead to refrigerator raids and an overload of food, which leads to obesity. Then there's the diet soda and ice cream sundae theory. Some people believe that by drinking diet beverages they're "saving" calories, which, subconsciously gives them "permission" to eat more.

TRIFECTA FOR AN ENERGY DRAIN

Finally, there's the heart disease connection. Aspartame is primarily made from three ingredients: *aspartic acid*, *phenylalanine*, and *methanol*. Methanol, an alcohol, breaks down in the body into formaldehyde, a poison if there ever was one.

Apologists for aspartame say that it doesn't create enough formaldehyde in the body to make a difference or cause any damage, but I'm not so sure. Exposing children to formaldehyde levels as low as 0.75 mg daily for several months has been shown to cause gradual toxicity. Plus, diet soda is frequently stored in hot warehouses, causing breakdown that goes undetected in the original safety studies that looked at "ideal" conditions.

Obesity, heart disease, toxicity—it's the trifecta for an energy drain.

Soda—regular or diet—is bad news. Period. For more energy and better health, dump the diet soda and drink more water.

#26

For Surprising Energy Benefits, Stay Hungry

A little bit of hunger can mean a whole lotta energy. Let me explain.

People who remember Arnold Schwarzenegger from his pre-Governor, pre-*Terminator* days might recall a 1977 movie called *Pumping Iron* that introduced the young Austrian bodybuilder to American audiences. But what they may not remember is that *Pumping Iron* wasn't Arnold's first movie. That honor went to a Bob Rafelson film made the previous year. It told the fictional story of a bunch of young bodybuilders in Southern California who were willing to do anything to become champions. The prophetic title of that long forgotten film? *Stay Hungry*.

The young Arnold and his fictional band of merry men were on to something. It's not an accident that there's a cliché that goes "lean mean hungry machine." When you hear that, you sure don't think of someone with fatigue, dragging through his day, do you? More likely you think of some up-and-coming middleweight fighter, ripped to the bone, bursting with energy (at least that's what I think of, but that's just me). Point is, hungry isn't always bad.

A little hunger can also mean a lot more energy. It may even mean a whole new lease on life, if you're interested in such things. (I'm kidding. I know you are.) Consider this: The only strategy that's ever been shown in research to extend life span is eating less food. The absolute truth is that eating less food extends the life span of every species ever tested—from yeast cells to rodents to fish to fruit flies to worms to monkeys. Maintaining a healthy weight reduces all sorts of metabolic stresses on the body, but you already know that. What you might *not* know is that staying just a little bit hungry—pushing away from the table when you're, say, 75 percent full instead of 100 percent—can also boost your energy like rocket fuel. There's a fabulous Confucian-inspired phrase used by the long-lived, high-energy people in Okinawa that goes like this: *"Hara hachi bu."* Literally translated, it means: "Eat until you are 80 percent full."

It works for me!

A LITTLE BIT OF HUNGER ISN'T A BAD THING

I remember once talking with the irascible and brilliant C. Leigh Broadhurst, Ph.D., at one of Robert Crayhon's legendary Boulderfest nutritional medicine conferences. Broadhurst is a scientist at the U.S. Department of Agriculture, who, in addition to being one of the smartest people on the planet, also happens to be a bodybuilder with about 1 ounce of body fat on her 6-foot athletic frame and enough energy to power a small city.

Broadhurst was holding court on the obesity epidemic in this country at the conference, and was scoffing at what she perceived as the wimpiness of the average American dieter.

"You need to learn to go to bed hungry," she said. "It's not going to kill you. Most of the world does it every night."

Okay, so Broadhurst, genius IQ and all, isn't going to win the Richard Simmons award for compassionate encouragement. But she's on to something. The key to eating less to increase your energy is doing it properly, making sure what you do eat is loaded with nutrients. (We call that low-calorie, nutrient-dense eating.) Eating less as in "I only had half a slice of bread for breakfast" is exactly what I am not talking about.

When you load up on protein, a little fat, and a ton of vegetables, you'd be surprised at how few calories can actually sustain you, and how little it takes to have super energy. (Come to think of it, I don't know a lot of high-energy people who are consuming 4,000 calories a day unless they're professional athletes.) A good place to start: Reduce calories by 25 percent a day. You get bonus energy points for eliminating those 25 percent calories from the least important foods, such as desserts, sodas, sugar, cereals, breads, rice, and pasta.

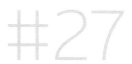
#27

Identify the Food Sensitivities That Slow You Down

Here's how I discovered the effect food sensitivities have on energy. It was around 1990 and I had recently started my career in health and fitness at the Equinox Fitness Clubs in New York City. I had a small basement office in the beautiful Equinox building in the Flatiron district of New York, where I was seeing clients for nutritional counseling.

A client named Mary came in. "I'm really fit," she said, "and I eat really well. But I simply can't seem to lose weight. Oh, and by the way, I've had these headaches ever since I was a little girl. They come and go, they drain my energy, and I can never work out when I have them. Got any ideas?"

Well, my first idea is usually this, especially when weight loss is stalled: Go back to basics. Eat food you can hunt, fish, gather, or pluck—i.e., food that isn't processed. Then see what happens. Mary tried an elimination diet: no wheat, dairy, or sugar. No bread, no milk, you know the drill.

Fast forward a couple of weeks. Mary came back in, happy as a proverbial clam. "I got off my plateau and started losing," she told me excitedly. And then, almost as an afterthought, she added: "Oh, and by the way, the weirdest thing happened. I haven't had a headache, and my energy is through the roof!"

DEATH TO ENERGY RESERVES

So here's the deal. Allergies are only one small piece of the pie when it comes to your body telling you about foods it doesn't like. Only about 5 percent of the population has what's considered classic food allergies, where there is an immediate, measurable, observable, physical response to a food or substance (if you prick their skin with the substance, you will almost immediately see a rash develop). But a huge percentage of people have something else—delayed food sensitivities. And those are death to your energy reserves.

The difficulty in identifying delayed food sensitivities is that they are exactly as advertised—delayed. You might eat the offending food at lunch, and then early in the evening (or even the next day) find yourself dragging, or feeling bloated, or having brain fog where you can't seem to shake yourself alert. But by then, you no longer associate the low-energy feeling with the food that triggered it (if you even remember eating it in the first place!).

Symptoms of food sensitivities run the gamut from the abovementioned items to annoying muscle aches and headaches (as in Mary's case). They almost always sap your energy, sometimes immediately, sometimes later, sometimes mildly, sometimes a lot.

What to do, what to do?

START WITH THE USUAL SUSPECTS

Nutrition and holistic health professions abound with partisans of various kinds of food testing and "allergy" (actually delayed food sensitivity) testing. Some are really good (the ALCAT test and the LEAP test in particular; see resources), and some are not so good. Many are expensive and frequently need someone to help you interpret them. ("But, doc, this says I'm highly sensitive to asparagus and I *never* eat asparagus!")

Fortunately, there's a really easy, low-tech way to test yourself for food sensitivities. And guess what? It doesn't cost anything.

You start with what I call "the usual suspects." My friend Elson Haas, M.D., author of *The False Fat Diet*, calls them "the sensitive seven." They're the usual suspects because the majority of people (not all, but most) who have food sensitivities find that one of these (or *several* of these) is the offending food or ingredient. (If that's the case, bingo! Case closed!)

If, however, eliminating these seven doesn't improve your energy, you might want to consult with a health professional about more extensive food sensitivity testing if you believe that food sensitivities are at the bottom of your lowered energy state. But I can tell you this—a huge, double-digit percentage of people will see their energy improve *a lot* by eliminating these seven foods and food groups.

Here's the list of what Haas calls the "sensitive seven":

1. Wheat (and/or all grains)
2. Dairy (especially milk and cheese)
3. Sugar
4. Soy
5. Corn
6. Chocolate
7. Citrus fruits

Now a word about number one on the list—grains. I know what I'm about to say may sound like heresy in a world that gets most of its calories from grains, and in a country whose nutritional policy is based on a food pyramid that puts grains at the center of any healthy diet. But I've never shied away from controversy, and I'm not going to start now: Grains are just not a great food for many people. If you're one of them—and there are many more of you than you might think—eating grains is going to be an energy disaster.

Here's why. Most grains* (wheat, barley, rye, spelt, durum, and semolina) contain a sticky, gluey substance called *gluten*. If you're gluten-sensitive and you eat gluten, watch out. You certainly won't have optimal energy, and you may have a host of other unpleasant (or even worse) symptoms as well.

There is a serious digestive disease called celiac disease that is pretty much defined by a complete intolerance to gluten. Celiac disease is an autoimmune disorder that damages the small intestine and interferes with the absorption of nutrients. We used to think it was rare; we now know it occurs in approximately 1 percent of the world's population, and in even higher rates in some countries (about 1 in 133 people in the United States).

Even without full-blown celiac disease, you may have gluten sensitivity. My great friend, the nutritional scientist Shari Lieberman, Ph.D., C.N.S., has written the definitive book on the far-ranging symptoms that can be triggered by gluten sensitivity (*The Gluten Connection: How Gluten Sensitivity Can Be Sabotaging Your Health—And What You Can Do to Take Control Now*). To those who are sensitive to gluten, "bread is not the staff of life," Lieberman says, "it is a slow-working poison."

Personally, I've seen some major action on the energy front when people just remove grains and dairy from their diet (and even more action energetically when they remove sugar as well). Give it at least two weeks (three is better) and see what you think.

I'm willing to bet it'll make a great difference in your energy.

According to Lieberman, oats don't actually contain gluten, but because of widespread cross-contamination from fields in which wheat has been grown, or processing in plants that refine wheat, they may not be safe for gluten-sensitive individuals unless certified to be gluten-free.

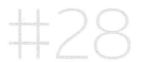

For More Energy, Eat Right for Your Type

Ever notice how some people bounce off the walls with energy when they eat a high-protein diet, while other folks feel lethargic on the same meal plan? Or how some people seem to have boundless energy when they switch to a vegetarian diet that makes their pals feel fatigued and listless?

For decades, various researchers have taken a stab at the elusive holy grail of matching people to their perfect diets. And doesn't it make perfect sense? It's absolutely elegant: A type X would have great energy and health on a high-protein diet, a type Y would thrive on raw foods, and a type Z would function just fine on nothing but Cherry Garcia.

Recognizing the vast diversity in genetics, hormones, metabolism, ancestry, and a million other variables, many nutritionists and other health professionals have correctly intuited that it would be oh-so-wonderful if only we could identify those "types" so that we could determine what sorts of people would do best on what sorts of diets.

And indeed it would. There have been numerous tests, from saliva tests to blood tests to sophisticated questionnaires, developed in an attempt to identify certain characteristics in a person's makeup that would make it more likely that he or she would thrive on a certain kind of diet. William Wolcott's metabolic typing is one such system, and Peter D'Adamo's blood type system is another. (In the blood type system, for example, people with type O blood are believed to do much better on diet higher in meat than, say, a person with type A blood. This is a huge oversimplification, but hopefully gets the point across.)

These systems have both their proponents and their critics. The practitioners of these systems devote a great deal of time, energy, and study to refining them so that they can help their clients pick the foods that support them in health, and avoid those that don't. One thing all these typing systems have in common is the belief that it's not enough for a food to just be healthy—if you're not suited to that food, it's not healthy for you, even if it's great for someone else. (An easy-to-understand example that doesn't require any typing system to comprehend is a food allergy. Foods can be amazingly healthy, such as citrus fruits, tree nuts, and eggs, but if you're allergic to them, they're all wrong for *you*.)

THE NUTRITIONAL TYPING SYSTEM

The system I like best so far for identifying what type of diet is most likely to give you the most energy was developed by my good friend Glen Depke, N.D., and is called nutritional typing. Depke, a traditional naturopath and the chief nutritionist at the Mercola Optimal Wellness Center in Illinois, has developed a terrific basic questionnaire that you can use to determine whether you are a "veggie type," a "mixed type," or a "protein type." He has generously allowed me to reproduce that questionnaire here. It's a simplified version of the nutritional typing test they use at the Mercola Center.

Take the test, and use the results to determine where you should start for your optimal high-energy diet plan, realizing that you may have to tweak it depending on your needs. Nonetheless, the two sample diet plans below should give you a great place to start once you know which type you are.

NUTRITIONAL TYPING TEST

Choose your answer and keep a tally of your score according to the number of points assigned.

1. If you had to be at your best throughout the morning with high physical, mental, and emotional energy and did not have a chance to have anything but water from breakfast to lunch, which meal would you choose for breakfast?
   - Yogurt mixed with fruit –2
   - Steak and eggs with a small amount of hash browns +2
   - Almost any food would work for me 0

2. Do you crave salt or snacks with salt, such as potato chips?
   - Yes +1
   - No –1
   - At times but not consistently 0

3. Do you do well with a juice or water fast? (If you've never done one, take a guess at how you might feel.)
   - No +2
   - Yes –2
   - Can fast if need be 0

4. If you had to be at your best throughout the afternoon with high physical, mental, and emotional energy and did not have a chance to have anything but water from lunch to dinner, which meal would you choose for lunch?
   - Large salad with a small chicken breast –2
   - Beef tenderloin with a small spinach salad +2
   - Almost any food would work for me 0

5. If eating dessert, what would you prefer? (Remember, this is based only on your desire, not what you think is better or worse for you. What would you eat if no one were looking?)
   - Cheesecake +2
   - Mixed berries with low-fat yogurt –2
   - Almost any desert would appeal to me 0

6. If you had to be at your best throughout the evening with high physical, mental, and emotional energy and did not have a chance to have anything but water from dinner to bedtime, which meal would you choose for dinner?
   - Rib-eye steak with cauliflower topped with cheese sauce +2
   - Tilapia with a large Caesar salad –2
   - Almost any food would work for me 0

7. How would you react if you were forced to skip a meal?
   - I would have no problem –2
   - I would react very poorly +2
   - I could skip a meal if necessary but would really prefer not to 0

8. If you drank a glass of fruit juice on an empty stomach, how would you react?
   - Poorly +2
   - I would respond well –2
   - This would have no noticeable effect on me 0

Add up your score to determine your estimated nutritional needs.

–15 to –5	Veggie type
–6 to +5	Mixed type
+6 to +15	Protein type

If you're a veggie type, it would be best to include higher amounts of vegetables in your diet, cut back on red meat, focus on lighter fish and white meat fowl, and use fat sparingly.

If you're a protein type, increase quality organic red meat (I recommend only grass-fed meat), wild-caught fatty fish, and dark meat fowl in your diet and consume higher amounts of quality fats and slightly lower amounts of vegetables.

If you fall into the middle, you're probably a mixed type. Start with an assortment of quality meats and vegetables and a fair amount of fat.

To further your understanding of your true nutritional type, visit www.mercola.com, click on the store, then membership programs, and finally the nutritional typing test. The full version of the nutritional typing test includes meal plans, instructions, meal planning ideas, and a free one-month membership to the nutritional typing forum. Highly recommended! You can also contact Glen Depke at www.depkewellness.com.

HIGH-ENERGY EATING PLANS

The following are sample meal plans suited to each nutritional type. Note that specific amounts will vary from person to person, depending on your height, weight, gender, activity level, etc.

Veggie Type—Two-Day Sample Meal Plan for Optimal Energy

DAY 1
BREAKFAST
- Grapefruit
- Oatmeal topped with plain yogurt, apple, and cinnamon

LUNCH
- Organic mixed green salad with tomato, cucumber, and dressing of freshly squeezed lemon or apple cider vinegar
- Low-fat organic cottage cheese
- Fresh cantaloupe slices

DINNER
- Lightly steamed or sautéed zucchini with freshly squeezed lemon
- Chicken breast
- Small organic baked potato

DAY 2
BREAKFAST
- Veggie juice
- Low-fat plain organic yogurt with organic blueberries

LUNCH
- Raw cucumber, green pepper, and carrot slices
- Turkey breast slices
- Organic grapes

DINNER
- Lightly steamed broccoli with freshly squeezed lemon
- Baked codfish
- Organic apple

Protein Type—Two-Day Sample Meal Plan for Optimal Energy

DAY 1
BREAKFAST
- Turkey sausage
- Omelet with spinach and feta cheese
- Small handful of raw walnuts with an apple

LUNCH
- Roast beef slices
- Celery sticks with whole-fat cottage cheese
- Small handful of raw Brazil nuts with half of a pear

DINNER
- Sirloin burger with cheese
- Baby spinach salad with sliced avocado, mushroom, and olive oil
- Winter squash with butter

DAY 2

BREAKFAST

- Steak with mushrooms
- Soft-boiled or sunny-side-up egg
- Oatmeal with butter or coconut oil, cinnamon, and diced apple

LUNCH

- Whole chicken leg (includes leg and thigh)
- Lightly steamed asparagus with a hard-boiled egg
- Raw carrot sticks dipped in organic ranch dressing

DINNER

- Wild-caught salmon
- Green beans drizzled with olive oil
- Brown rice with coconut oil* or butter

Mixed Type—Two-Day Sample Meal Plan for Optimal Energy

DAY 1

BREAKFAST

- Veggie omelet with tomato, spinach, and Swiss cheese
- Organic plain yogurt with fresh organic raspberries

LUNCH

- Roast beef rollups stuffed with cucumber slices, cheese, and mustard
- Fresh pineapple with cottage cheese

DINNER

- Baked tilapia
- Spinach and mushroom salad with dressing of apple cider vinegar and olive oil
- Small handful of raw pumpkin seeds with an apple

DAY 2

BREAKFAST

- Chicken sausage cooked in butter or coconut oil
- Hard-boiled egg with sliced tomato
- Fresh grapefruit

LUNCH

- Lettuce wraps with romaine lettuce, turkey breast, ham, and cheese
- Apple with organic peanut butter

DINNER

- Pork chop
- Organic mixed greens drizzled with olive oil and apple cider vinegar
- Small organic sweet potato with skin

Remember, these plans are not set in stone; they're merely suggested starting points. The idea here is to be more mindful of the effect food has on your mood and energy. If with these plans you're flying high, then bingo. If you need to fine-tune them, so be it. The point is not to slavishly follow a diet plan but to use your natural inclinations—what Depke and the folks at the Mercola Center would refer to as your nutritional type—as a place to start, a place from which to expand and develop your own personal high-energy eating plan. With a little experimentation and mindfulness, you'll soon discover your own personal formula for blasting through any day with optimal energy and well-being.

*To read why coconut oil is such a good oil, see my book The 150 Healthiest Foods on Earth.

More Processed Carbs Equals Less Energy

One thing is fairly certain: Whatever the proportions of protein, fat, and carbohydrates you eventually come up with as being ideal for your type, the fewer processed carbohydrates on your plate the better.

Ideally, the highest energy diet will include food as close as possible to that which our Paleolithic ancestors could have hunted, fished, gathered, or plucked from a tree. That means meat (grass-fed or wild game), fish, vegetables, fruits, berries, and nuts, with some modern high-tech versions of those staples, such as whey protein powder or coconut oil thrown in for good measure.

That's a prescription for high-energy eating if ever there was one.

29

Choose the Right Energy Drink (or None at All)

Caffeine- and taurine-containing drinks such as Red Bull have been on the European market for more than a decade. And the whole category of energy drinks is exploding. As of this writing (June 2008), here is just a random sampling of the ones lining my local convenience store: BPM Energy, Beaver Buzz, Blue Charge, Hype Energy, Full Throttle, Rockstar, Jolt Cola, Spike Shooter, Lightning Bolt, Boost, and Monster Energy. (Let no one accuse the manufacturers of too much subtlety.)

The basic ingredients of the most successful ones are caffeine, taurine, and glucuronolactone (a naturally occurring carbohydrate in the body that is believed to help fight fatigue and increase well-being). Plenty of studies show that caffeine can be a mild energy booster, albeit not one without some side effects—such as jitteriness—that depends largely on both the dose and the sensitivity of the person taking it. (See page 72 for a discussion of the most famous caffeine-containing drink on the planet, plain old coffee.) But what are these other ingredients? Do they work? And more important, can I recommend them?

Let's go to the videotape.

TAURINE: MIXED REVIEWS FOR ENERGY ENHANCEMENT

Taurine is a conditionally essential amino acid, meaning that in certain times, such as during high stress, the body doesn't make it very well, so it has to be provided by the diet. It's somehow managed to get a reputation as an energy supplement, largely because manufacturers now routinely add it to most drinks that are in the class of beverages known as energy drinks. The evidence for taurine as an energy booster is, to say the very least, mixed. But some preliminary research seems to show that it *might* have a place in your program.

If you're a serious endurance athlete, taurine makes sense. Long, stressful exercise absolutely depletes taurine, and it makes sense to supplement with it if you want to keep performance up. Question is, does it help fight fatigue and increase energy for normal folks who aren't running marathons? The jury is still out on that.

A number of animal studies seem to show that if animals are taurine-depleted, they don't have much energy. Because animals can't actually tell us how they feel, scientists use objective measures of energy, such as the ability to produce force, or the length of time they can run on little mouse treadmills, or other similar measures. It's pretty clear that with less than optimal levels of taurine,

lab animals aren't winning the equivalent of the Australian Grand Slam, and that when researchers give them taurine, their performance improves significantly.

And it's not just animals. There are some human studies that are also promising. Problem is, some of these studies use popular drinks such as Red Bull, which mixes three potentially fatigue-busting ingredients (caffeine, taurine, and glucuronolactone), so it's less clear which ingredient is having the fatigue-fighting, performance-enhancing effect.

One study looked at the effect of taurine supplementation on visual fatigue in college students and found that taurine supplementation for twelve days significantly reduced the visual fatigue brought on by long, boring tasks in front of a computer. Another study, published in the *International Journal of Sport, Nutrition and Exercise Metabolism* in 2007, found that a supplement containing a combination of amino acids, creatine, taurine, caffeine, and glucuronolactone did modestly improve high-intensity endurance. Yet another study showed that a typical energy drink preparation with those same three ingredients (taurine, caffeine, and glucuronolactone) given to very sleepy participants improved their driving performance and reaction time as measured in a driving simulator.

It's pretty clear that with less than optimal levels of taurine, lab animals aren't winning the equivalent of the Australian Grand Slam.

One study from the University of Vienna in Austria tested that same mixture of the three ingredients found in Red Bull and found that it had positive effects on both mental performance and mood. Red Bull was also studied in the psychology department of the University of the West of England in Bristol, and it was found to significantly improve both aerobic endurance and anaerobic (speed and strength) performance on cycle ergometers. That study also demonstrated significant improvement in mental performance, including reaction time, concentration, memory, and alertness.

So if I'm the manufacturer of Red Bull, this news is making me very happy.

OCCASIONAL ENERGY BOOSTS

However, I'm not the manufacturer of Red Bull. I'm someone advising you on your health and energy. Although Red Bull and its clones might get you through the occasional rough patch of low energy, it's really hard for me to recommend them as a regular supplement.

For one thing, they're loaded with sugar (or aspartame, if you get the sugar-free kind). For another, many drinks in this category are packed with artificial chemicals and colors. The drink doesn't hydrate the way regular sports drinks do (see page 71 for Accelerade). One (admittedly small) study linked overconsumption to high blood pressure. For all these reasons, I'm extremely hesitant to recommend that you start relying on Red Bull or its clones.

That said, it's clear that energy drinks *can* make a difference and might be a good emergency measure, one that you want to keep in your back pocket for those special times when you

really need a little boost. But don't make it a habit. I'd still rather see you increase your energy naturally with good lifestyle choices that will make it less necessary for you to reach for the Red Bull in the first place.

#30
Snack on Seeds to Sustain Stamina

Ever wonder how trail mix got its name? Well, I'll tell you. It was originally designed for hikers. (Get it?) Back in the day, before it was sold in every health food store as a premix, my friends and I would make up a big bunch of the stuff using nuts, seeds, raisins, and sometimes carob chips, mix it all together, throw it in our backpacks, and go do a four-hour trek on the Delaware Water Gap hiking trail in New Jersey. Trail mix was the ultimate energy food.

One standard component of trail mix is seeds—sesame seeds, pumpkin seeds, it hardly matters. All are good, for much the same reason nuts are—they contain fiber, protein, nutritious fat, and a high content of minerals needed for every metabolic process. They can be a great addition to any energy snack, or you can eat them alone. (Just don't eat the whole bag, especially if you're trying to manage weight and especially if you're *not* hiking a four-hour trail!)

The key to using seeds—and nuts—for energy is to keep the quantity low, just enough to give you an edge, not enough to slow you down. The beauty of trail mix is that you don't need to be too exact about measurements. For example, start by taking equal portions (say 1 tablespoon, or 15 g) of oats, nuts, raisins, pumpkin seeds, and cranberries. Later, you can have a little less of one, a little more of another, and maybe add some special ingredients such as goji berries or carob chips. It's fun, and it's all about your own personal taste.

Pumpkin seeds in particular are good for men (though fine for women as well). Why? Because they contain chemicals called *cucurbitacins* that seem to interfere with the production of a metabolic by-product of testosterone called DHT (dihydrotestosterone), which can cause hair loss in both men and women. (A lot of energy is spent worrying about said hair loss and opening stupid emails promising a cure for baldness. Use your energy for better things!)

Roasting your own pumpkin seeds is easy and multiplies their health benefits even further, especially when you season them with turmeric, garlic, or cayenne pepper. Just melt some organic butter, macadamia nut oil, coconut oil, or olive oil in a frying pan and toss in the seeds. Stir them around for 2 to 3 minutes, or until they're slightly browned. Then spread them on a baking sheet, spice them up with seasoning, bake them for a few minutes until they're crisp, and enjoy!

TRY SOME TAHINI

Tahini is made from sesame seeds, which contains plant chemicals called *lignans*, in particular *sesamin* and *sesaminol*. I love tahini as a spread, and use it all the time as a stand-in for peanut butter, almond butter, or any other kind of spread. Sesame butter, a close relative of tahini, is an even less processed version, made from whole roasted sesame seeds. (Tahini is made from hulled seeds.) Animal studies show that sesame lignans enhance fat burning by increasing liver enzymes that actually break down fat. Sesame seeds—in tahini or otherwise—are also a rich source of minerals, fiber, and protein, making them a terrific energy snack. They can be roasted or toasted in a dry skillet over medium heat. Toss them until they're golden brown, and then enjoy. Or spread tahini (or sesame butter) directly onto celery, apple slices, whole-grain bread, or anything else you'd use nut butter on. It's great!

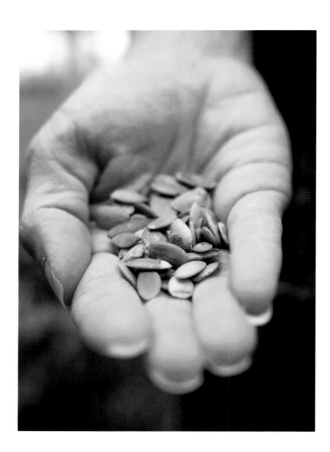

#31

Choose Oatmeal, Quinoa, and Amaranth for Energy!

In general, grains are the last category of food in which I'd look for an energy booster. More people than you might think have food sensitivities to gluten (a component of rye, barley, wheat, and oats, most grains are pretty high glycemic (even those that are marketed—often duplicitously—as "whole grains"), and most of the grains we actually consume are in the form of junk cereals frequently marketed as "healthy" while being anything but.

That said, I make a big exception for oatmeal, quinoa, and amaranth. Oatmeal is a high-fiber food that also contains protein, and its very low glycemic load ensures that it won't play havoc with your blood sugar and cause your energy to crash a half hour after you eat it. It's a great, energy-boosting breakfast—bodybuilders have combined oatmeal with eggs for years.

To this day, you can't walk through Gold's Gym in Venice, California (known as "the Mecca" for serious bodybuilders), without tripping over at least ten huge guys (and an equal number of "Ms. Fitness" types) eating a homemade mixture of oats and eggs out of the resealable containers they frequently bring with them to the gym. (And considering that most of these men and women do four-hour workouts, it's reasonable to assume that they know something about energy!)

One try of the eggs and oatmeal mix and you'll see why. Throw some raisins on and season with cinnamon, which helps modulate blood sugar. The key to the whole thing is using real, slow-cooking oatmeal. The parboiled, precooked kind does nothing for you.

One warning: More people than anyone would guess are gluten-sensitive, which means they don't react really well to a protein in grains called *gluten*, or a substrate of gluten called *gliadin*. Gluten is found in wheat, rye, barley, and, to some extent, oats. If you're a gluten-sensitive person, these grains can make you tired and bloated, and you might have to pass on the oatmeal, great food that it is. If you're not gluten-sensitive, it's a great energy food.

ANCIENT GRAINS FOR MODERN ENERGY

Quinoa, on the other hand, looks like a grain, cooks like a grain, and tastes like a grain, but is actually a seed. Who cares? Quinoa (pronounced keen-wah) has the highest protein of any "cereal," and it's gluten-free to boot. It's a great energy food either as a breakfast or as a snack.

Legend has it that the Incan armies marched for days at a time fueled by a mixture of quinoa and fat known as "war balls." 'Nuff said. (If it could get the Incan armies through their day, it should be able to do the same for you.) Quinoa also contains a fair amount of iron, not to mention 5 grams of fiber per $\frac{1}{2}$ cup.

Finally, there's amaranth. This grain has been around for 8,000 years and was a staple of the Aztecs. As cereals go, it's pretty high in protein and fiber, both of which are energy-sustaining ingredients that are in surprisingly short supply in most breakfast cereals. The protein in the amaranth grain is of an unusually high quality, and it's high in an essential amino acid called lysine, which is lacking in most grains. And amaranth is completely gluten free. It usually comes in the form of cereal.

#32

Drink Purple Juices for More Pep

These days, you can't walk into a convenience store without being overwhelmed by the offering of energy drinks. Of course, the big daddy of popular energy drinks is Red Bull, which originated in Thailand and is still the category leader. By 2006, it was sold in more than fifty countries, more than 3 billion cans a year were consumed worldwide, and sales had reached well over 2.5 billion Euros (about 3.9 billion US dollars). However, I think you can do better than caffeinated soda pop. Start by trying the following energizing alternatives.

NONI JUICE: A CROWD FAVORITE

Noni juice is made from the *Morinda citrifolia* fruit, and it's a good energy drink when consumed properly. Don't drink it straight because it's far too expensive and somewhat bitter tasting. But do throw an ounce or two into a glass of water, or add it to a smoothie. (I frequently mix it with my green drink in the morning.)

Like a lot of antioxidant-rich beverages— mangosteen comes to mind, as does the acai berry juices such as XanGo and Mona-Vie—people swear by it. Although there's no rigorous science to back up noni's use for energy enhancement (nor for any of the other exotic beverages mentioned above), thousands of fans can't all be wrong.

POMEGRANATE JUICE: A SUPERFOOD STAR

If juices were Hollywood stars, pomegranate juice would be on the cover of *People*. It's a rising star in the superfood community, and for good reason. Its combination of nutrients and low sugar is a

perfect prescription for more energy. According to research at the Technion-Israel Institute of Technology in Haifa, long-term consumption of pomegranate juice may help slow, as well as possibly protect against, both heart disease and cancer. Flavonoids, a fantastic class of healthful plant chemicals, are more concentrated in pomegranates than in grapes, and the antioxidant capacity of pomegranate juice is two to three times that of red wine or green tea. That's a pretty impressive resume.

Because sexual energy is closely related to energy in general, it's worth noting that pomegranate has been called a "natural Viagra." Research in the *Journal of Urology* suggested that long-term intake of pomegranate juice may have a positive effect on erectile dysfunction. And for you ladies, it's worth noting that the pomegranate itself has long been associated with love, erotica, and energy. In Turkey, the bride throws the fruit to the ground because traditional beliefs hold that the number of seeds that pop out will predict how many kids she's going to have. Enough said!

JONNY'S "ROLL YOUR OWN": AFFORDABLE AND HEALTHY FOR EVERYONE

This isn't the place to go into the absolutely outlandish claims of some of the multilevel marketing products such as XanGo and Mona-Vie, which are basically extremely overpriced, albeit high-antioxidant, juices. I'll leave that for another place (such as my blog on the *Huffington Post*). But I will tell you this: You can make your own high-antioxidant, energy-enhancing juice mix for about one-sixth the price of any of these products, and it will be just as good.

Some of the juices I personally keep on hand for a high-energy boost include blueberry, goji berry, acai berry, cranberry, black cherry, and the aforementioned pomegranate and noni. The beauty of making your own (besides the enormous savings in price) is that you can mix and match to your taste. One recipe I like is 2 ounces (60 ml) blueberry, 2 ounces (60 ml) black cherry, 1 ounce (28 ml) goji, 1 ounce (28 ml) noni, and 4 ounces (120 ml) pomegranate juices mixed together with 10 to 16 ounces (285 to 475 ml) of pure (filtered or artesian) water. (Again, there's no right and wrong here; just mix and match any way your taste buds dictate.)

Three things are important here: One, get the brands that are pure juice, and skip the "cocktail" juices. The pure juices are more expensive (though not even close to the price of the multilevel marketing stuff), but they have no sugar added and aren't diluted with cheaper juices. They're also a tad more bitter. Real juice has a certain natural sweetness, but nothing like the juice "cocktails" that are mostly sugar.

Second, dilute with water. You don't need to drink them straight. (How diluted is up to you. Some athletes, for example, like to mix one part juice with five parts water. My friend Ann Louise Gittleman, Ph.D., sips her "fat flushers" drink of cran-water all day long. It's a mixture of one part pure cranberry juice and three parts water.)

Third, feel free to sweeten these drinks with something such as stevia, xylitol, Lo Han, or even a drop of agave nectar (a natural sweetener). If that makes it more palatable for you, fine. You'll be getting the health and energy benefits of some of the most nutritious fruits on the planet without the energy-robbing high-sugar content of the expensive commercial mixes.

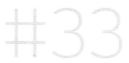

Try Accelerade to Reclaim Your Energy After a Workout

When it comes to energy, carbohydrates used to corner the market.

Not anymore.

For years—decades, even—carb loading dominated the field of sports nutrition. Standard operating procedure was to load up on pasta before a big run, and use carbohydrate drinks to recover from a hard bout of energy-draining exercise. With the advent of low-carb diets, the discussion about carbs and energy grew more sophisticated and nuanced.

We now know that a high intake of carbs can actually *drain* your energy by increasing both blood sugar and insulin, setting you up for an energy crash (not to mention weight gain and mood swings). Although the spectrum hasn't swung full circle away from carbohydrates, the bloom is off the rose. There are more sophisticated, and effective, ways to reclaim your energy after a workout.

BALANCING CARBS AND PROTEIN FOR RECOVERY

When I was a personal trainer, there was much talk about the so-called "golden window," a period of about 45 minutes right after exercise when your muscles would just soak up nutrients and energy, and your body would be primed for storing glucose (energy in the form of stored carbohydrates is called *glycogen*). Replenishing glycogen stores after exercise was the name of the game—that and repairing, rebuilding, and growing muscles that were broken down by a hard workout. Drinking or eating carbohydrates after a workout is a time-honored way to restore the lost energy and make sure you have enough for the next day.

Now, interesting research has caused us to rethink that ancient wisdom. We now know that it's critical to also take in some protein, and manufacturers are wisely paying attention to the ongoing and emerging research on just what the perfect mix of carbs and protein might be for maximum energy (and recovery). Exercise physiologist John Ivy, at the University of Texas in Austin, is one of the leading lights in this research. He has his own theory about what the right balance is.

"Our work indicates that a ratio of 2.6 grams of carbohydrates to 1 gram of protein works extremely well to replenish glycogen and speed muscle healing," he told the *New York Times* in an interview.

And that's just what you need to do to maintain, and increase, energy reserves.

DRINK BACK YOUR ENERGY

Robert Portman, PhD, is an exercise physiologist and biochemist who believes that the "sweet spot" for an energy or sports drink is a perfect combination of protein and carbs. So he and his research team at Pacific Health Laboratories in New Jersey went out and created it. It's called Accelerade.

Recent research in the highly respected journal *Medicine and Science in Sports and Exercise* found that cyclists who drank Accelerade were able to crank out about 30 percent more miles with more than 80 percent less muscle damage than those who drank conventional energy or sports drinks. The authors concluded, albeit with typical scientific reserve and caution, that Accelerade "could significantly benefit athletes in sports where endurance and recovery are important."

Accelerade also comes in a gel pack, called Accel Gel. A number of studies have shown that people who consume Accel Gel have had more energy for workouts, as demonstrated by improved swim times, improved cycling times to exhaustion, and even improved training run finish successes in slalom ski races. And Accelerade (the drink) has improved muscle recovery in runners, cyclists, and collegiate hockey players.

Remember, when athletes and exercise physiologists talk about "recovery" and "performance" they're really talking about *energy*. Granted, you have to use these drinks as intended—after working out—but many people reading this book work out regularly and are frequently exhausted. If you find that your workouts are draining you of energy and that you're not recovering fast enough, Accelerade or Accel Gel may be just what you're looking for.

#34

Drink Your Java for a Jolt

I'm probably going to lose a lot of friends in the natural health community over this one, but I think drinking coffee isn't the worst thing you could do if you need a quick energy boost.

I probably don't have to tell you about the energy-enhancing effects of coffee, but here they are in a nutshell: Coffee sits in the receptors for a brain chemical called *adenosine*, a chemical whose job it is to signal calmness. By occupying those parking spaces, the adenosine message—"you're tired"—gets interrupted or overruled. Although this is definitely *not* a good thing long term, it can have some benefits in the short term.

Coffee makes you feel perky, and used judiciously, it can be a great lubricant for mental performance, social interaction, and even athletic performance.

If all this information were a secret, there probably wouldn't be 11,000-plus Starbucks stores worldwide. But coffee is probably a guilty energy pleasure for you because you've heard so much about how bad it is. So let me assuage your guilt—at least a little.

I'm a contrarian on a lot of subjects having to do with nutrition, health, and diet, and I usually find myself at odds with conventional dietitians on a wealth of subjects. But I'm an equal-opportunity contrarian—on some issues, I find myself on the other side of the fence from even my most esteemed and respected colleagues on the "left wing" of nutritional medicine. Coffee is one of those subjects.

I may be a contrarian, but I'm not a hypocritical one. I drink coffee. Practically every day. I love it. And yup, I think it can contribute to energy in a healthy way, and nope, I don't think it's the big huge health risk many of my respected friends think it is. Of course, that endorsement comes with some caveats, so read on.

COFFEE: THE NEWS IS *NOT* SO BAD!

First the good news: Coffee has a lot of antioxidants. There's been a ton of research done on it—some 19,000 studies according to WebMD. "Overall, the research shows that coffee is far more healthful than it is harmful," says Tomas DePaulis, Ph.D., a research scientist at Vanderbilt University's Institute for Coffee Studies. "For most people, very little bad comes from drinking it, but a lot of good can result."

Research shows that people who drink coffee regularly are up to 80 percent less likely to develop Parkinson's, are 25 percent less likely to develop colon cancer, have an 80 percent reduction in their risk for liver cirrhosis, and have an almost 50 percent lower risk for gallstones. A widely reported 2004 study published in the *Annals of Internal Medicine* by Harvard researchers shows that long-term coffee consumption substantially and significantly reduces the risk for type 2 diabetes.

Even the aroma of coffee can have some benefits by positively affecting both genes and brain proteins, according to a 2008 study in the *Journal of Agriculture and Food Chemistry* (giving new meaning to the old saying "Wake up and smell the coffee!"). Researchers from Seoul National University found that merely sniffing coffee actually affected seventeen different genes in the brain, at least in rats. Levels of some brain proteins also changed in ways that could increase antioxidant function and have a soothing effect on stress.

The bad news is that many people abuse this potentially beneficial substance, literally running their empty engines on the false fuel of caffeine. Instead of using it as a pick-me-up and mild energy enhancer, they depend on it to overrule any brain messages telling them to slow down. For some susceptible people, the increase in blood pressure (though usually temporary) can be a problem. Plus coffee is an acidic beverage, something most of us don't need more of in our diet.

The best solution? Use your judgment. I don't think coffee is a health hazard, and truth be told, I wouldn't be without it. (Full disclosure: Espresso is my favorite.) But you really don't want to drink coffee late in the afternoon (it stays in your system way longer than you might think, decreasing the effectiveness and quality of your sleep), and you don't want to drink too much, ("too much" being defined as the amount that makes you feel jittery and keeps you awake at night). I also highly recommend organic, because coffee can be a highly sprayed crop loaded with toxins.

However, for a quick energy boost, or a before-exercise performance enhancer, you can't beat it. "People who already drink a lot of coffee don't have to feel guilty as long as coffee does not affect their daily life," says Harvard researcher Frank Hu, M.D. "They may actually benefit from coffee habits in the long run."

Amen to that.

crackers such as Wasa bread (or, in a pinch, you can eat them out of the can with a plastic fork). If you're in somewhat more relaxed circumstances than we were, sardines over any kind of green salad makes the perfect low-carb meal.

You simply cannot beat those little fish for a quick, easy, inexpensive source of first-class protein and omega-3 fats, both of which are essential for energy and metabolism (not to mention overall health). The best kind of sardines, if you can find them, are packed in sardine oil. Do not get the kind in soybean or cottonseed oil, because these are way too high in inflammatory omega-6s.

#35

Grab a Can of Energy

Here's a riddle for you: What's the best energy food in the world that comes in a can?

Here's a hint: It's not a drink, it's easy to find, and it's easy to eat.

I learned about the perfect "energy food in a can" while traveling around in Florida with my dear friend, the famous New York nutritionist Oz Garcia. Oz and I were giving seminars and had a brutal schedule, traveling from place to place with almost no downtime to grab a bite to eat. Whenever Oz, who, by the way, is one of the most high-energy people on the planet, felt his blood sugar dropping or his energy dipping, he would stop the car, run into the nearest convenience store or bodega and grab . . . a can of sardines.

That's how I learned firsthand how energizing and satisfying this food can be, right out of the can! You can eat sardines with some low-carb, low-sugar

#36

Eat Beans and Lentils to Get Through the Day

Beans and lentils are absolutely great for sustained energy. The high fiber content ensures that the sugars in them are released slowly into your bloodstream, resulting in a nice, even flow of energy rather than the quick spike and drop associated with, say, a candy bar (not that you'd ever eat one of those things!).

The protein in beans and lentils is filling, and the carbs in them provide a great, slow-burning source of fuel. Eat beans on a Monday morning and your blood sugar won't drop again until Tuesday afternoon. (Just kidding—but you get the idea.) Garbanzo beans and lentils are particularly high in fiber, 12.5 grams and 16 grams per cup, respectively. You can't do better than that!

I recently interviewed Dan Buettner, the *National Geographic Explorer* whose *New York*

Times best-selling book *The Blue Zones* chronicled the lifestyles and diets of people in four areas around the world ("blue zones") where there are the highest numbers of healthy centenarians. These folks, who are scattered around the globe in the far-ranging places of Sardinia, Italy; Loma Linda, California; the Okinawa prefecture in Japan; and the Nicoya Peninsula in Costa Rica, are among the healthiest, leanest, and most energetic in the world. Many of them are still active in their early hundreds!

Buettner told me one of the features shared by all their diets was a high intake of beans. "Beans, whole grains, and garden vegetables are the cornerstone of all these longevity diets," he said. The Seventh-Day Adventists in Loma Linda who ate legumes (such as peas and beans) three times a week had a 30 to 40 percent reduction in colon cancer. The Okinawan diet is high in bean curd (tofu), and the classic Sardinian and Nicoyan diets are also high in locally grown beans.

Something to think about.

#37

Try Superfood Maca

You may have noticed an underlying theme in this book: All sources of energy are related. When your energy is depleted physically, it's also usually depleted mentally, sexually, and spiritually. Activities, foods, lifestyle changes, or supplements that help in one area tend to help in others.

Which brings me to the energy superfood maca.

I first heard about maca back in the 90's, when I interviewed a researcher who had discovered

that maca produced spontaneous erections in rodents. (Her study was published in the *Journal of Urology* in 2000.) I wrote about it in *The Most Effective Natural Cures on Earth* as part of a natural prescription for sexual vitality and health. My friend Chris Kilham, also known as the Medicine Hunter, has long touted this herb for its aphrodisiac and energy-increasing powers, and points out that it's also known as Peruvian ginseng.

Maca deserves the name superfood. It's a cruciferous plant, putting it in the same distinguished family as broccoli and watercress. It's rich in sugars, protein, starches, and essential minerals, especially iodine and iron, as well as tons of other biochemically active ingredients. It's used traditionally not only to increase sexual energy but also to increase stamina and well-being.

Traditionally, maca is believed to simulate metabolism, regulate hormones, and improve memory, although empirical scientific research has not yet been done to substantiate these uses. Nonetheless, I believe maca belongs on anyone's short list of superfoods for improving energy.

The blue-ribbon research committee that authored the National Institutes of Health's prestigious *Encyclopedia of Dietary Supplements* says maca has been established as a nutritionally valuable food and food supplement.

Maca is known to be an adaptagen, which means it provides more energy if needed, but won't overstimulate you. My preferred form of maca is as a food rather than as a supplement. One company that makes a superb product is David Wolfe's Sunfood Nutrition (www.sunfood. com). I buy the 1-pound (455 g) raw, certified organic package, and mix a tablespoon or two (14 to 28 g) into any number of energy drinks, from protein shakes to smoothies.

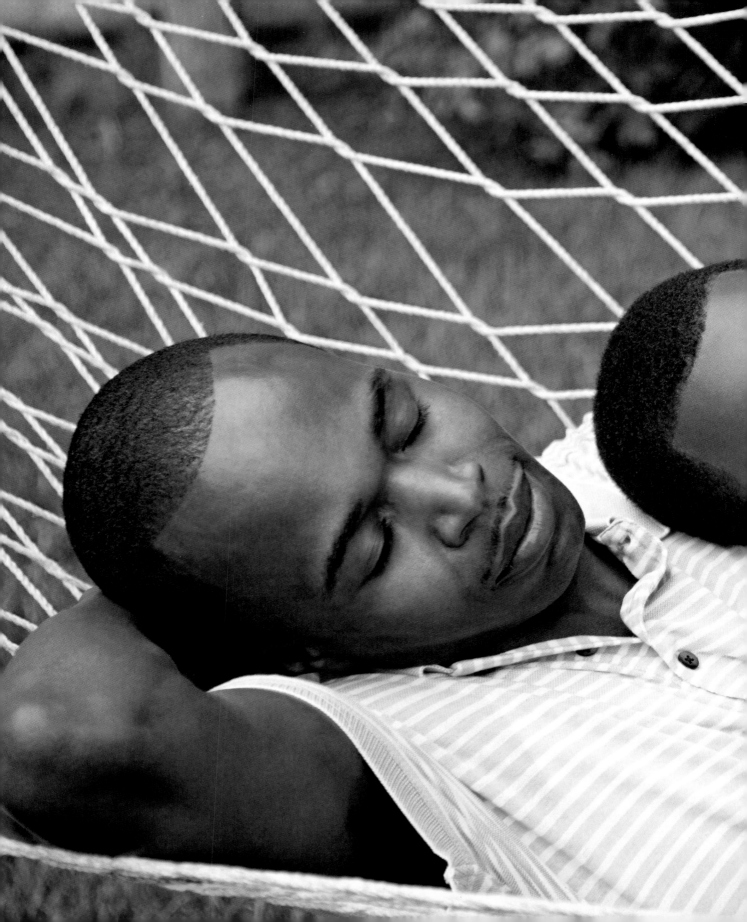

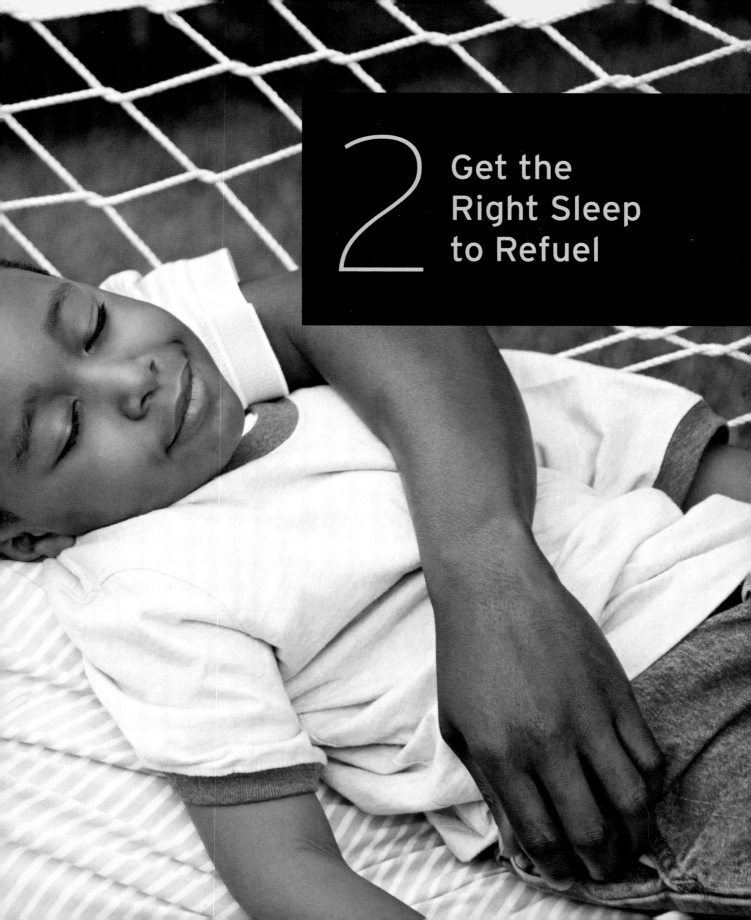

2

Get the Right Sleep to Refuel

There's a saying one of my psychology professors was fond of using, and it's stayed with me for the better part of three decades: "When you hear hoofbeats, don't start looking for zebras."

That saying, which every medical student is familiar with, is a clever reworking of Occam's razor, a principle that, roughly translated, means: "All things being equal, the simplest explanation is the best one." Hoofbeats *usually* mean horses—at the very least, that's a darn good place to start when you're searching for an explanation for that galloping sound you hear outside your window. "Don't start by looking for zebras" is a philosophy that's informed most of the work I've done in nutrition for the past fifteen years or so.

Which brings me to sleep.

There are obviously a slew of reasons to explain why so many of us are fatigued, drained of energy, and unable to get through our day on full steam. To paraphrase Elizabeth Barrett Browning, let me count (some of) the ways: Bad food choices. Too little exercise. Toxic relationships. Financial insecurity. Medication side effects. Depression. The list might not be endless, but it sure is long. But without question, the simplest, most obvious, sound-of-the-hoofbeats explanation as to why we are chronically, constantly fatigued, is this: *We just don't get enough sleep.*

When I lived in New York, I knew people who liked to flaunt their lack of sleep like a badge of honor. It was like their own personal gold star of productivity, their personal statement that their time was simply *much too valuable* to waste sleeping. ("I'll sleep when I'm dead" was a common refrain. Together now, let's all roll our eyes.) To these folks, habitual eight-hour-a-night snoozers were people with nothing more important to do with their nights than sleep.

Those masters of the universe, financial wizards though they may have been, didn't appreciate that sleep is not just a valuable commodity, it's literally the currency our body runs on. Studies have shown time and time again that to be our most productive, a good night's sleep is essential. So if we want to stay healthy and energetic, there is nothing better we can do with our late nights than climb into bed and get a good, sound sleep.

It's not a luxury—it's a necessity. Plain and simple.

FLAGGING ENERGY COULD SIGNAL A FAULTY FOUNDATION

Call me crazy, but I'm certainly not the only person who thinks so. I asked a dozen of the academic boldface names in my Brain Trust Contact List what would be the first thing they'd look for when a patient or client complained of flagging energy. Every one—every *single* one—said sleep problems.

This book is filled with suggestions and plans for what you can do to increase your energy. But all the tips in the world won't keep you energized if you keep cheating yourself on sleep.

That's not sexy, hip, trendy, or fun, but, unfortunately, it's 100 percent true.

Good sleep habits are the structural foundation of energy. If that structure is weak, then eating well, exercising regularly, managing stress, and following all the other strategies offered in this book will be like spackling and painting the cracks on the wall of a house with a faulty foundation. It might look good for a while, but the house will still be crumbling underneath. Unless you attend to the cause of those cracks, you'll never have a sound structure.

Keep depriving your body of the sleep it needs (and deserves) and eventually—like the house with the faulty foundation—it'll simply collapse.

FATIGUE-RELATED DISASTERS

The media and the public seem to be finally waking up to the importance of sleep and the role it plays along with stress management, good nutrition, and regular exercise in the energy equation. And not a moment too soon.

As I write this, the National Transportation Safety Board (NTSB) is investigating whether the pilots of a go! airliner in Hawaii overshot their intended destination and failed to respond to repeated calls from air traffic control because they were asleep in the cockpit. I don't know about you, but when I think of a high-energy airline pilot, I don't picture him or her nodding off in the cockpit.

Underscoring the concern about pilot fatigue was a story that appeared in *The Christian Science Monitor* shortly after that incident. The paper obtained a series of confidential safety reports made by pilots, listing potentially dangerous fatigue-related incidents. "They range from failure to level off at assigned altitude to inadvertent taxiing onto active runways to actually falling asleep at the flight controls. In one report, a captain who accidentally crossed onto an active runway wrote that his copilot tried to warn him, but he 'was tired and didn't listen.'"

Fatigue-related errors have been a factor in some of the biggest disasters of recent times, including the Exxon Valdez oil spill, the Three-Mile Island and Chernobyl nuclear accidents, and the explosion of the space shuttle Challenger.

Although those cases are some of the most dramatic consequences from sleep loss, millions of us operate with some level of impairment and energy depletion because we don't get adequate sleep. Sleep affects how we work, how we relate to other people, how we make decisions, and how we feel in general.

"Our culture has forgotten what it means to be awake," said Robert Stickgold, Ph.D., of Harvard Medical School's Division of Sleep Science. "I think we spend most of our days a little bit groggy and a little bit inefficient." Ya think?

Cheating sleep makes you more prone to diabetes, cardiovascular disease, depression, and anxiety. It resets our internal clock, throwing off our endocrine, immune, and metabolic systems. And, oh yeah, lack of sleep makes you dull and fat. By getting adequate sleep, you'll perform better and feel better, and your energy levels will soar.

Isn't it about time we remember what it means to be awake?

Good sleep habits are the structural foundation of energy. If that structure is weak, then following all the other strategies offered in this book will be like spackling and painting the cracks on the wall of a house with a faulty foundation.

#38

Go to Sleep an Hour Earlier

If you think for a minute about what energy really is, you'll find that on some level it's about a sense of feeling alive and awake. In fact, the sense of vitality that comes from experiencing something new and exciting, whether it's rafting down a river, taking on a challenging project, or going out on a first date, is what being alive, being truly awake, is all about.

Humans are hard-wired to face stress—both the positive and the negative kinds—with a rush of energy. And we need restful sleep so the brain will flip the switch to the neurological systems that produce high energy and a positive perspective. I don't know about you, but I don't need a study to tell me how lack of sleep can make a person irritable (though there have been plenty of studies that show exactly that). At one time or another, most of us have probably experienced some degree of the increased anxiety, anger, and foul mood that comes from inadequate sleep. When you've had inadequate sleep, there's no way you can be at the top of your energy game.

Sleep deprivation, which sounds like a form of torture used on prisoners of war, is endemic in modern life, whether it refers to a lack of sleep or a lack of uninterrupted sleep. (See The Hard Numbers on Sleep Deprivation on page 81 for statistics.) This cumulative lack of sleep adds up to what sleep scientists call "sleep debt," and just like the bill on your credit card, it comes due.

With interest.

The best way to wipe that sleep credit card clean is to go to bed one hour earlier. (More on that in a minute.)

A LITTLE LOST SLEEP CAN MEAN A LOT OF LOST ENERGY

Sleep debt, even moderate sleep debt, can interfere with your stamina, judgment, coordination, mood, and immune system. (It can also affect your weight, which can indirectly affect your energy as well.)

See, when you're sleep deprived it seems like there's a big fog that permeates your brain. It's almost like being drunk. In fact, it's *exactly* like being drunk. Studies show that people with sleep loss respond physically and mentally as if their blood alcohol level were .05, which is actually the legal limit for driving in many countries. Being even a little sleep deprived is equivalent to drinking two glasses of wine. And although drinking a couple of glasses of vino might be a nice way to end a night, it's not exactly the first thing you'd think of doing if you were trying to boost your energy.

Statistics support the druglike effect of even minor sleep deprivation. According to the National Highway Safety Administration, driver fatigue is the cause of more than 100,000 motor vehicle accidents, 71,000 injuries, and 1,500 deaths a year. And guess what day of the year has the highest number of car accidents? It's the day after we spring forward for daylight savings time, when most of us have lost an hour of sleep time. Just *one hour less sleep* can make that big a difference.

ERASE YOUR DEBT TO BOOST YOUR ENERGY

That's what I mean by sleep debt. And by the interest that comes due when you incur it. The sleep deprived are at higher risk for depression, hypertension, stroke, cardiovascular disease, diabetes, and obesity. Studies also find that short sleepers are more likely to be sedentary, to smoke, and to drink to excess.

No wonder William Dement, M.D., Ph.D., stated at a congressional hearing, "We are not healthy unless our sleep is healthy." It was Dement, a Stanford professor and pioneer in sleep research, who coined the term "sleep debt," which he cleverly (and accurately) says awakens what he calls "nature's loan shark." As Dement explains, the body keeps careful tabs on just how much sleep it's owed and ultimately, just like a real loan shark, it demands payment.

Every time you ignore your body's demand for payment, the sleep loan shark goes behind your back and grabs payment from your energy stores. Meanwhile, like inveterate gamblers, we continue to ring up the charges. To complicate matters, we're lousy judges of how much we owe. Several studies have shown that subjects overreport the amount of sleep they get and underreport the effect that it has on them (much like calories, come to think of it).

While you can make up sleep debt—to a point—it's a pay-as-you-go system, so building up a reserve of sleep won't avoid future debt.

Which brings me back to the solution: *Go to bed an hour early*. For whatever reason, "sleeping in" just doesn't work, not when it comes to paying back sleep debt and getting back on a "sleep budget." Going to sleep earlier does. We're pretty hard-wired to wake at the same time, and in any case, even if you manage to sneak in a couple of extra hours on the weekend, the fact is that during the week most of us are on a schedule that doesn't allow that kind of flexibility. If you need to wake up at 6:00 a.m. to take the kids to school,

you're going to wake up at 6:00 a.m.—sleep debt be damned. We've got a lot more options when it comes to retiring early.

When it comes to sleep—and its effect on energy—the choice is clear: Pay me now or pay me later. Either way, if you owe the sleep loan shark, you're going to pay up in lost energy. You might as well wipe the slate clean and then do your level best to keep it that way.

The Hard Numbers on Sleep Deprivation

Each year more than 50 million Americans suffer chronic, long-term sleep disorders, and 20 million more experience occasional sleeping problems.

More than two-thirds of women frequently experience sleep problems, and more than one-third of adults suffer from insomnia *every single* night. (Daytime sleepiness, anyone?) The National Sleep Foundation tells us that 75 percent of adults experience it, with a third of those saying they have actually fallen asleep at work or come darn close to it.

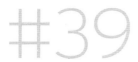

#39

Race Through the Day by Taking Melatonin at Night

You are not going to be in top shape energetically if your immune system isn't running on all cylinders, if you're not managing stress, and if you're not sleeping properly. Melatonin can help with all of the above.

You may know melatonin from its reputation for being the go-to supplement for travelers experiencing jet lag, but the benefits of melatonin go well beyond its positive effect on sleeping patterns. Melatonin is actually a hormone, made in the pineal gland (a gland about the size of a pea that's buried deep in the brain and located right above the brain stem). And this vitally important hormone has many functions, among them helping to regulate immunity and stress response. It's also a powerful antioxidant that easily gets into the cells and can help protect nuclear DNA. All told, not a bad resume!

Although melatonin isn't a sleeping pill, and is far from a panacea for all the things that might be keeping you awake at night, there's good evidence that it may help you sleep. Its main function in the body is to control circadian (those day-night) biological rhythms. Turn off the lights and you send a signal to the brain to turn on the melatonin production factory and get ready for sleep.

MELATONIN FOR SLEEP, SLEEP FOR ENERGY

Melatonin has some far-reaching effects on the body independent of its effect on sleeping rhythms and jet lag. One of the reasons that massive deregulation of our natural light-dark cycles by artificial means, such as computers and electricity, has wreaked havoc with our health has to do with the disruption of melatonin production. If you so much as turn the lights on in the middle of the night when you go to the bathroom, it's a signal to your brain to turn off the melatonin spigot.

Your brain makes melatonin in a series of sequenced steps that begin with L-tryptophan, an amino acid found in protein foods, including eggs, poultry, beef, and even tofu. "Cofactors" (helpers) such as vitamin B_6 turn L-tryptophan into something called *5-HTP* (5-hydroxytryptophan) and then into the famous "feel good" neurotransmitter, serotonin. Two more biochemical steps, and voilà, serotonin turns into melatonin. A lack of any of these precursors or building blocks—such as L-tryptophan or B_6—can compromise your body's melatonin production, as can excessive stress; high levels of adrenaline, caffeine, or alcohol; or lack of complete darkness.

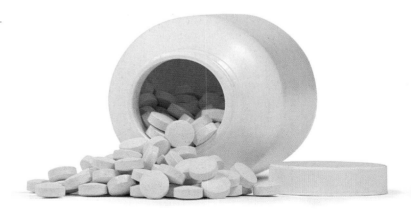

Why should you care? Because lack of melatonin can seriously compromise sleep quality, meaning bye-bye energy. A number of studies have shown that supplemental melatonin taken about 30 minutes before bedtime can help reduce the time it takes to fall asleep (called *sleep latency* by scientists). There's good scientific evidence that it can help with insomnia in the elderly and may help with sleep quality in healthy people in general.

Raising blood levels of melatonin (through supplements) to those that approximate normal nighttime levels can help induce and sustain sleep in many people. And there's excellent scientific evidence that it can help with jet lag (see my book *The Most Effective Natural Cures on Earth*).

Under normal conditions, the body secretes melatonin for a few hours every night, an effect that can be duplicated best with time-release supplements. A regular supplement will work well also, especially if you take it half an hour before you fall asleep. Most studies have typically used small doses ranging from 0.3 to 3 mg, though higher doses have been recommended. I myself have previously recommended 6 mg as a good dose for insomnia, which may be absolutely fine for many people, but you can probably start with a smaller dose (say, 3 mg). A lot of studies show the low dose works fine.

Don't make the mistake of taking melatonin during the day. It will send conflicting signals to your body—*It's light out, yet this darkness hormone is floating around the bloodstream! Something's not right here!* Supplemental melatonin works best when you take it at the time your body expects it—sleep time, when it's dark outside (and inside). Because melatonin is part of the body's internal signal system that prepares for slowing down, dropping body temperature, and hibernating for the night, it's conceivable that taking melatonin during the day could have adverse effects, including grogginess, tiredness, or even depression.

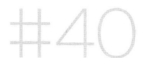

#40
Take a Nap

What do Winston Churchill, Albert Einstein, and Eleanor Roosevelt all have in common?

Give up? They were all known to enjoy an afternoon snooze.

These folks must have known intuitively what studies now confirm: Catching twenty (minute) winks during the day can improve productivity, bolster memory, lower stress, and improve learning and skill development—energy-dependent activities all. In fact, one group that relies on the energy of its participants for its success has done studies showing that a short siesta can increase performance by 34 percent and alertness by a whopping 54 percent. That group? None other than NASA—the National Aeronautics and Space Administration.

Lack of melatonin can seriously compromise sleep quality, meaning bye-bye energy.

Although naps don't take the place of a good night's sleep, they can be restorative and help counter some of the impaired performance that results from not getting enough sleep at night. Naps can actually help you learn how to do certain tasks quicker. Napping is also good for your heart. According to studies at the Harvard School of Public Health, a 20-minute snooze three times a week can reduce the risk of heart disease by 37 percent, not a bad side benefit of this natural and easy energy booster.

It always amuses me that when health professionals talk about the health benefits of the Mediterranean diet, they make it sound as if it's all due to the olive oil (leading some nutritional wits like Robert Crayhon to wryly remark, "Well, I guess all we've got to do is pour olive oil on our sugared cornflakes and we'll be fine"). We often forget that the folks over there in Crete and Cyprus and all those gorgeous areas by the Mediterranean Sea aren't healthy just because they consume a ton of olive oil. They're healthy because of the overall Mediterranean *lifestyle*, which, to be sure, includes olive oil, vegetables, and fish, but also working outdoors, spending time in the sun, laughing a lot, eating the biggest meal midday, and ... napping! (Try shopping after lunch on a Caribbean island such as St. Martin, where they're heavily influenced by European traditions. You can't. They close their stores from around 1:00 p.m. to 3:00 p.m. Guess why?)

Experts suggest catching up on your zzz's either late in the morning or early in the afternoon, and limiting naptime to about 20 minutes to avoid falling into a deep sleep (our circadian rhythms make that harder to avoid in late after-noon). If you have the time and inclination to snooze longer, make it a full sleep cycle, say 90 minutes, which will get you in and out of deep sleep.

Some companies now offer sleep-deprived employees time and space for napping. If you work at a company whose workplace culture isn't that evolved (which probably means anywhere but Google), look for someplace dark and quiet. Since body temperature drops when we sleep, cover yourself with a blanket (or makeshift blanket).

THE CITY THAT NEVER SLEEPS NOW NAPS

In New York (and other large cities), napping is serious business. For a price you can catch up on your zzz's by booking time in a slumber station, such as the ones at Yelo (www.yelonyc.com). For just a few bucks you'll get 20 minutes in a beehivelike cab, where you can sink into an adjustable leather lounger, cover up with a cashmere blanket, nod off to the soundtrack of your choice, and awaken to a simulated sunrise. (Add a pre-nap reflexology session and your bill will come to $77.)

Paying for naptime might seem ridiculous, though don't tell that to the 3,200 people who packed Yelo's facilities in the first year it opened, or to owner Nicholas Ronco, who's currently planning to expand to 500 locations nationwide. Twenty minutes of naptime: $12. Catching up on sleep: priceless.

——————— **WORTH KNOWING** ———————

Napping is a refreshing way to make up a little sleep debt and face the afternoon if you have no trouble getting—and staying—asleep once you hit the mattress. But if it's getting to sleep in the first place—not getting to bed—that's your problem, then skip the afternoon nap—it's more likely to make things worse.

Why Sleep Matters

It feels good to be aroused, whether it's sexually, intellectually, or spiritually. Anyone who's ever been in love knows that, as does anyone who's ever been on upper drugs (not recommended) or been excited by a new adventure.

The term *adrenaline junkie* was coined to describe this common feeling of coming alive when something new, exciting, and stimulating is happening to us, whether it be a new project or a first date. One of the many roles of sleep is that it sets us up for that stimulation that everyone seems to want. That sense of vitality, well-being, and excitement is what being alive—being awake—is really all about.

As sleep expert William Dement, M.D. Ph.D. of Stanford University points out, the human organism is hardwired to be energetic when it's faced with challenges. Good and restful sleep sets up the brain for high energy and the positive feelings that goes with it. Without restful sleep, we tend to view the world through foggy glasses. With it, the world is brighter, more stimulating, and more exciting.

So because sleep is so important, you'd think scientists would know exactly why we need to sleep, wouldn't you?

So would I. But truth is, it's an unanswered question. We know a lot about what happens *during* sleep, we know a lot about what happens when people *don't* sleep enough, we know a lot about what we can do to improve the *quality* of sleep, but the actual reason why people *need* sleep is a bit of a mystery. It's pretty clear, though, that it's necessary for our survival, and equally clear that it's directly, unambiguously, stunningly connected to our daytime energy levels and mood.

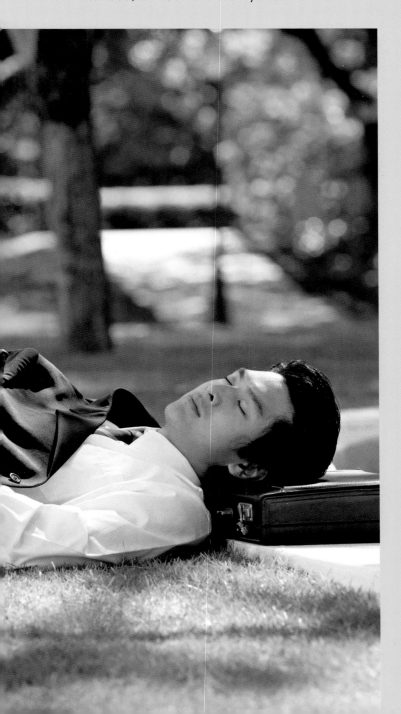

THE BODY'S BUILT-IN THERMOSTAT

Homeostasis—maintaining a constant internal environment—is like a thermostat. If it gets too hot, the thermostat turns itself down; if it gets too cool, it turns itself up. Let's say your sleep debt is zero, like a zero balance after you've paid off your credit card. Now every hour you stay awake is like putting small charges on the sleep debt credit card, and the homeostatic mechanism will demand that you pay that off, which, presumably in a perfect world, you would do at the end of the day with a nice, uninterrupted seven to nine hours of sleep. Then you'd be even again—at zero balance—and the cycle would start all over. That's homeostasis.

But if homeostasis were the only thing operating here it would be like a credit card that had to be paid off every time you went into the store to make a purchase. Every time you were up for a few hours, you'd owe yourself a few hours of sleep and have to go to bed. Obviously, life doesn't work this way. And the reason it doesn't is something called the biological clock.

NATURE'S BIOLOGICAL CLOCK— IT'S NOT JUST FOR WOMEN

The biological clock I'm talking about isn't the one that we hear about in romantic movies, where the thirty-something woman is getting nervous about being single and childless. It's a far more fundamental mechanism that regulates our sleep-wake cycle.

Animals have this biological clock built in, and they've never even read a book about it. Rats will get on their little exercise wheel at the same time every day, and they don't even have clocks! I know personally that I experience a little drop in energy around 4:00 p.m. and then a rise again around 6:00 p.m., and that seems to be fairly independent of what I do, eat, or drink, though it can certainly be made worse and much more dramatic by the wrong choices.

The rhythm of this internal biological clock is called a circadian rhythm. People who are at odds with it, such as night-shift workers, suffer serious health consequences, not the least of which has to do with their energy and performance.

The circadian rhythm is a cycle of roughly twenty-four hours (some say twenty-five) that is in the physiology of almost all living beings, from fungi to people. It was originally coined by a researcher at the University of Minnesota named Franz Halberg, and it comes from the Latin words *circa* (meaning "around") and *diem* (meaning "day"). A circadian rhythm, then, can be thought of as the ebb and flow of different metabolic and biological processes over the course of about a day.

It's pretty clear, though, that sleep is necessary for our survival, and equally clear that it's directly, unambiguously, stunningly connected to our daytime energy levels and mood.

Circadian rhythms seem to be generated internally—what scientists call endogenously—even though they can be affected or modified by outside cues such as light. But they are clearly observed in animals such as monkeys, even in the complete absence of external cues. They're more or less hardwired into our DNA.

So our biological clock, this circadian rhythm, regulates our cycle of sleep and wakefulness. Stanford researchers postulate that this clock has an active alerting function that keeps us up during the day, and then lets us sleep at night by simply turning the alerting function off, or at least that would be what would happen in the best of all possible worlds.

They also theorize that the daytime clock-dependent alerting occurs in two distinct waves—one in the morning when you first wake up, and the other late in the day (which totally accounts for my increased energy around 6:00 p.m.). Finally, they postulate that the second wave of alerting that takes place in the early evening is stronger than the first early morning wave, which makes total sense because by then we will have accumulated more sleep debt and will need a stronger alerting stimulus to overcome it and stay awake into the evening.

Now here's the good part, and it will blow your mind. In between those two peaks of what the Stanford group calls heightened clock-dependent alerting, the clock operator slacks off and takes, forgive the pun, a nap. Right in the middle of the day, right during the matinee, before it kicks up again for the evening show.

What happens to us around mid-afternoon? We feel tired. Our energy drops. According to the Stanford group, most people incorrectly assume that this is the result of eating lunch. Indeed, it can be made way worse by eating the wrong foods for lunch, and it frequently is. But it's not *caused* by eating lunch. In reality, says Dement, author of *The Promise of Sleep*, people are only feeling their accumulated sleep debt, but this time there's no surge in clock-dependent alerting to mask that feeling.

People who are not sleep deprived at all have accumulated virtually no sleep debt—their credit card bills are paid off. Therefore, when the alerting mechanism takes a nap in mid-afternoon and exposes them to the big bad sleep loan shark who comes to collect, they owe nothing. If on top of that, they also eat right and keep their bodies fit, their mid-afternoon energy slump should be . . . let's see now . . . roughly zero.

#41-53

For Better Daytime Energy, Try These Thirteen Insomnia Aids

Tattoo this underneath your eyelids: The number one, with a bullet, reason why you don't have energy is that you're not sleeping enough. In fact, to paraphrase the top three rules of real estate (location, location, and location), lack of sleep is the number one, number two, and number three reasons for folks not feeling at the top of their game.

Now you may think you get plenty of sleep, but you probably don't. Remember, eight hours *in bed* doesn't always translate to eight hours of *sleep* (even accounting for the time you subtract if you happen to get lucky). If you find yourself tossing and turning instead of falling asleep, try these tips and techniques that will condition your body and mind to become drowsy by the time you hit the bed.

#41

Exercise Early and Often

People who are in good shape tend to have good sleep, and working out on a regular basis can help you accomplish both. But because exercise actually raises cortisol levels, which in turn "turns on" the mechanism that keeps you awake, separate your training routine from your bedtime routine by at least three hours. I've met very few people who can finish a hard workout at 9:00 p.m. and then fall asleep by 10:30 p.m. There may be some, but you're probably not one of them. Neither am I.

#42

Clear Your Mind

In a lot of healing practices, you're told to write down a list of the worries you want to let go of and then burn them, a symbolic way of releasing them. But maybe you don't actually have to build a fire to get the mind-clearing benefits of releasing your worries. Try this little trick: An hour or two before sleep, write a list of everything you're worried about or all the things you need to do, and then just put it away—physically and emotionally. Allow it to live on the paper; it'll be there when you pick it up in the morning. But for now, let it go.

#43

Have a Snack

This tip is a tricky one, because eating before bed is a double-edged sword and you have to balance conflicting needs. On the one hand, you want to sleep soundly; on the other hand, you don't want to wake up fat. (Remember, on page 57 I told you to embrace hunger—a great idea for overall energy, but one that takes some getting used to, at least as far as sleepy time goes.)

So although you definitely want to avoid big meals close to bedtime, if your stomach is growling to the point where it's going to keep you up, a light snack before bed may help you sleep more soundly. (Notice I said if your stomach is growling, not "if your mind is craving Häagen Dazs.") There's no consensus on what constitutes the best bedtime snack, so just make sure it's something you can easily digest.

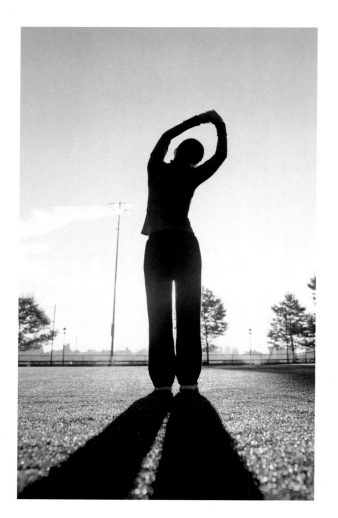

Remember, you're balancing conflicting priorities here. A high-carb snack may make some people fall asleep faster (though not necessarily sleep well), but it will also raise insulin levels, making "fat burning" an impossibility during the night. It's best to train yourself to put a few hours between your last feeding and sleepy time, but a snack may help on occasion while you make the transition into the world of no nighttime snacking. Remember, going to bed just a little bit hungry isn't the worst thing in the world.

#44

Skip the Nightcap

Contrary to movie images of drunken frat boys snoring loudly and merrily oblivious to the world, alcohol usually winds up disrupting your sleep cycles. Badly.

Alcohol is, after all, a depressant, so although a drink before bed may help you *fall* asleep, a few hours later it has the opposite effect, and part of your brain thinks it's party time (though the part that's paying attention to your headache may not agree). Even if you only had a couple of drinks, you're likely to wake up with a hangover. Limit alcohol consumption to no more than one or two drinks a day, and three hours before bedtime, enforce a prohibition.

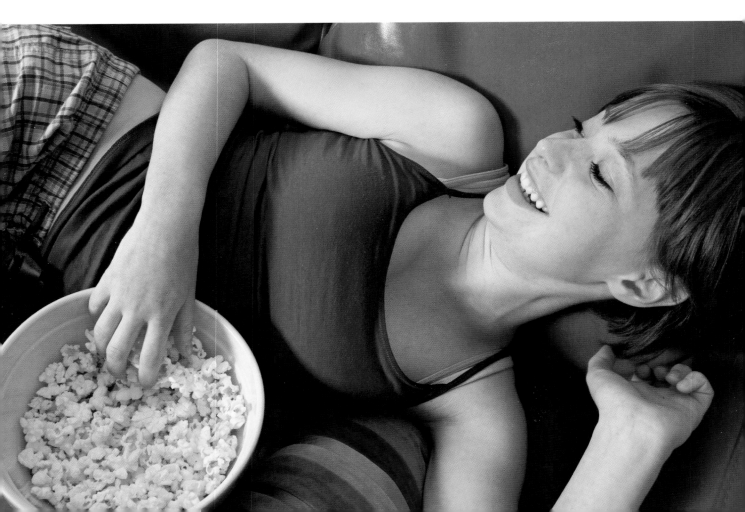

#45

Put a Nighttime Ban on Cigarettes

As if you need another reason to kick the habit, nicotine disrupts sleep. Anyone who's tried to kick the habit using a nicotine patch knows that once you put the patch on, you may as well get out of bed because sleep won't be coming anytime soon. (I once, in an ill-advised attempt to understand what my girlfriend, who was kicking cigarettes, was going through, put on a nicotine patch for a day. I was sick, jittery, and nauseous for more than twenty-four hours, and sleep was out of the question.)

If you're an unrepentant smoker, the idea of getting better sleep probably isn't going to motivate you enough to give up the habit, but if you're thinking about giving it up anyway, better sleep is an added benefit to dumping the smokes.

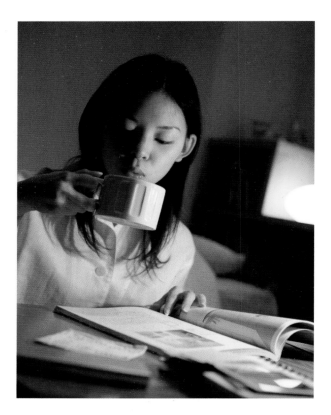

#46

Kick the Caffeine

As any double latte drinker knows, caffeine wakes you up, which is why we love it so much. Coffee, chocolate, some colas, teas, and pain relievers will leave you, well, caffeinated.

Caffeine actually sits in the receptors of a calming neurochemical called adenosine; because caffeine literally occupies the parking spaces reserved for adenosine, adenosine doesn't get to send its normal signals to the brain, signals that would normally say, "Relax! It's time to rest." The result? You get to stay awake. Sometimes that can be a good thing, but around bedtime—not so much. Ban the stimulant at least six hours before bedtime. It hangs around in your system way longer than you think it does.

#47

Set Your Internal Clock

Much as you might hate sticking to a schedule, your body disagrees—it actually loves regularity. Try going to bed and waking up at the same time each day, even on weekends. Sticking to a sleep schedule (preferably one that allows you eight hours of sleep) will get you back into the rhythm of your internal clock and really make a difference in daytime energy. Seriously. In fact, there's no greater way to reset your clock than by waking up at a consistent time each morning.

Daylight is key to regulating daily sleep patterns. To help reprogram your body's responsiveness to circadian rhythms, try to get outside in natural sunlight for at least thirty minutes each day.

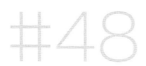

Don't Flush

I'm a great proponent of hydration, but deciding to detox your system with five cups of water just before you hop into bed is asking for trouble. (You know exactly what I'm talking about, too, especially if you're older than forty.) We don't need any extra reasons to visit the bathroom more than we already do.

Drink enough that you don't wake up thirsty (or keep a glass by your bedside in case you do), but curtail fluid intake close to bedtime, unless you plan on making a half dozen trips during the course of the night, annoying your sleeping partner and virtually guaranteeing you won't get the quality or quantity of sleep you need for super energy. (You may even be banished to the couch, which won't help your ability to follow tip number 144, Have More Sex.)

#49

Prepare to Sleep

Remember when you were a child and you couldn't get to sleep without a bedtime story? That was a bedtime *ritual*. Rituals are like stories—they're comforting, and they add security and stability to a fragmented, stressful life. Rituals make people feel grounded and connected, which is why cultures are built around them. Your body remembers—and still craves—rituals, and they're a great tool for helping you sleep like a baby.

So here's your homework, boys and girls: Establish an adult version of *Goldilocks*. Each night, thirty to sixty minutes before going to bed, follow the same routine. You might take a warm bath, listen to soothing music, or read a book. It doesn't matter what it is, as long as it's not stimulating (which probably, for most people, rules out watching the news or leaving the TV on at all).

By creating a comfortable, and *comforting*, bedtime ritual, you'll condition your body to become drowsy. Brush and floss, turn down the heat, shut off the lights, and get under the covers. (There's a reason they call that big fluffy white blanket a comforter.)

#50

Change Your Environment

If you're having trouble sleeping, one reason may be because you've turned your bedroom into a second office. Get over it—you're not Hugh Hefner. Most of us would be better off keeping the bedroom off-limits for work, and reserving it as a place of refuge and relaxation (and maybe even pleasure, if we get lucky). What it should *not* be is a glorified workstation with a bed.

Set the scene for sleep by making sure your bedroom is dark, cool, and well ventilated. Light is your body's wakeup cue, so use heavy curtains, blackout shades, or even an eye mask to achieve darkness. Those old-time movie actresses knew what they were doing.

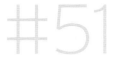

Turn It Off

Don't sleep with the TV on. If you're used to falling asleep that way, get unused to it. It's a huge mistake to have the television on while you're sleeping, one I've made more than once, sometimes by accident (as when I roll over on the remote control). Then the soundtrack of those 3:00 a.m. infomercials starts intruding into my brain and I find myself with unpleasant, restless dreams that seem to be filled with folks selling thigh masters and real estate. And it's not just me. Studies have shown that that stuff penetrates through to your consciousness, even when you're in a deep sleep. Avoid noise of all kinds when you sleep, whether it comes from the TV or any other source. A fan or other white noise device can be a lifesaver.

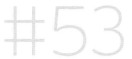

Get Up

If there's anything worse than insomnia itself, it's *worrying* about insomnia. Insomnia is a little like erectile dysfunction in one regard—the more you worry about it, the worse it gets. If, after twenty minutes, you haven't fallen asleep, just surrender to it. Get up, go into another room, and do something relaxing, such as listening to music or reading.

If you're just not sleeping, you might as well get up and do something else until you actually feel like hitting the pillow. And if you wake up in the middle of the night, the twenty-minute rule still applies. Stay up until you feel like going back to bed. Don't force it. Werner Erhard, a great teacher of mine, used to say, "What you resist, persists." Never was it truer than for when you can't sleep.

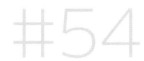

Get the LED Out

Turn the face of your clock—and its light-emitting diodes (LED)—away from you. Sleep researchers believe that even small amounts of ambient light can interfere with the production of melatonin and disrupt sleep cycles, particularly in sensitive people. Plus the fact that there's nothing more frustrating than watching the minutes tick away as you try to sleep.

Be sure to keep the lights low. When it comes to sleep, darkness rules. You don't need that nightlight anyway. As Julia Roberts said to a suitor in the 2004 movie *Closer, "What are you, twelve?"*

Replace Your Alarm Clock with a Dawn Simulator

I don't know about you, but in the old days, when I still used an alarm clock, the sound of the alarm had the power to ruin my day and zap my energy for hours after waking.

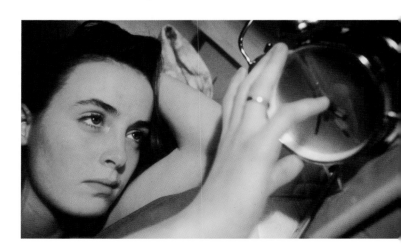

Of course, like most people, I probably didn't recognize that this was one of the causes of my being tired so much, but just because it's a hidden cause doesn't mean it's not a real one. Loud, jarring, and angry sounds waking you from what's supposed to be restorative sleep will send a jolt of stress hormones careening through your body, leave you in a foul and resentful mood, and ruin your energy for hours afterward. Maybe even your whole day.

Fortunately, there's an energizing solution. It's called a dawn simulator. It works just as the name suggests, by gradually brightening a room over the course of about 30 minutes. It simulates the warming appearance of the gentle dawn, and slowly, gently brings you out of deep sleep, finally waking you with a simulation of natural sunlight that's bound to set the tone for your day and boost your energy for hours after you get out of bed. (Who wants to waste all that precious energy being mad at the world because your alarm clock woke you with all the subtlety of a bucket of ice water?)

The dawn simulator is one of my favorite devices. I bought one of these for my beloved partner, Anja, who, when I met her, was still using an alarm clock from the era of the Hun Dynasty, which woke you with a noise so annoying and intrusive it could frighten a herd of wildebeests. Not a great way to start the day if you want lots of energy.

Dawn simulators appear to help people wake up more easily in the winter. Many people use them as a supplement to a light visor, light box, or desk lamp program. More information can be found at the website of the Circadian Lighting Association (www.claorg.org), which also lists many reliable companies that make these products.

#55

Try This Little-Known B Vitamin for Refueling Sleep

Let's review: You can't be at the top of your game energetically if you're not sleeping well. And you're not sleeping well if you're among the 60 million Americans suffering from chronic insomnia.

Inositol might help. A member of the B-complex family, inositol is a nutrient that has been used to treat anxiety. That's probably because of its relaxation effects, but many people also swear by its ability to promote restful sleep. Taking inositol is standard practice in my house—we use a heaping tablespoon (7g) in water almost on a nightly basis. "I find inositol to be highly effective in helping my clients get a good night's sleep," says celebrity nutritionist J. J. Virgin, Ph.D., C.N.S.

There are no great scientific studies supporting the use of inositol for promoting restful sleep, but you can go on the Internet message boards and find a million people singing its praises for just that purpose. As they used to say when I was a kid, "Fifty-thousand Elvis fans can't be wrong!"

Many of my colleagues use inositol for sleep, despite the lack of controlled scientific studies. It's been our collective experience that it works. I recommend starting with 500 mg before bed. Personally, I like the kind that comes in a powder, and since it is completely nontoxic, I'd start with at least a teaspoon, then add more if you need it.

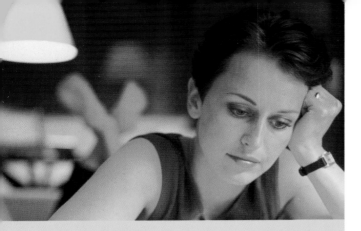

Ease Your Anxiety with Inositol

Inositol may be effective in treating many of the same disorders for which SSRIs (the major class of antidepressants) have been shown to be helpful, according to the *Physician's Desk Reference* (famous SSRIs include Prozac, Zoloft, and Lexapro). Interrupted sleep is a common symptom of depression and anxiety, and as I've stated before, you need solid sleep to refuel and face the day with enough energy.

In one study, patients with panic disorder who received 12 grams of inositol daily achieved significant improvement in both the frequency and the severity of panic attacks. In another, depressed patients receiving 12 grams of inositol daily for four weeks showed significant improvement in their depression scores. It also seems to have a positive effect on obsessive-compulsive disorder, which is often treated with SSRIs. All this makes sense, because one of the things inositol does is help reverse desensitization of the serotonin receptors. Remember, when serotonin is high, you usually feel happy and relaxed, not anxious.

The inositol powder I use is by Designs for Health and is available on my website (www.jonnybowden.com) under vitamins and supplements.

#56

Fly Free of Jet Lag

In the days when world travel meant crossing the sea in an ocean liner rather than by plane, our bodies would gradually cross time zones, and our internal clock would be in sync with the environment.

Well, we kissed those days goodbye a long time ago.

Now that we jet across time zones in hours rather than days, we experience an unsettling feeling called *circadian misalignment*, in which our internal clock is out of sync with the external environment. Because our internal clock controls many of the body's functions, jet lag can leave you with digestive problems, headaches, and of course, insomnia. As we know, insomnia always means low energy. It can also mean problems with memory, attention span, judgment, and communication, all especially troubling for business travelers.

The time of day that you travel, the direction, and, of course, the distance all factor into how jet lag might affect you. Traveling east to west tends to be easier on our bodies simply because we're heading into the sun. (Remember, light is the single strongest synchronizer for our internal clock.)

Generally our internal clock resets itself about one time zone per day. To help matters along (and minimize the loss of energy that comes from jet lag), here are some positive measures you can take.

- **Be well rested**. Don't start the trip with sleep debt. You'd be surprised how many people overlook this part of the anti-jet lag program and run themselves ragged right before leaving for vacation. I myself have done it, figuring, what the heck, I'll sleep on the plane. Not a great idea. Plan to have a few nights of quality sleep before you travel.

- **Drink wisely**. Since recirculated air is dehydrating (and dehydration equals a reduction in energy), drink water as you fly. How much?

Probably more than you think. A good idea is to drink at least a few of those small bottles the airlines give out. At the very least, keep refilling the glass. You won't drink it if it's not there in front of you. Limit caffeine and alcohol, as they can disturb sleep.

- **Ease into the zone**. If you are traveling eastward, try to follow your body's cues, avoid bright light when your internal clock thinks it's evening, and expose yourself to light sometime after 5:00 a.m. in your home time zone.

#57

Buy a New Mattress

Poor sleep equals poor energy. That's a no-brainer. And believe it or not, if you're not getting the sleep you need, an outdated mattress may be the culprit.

If you've hung on to the same mattress for more than ten years—or if you're waking up feeling stiff and sore—then it's time to go mattress shopping. A new mattress can do wonders for your ability to get high-quality sleep. Which, of course, can do wonders for your energy level. Finding the right mattress is like finding the right mate—what's perfect for one person is all wrong for the next. To underscore just how intensely personal mattress style is, *Consumer Reports* went through an exhaustive testing process to try to rate mattresses, and decided it was next to impossible. Because sleepers' reviews were all over the map, the magazine couldn't make a recommendation.

MATTRESSES MATTER

There is a dizzying array of styles, materials, and prices. Just going to the mattress store can drain your energy. But stick with it.

Innerspring mattresses are the most common, but there are also air beds and water beds and the exploding category of memory-foam mattresses (such as Tempur-Pedic). There's an energy-boosting mattress in there for you somewhere—you just need to take the time to find it!

Spend at least 15 minutes lying on a mattress in your normal sleeping pose, before shelling out your cash. If you share your bed, you and your mate should shop together. The right mattress takes your weight, sleeping style, and size into consideration. A good mattress and foundation will keep your spine aligned (it should look the same when you're lying down as when you're standing) and gently support your body. Pay special attention to how your hips, shoulders, and lower back feel. A lot of stores have a 30-day return policy—a good thing, because you may not really know how good (or bad) a mattress is until you actually sleep on it. So start shopping because choosing the right mattress means fewer muscle aches, better sleep, and more energy.

PILLOW TALK

Your pillow should offer enough support to cradle your neck and head. The optimum thickness depends on your sleeping style (and size).

If you sleep on your side, try a pillow that's between 4 and 6 inches (10 to 15 cm) thick; stomach sleepers should have one about 3 inches (7.5 cm) thick; and if you sleep on your back, your pillow should be about 4 inches (10 cm) thick. My personal favorite is the Primaloft Side Sleeper Pillow by Garnett Hill.

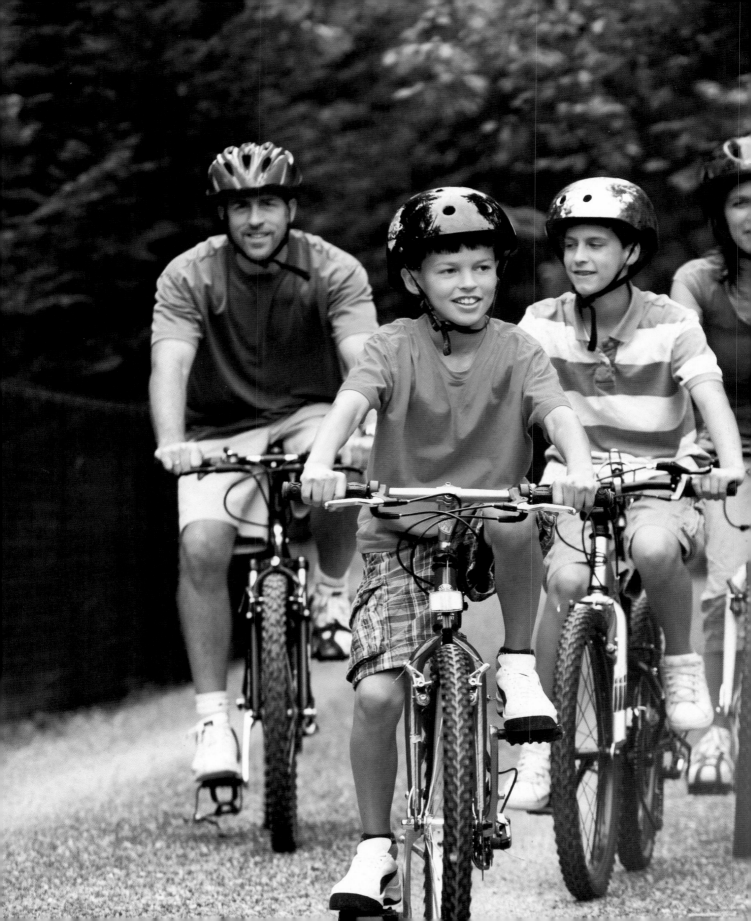

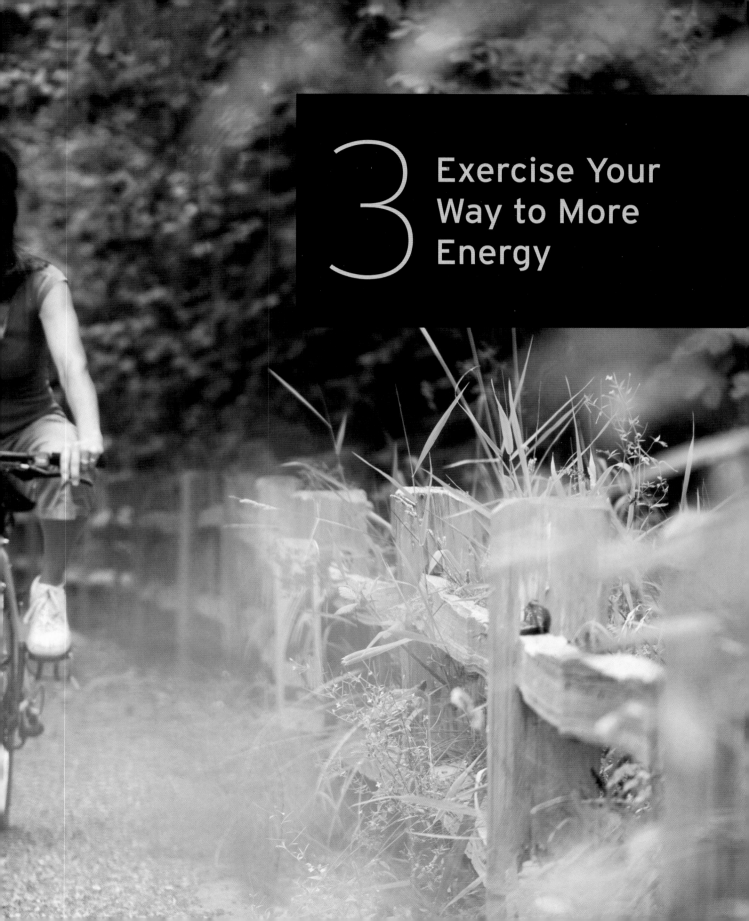

3 Exercise Your Way to More Energy

Back in the early 90s, when I was first starting my career in fitness (which morphed into the career that now allows me the privilege of writing books about health and energy), the "gym wars" were just heating up in New York City. I worked as a personal trainer at Equinox, a then fledging gym that has since turned into an American phenomena. At the time, new gyms were cropping up on every street corner. I was asked by a reporter for the New York Times to recommend the best gym in town.

My answer? "The one you go to."

It was, if I say so myself, one of my better responses to an interview question.

So, to answer the question of "What's the best exercise to do?" I'm going to steal from myself and answer it thusly: *The best exercise is the exercise you actually do.*

HOW THESE THREE TYPES OF EXERCISE BENEFIT YOU

Exercise gives you energy. It's that simple. Anything is better than nothing, and the more strategies for working out, the more likely you are to be successful in making exercise a regular routine and taking your energy to the next level.

That said, most of the neuroscience research on learning, focus, and attention refers to aerobic exercise (much as they love to spin around on their little wheels, it's hard to get mice to lift weights or stretch, so there's a lot more animal research on aerobic exercise than there is on, say, bodybuilding or yoga). High-intensity exercise, such as running, appears to provide the biggest bang for your brain. But even walking at a brisk pace will increase energy. Aerobic exercise also helps your heart and lungs function more effectively.

Resistance exercise builds more muscle mass, which, in turn, boosts your metabolism, always a good bet for increasing energy. Strong muscles also make it a lot easier to carry our bones around, especially important as we age. Studies show that strength training increases self-esteem and energy. Pumping iron three times a week, for example, can increase energy levels by up to 50 percent, even on days you don't lift, according to Mark Moyad, M.D., director of Preventive and Alternative Medicine at the University of Michigan Medical Center.

Flexibility exercise—such as yoga, tai chi, or stretching—can help alleviate muscle tension and decrease anxiety, both energy zappers. For overall health, well-being, and energy, you should incorporate all three types of exercise into your routine.

SKIP THE EQUIPMENT AND ENJOY WHAT YOU DO

So back to particulars. If it's been a while since you've exercised, then begin by walking. Aim for 30 minutes a day, and break it up into three 10-minute walks if that makes it easier. You'll notice the increase in energy in no time. As you get stronger and more energized, you may want to consider interval training (see page 105), the PACE program (see page 106), the Tabata Protocol (see page 109), or any of the other workouts in the pages that follow.

For people who are a little more in shape, or if you want to challenge yourself more, try stair climbing. Or stair running. And I don't mean getting on the stair-climbers you find at the gym (not that there's anything *wrong* with that). I'm talking about finding a flight—or forty—of stairs in your own environment and climbing them. Or running them.

And speaking of easy-to-do, no-cost, at-home creative ways to jump-start your energy with a short exercise break—jump some rope! Now truth be told, I've never been able to master the coordination of this, but when I used to take Aerobobox classes, I simply held the rope in one hand and slapped it to the ground while jumping in step with the rest of the class.

It's probably better if you can manage the coordination, but even without it, the jumping motion is stupendously effective for boosting energy. It gets oxygen and nutrients to the brain like nothing else, not to mention getting your blood circulating. You'll feel like your energy circuits just got a tune-up, and you'll be amazed at how long it lasts.

In sum, all these techniques are good. But just like the best gym in town is useless if you don't go to it, the best exercise program in the world means nothing to your energy if you don't actually do it. So whatever it is that gets you off the couch—be it biking, swimming, tennis, jogging, walking, gardening, weight training, skipping rope, running stairs, or running backwards—it's all good. At the risk of sounding like a Nike ad, just do it. Whatever "it" is.

It—meaning any kind of exercise at all—will boost your energy like nothing else in the world.

#58

Activate Your Brain's Miracle-Gro

Today, survival of the fittest is the credo for reality television. Yet when humans first inhabited the earth, it actually *was* reality.

The mind evolved to help our hunter-gatherer ancestors devise better strategies for survival so they could outrun, outwit, and outlast their enemies in the life and death competition for food, not just for bragging rights at tribal council on *Survivor*.

Movement, in other words, is a biological imperative, says John Ratey, M.D., a Harvard Medical School professor of psychiatry and author of *Spark: The Revolutionary New Science of Exercise and the Brain*.

If this book were one of my workshops or lectures, now would be the time when I'd stop for a minute and tell a joke. Bear with me, it has relevance. (Plus, it was a favorite joke of my Jewish mother.)

A Beverly Hills mother and her son arrive at a swanky hotel for a family vacation. She gets out of the limousine, followed by a butler, who then proceeds to lift the son up and carry him across the lobby to the check-in desk. The clerk, observing this scene, clucks sympathetically, and says to the mother, "Oh, how sad. I'm sorry to see your son can't walk." "Oh, he can walk," the snotty mother sniffs, "but thank God he doesn't *have* to."

Okay, I didn't promise that it was worthy of Jon Stewart, but it does illustrate a point. Although we haven't evolved much genetically since the caveman era, our lifestyles have all but wiped out the need for movement. Our sedentary ways are "disrupting a delicate biological balance that has been fine-tuned over half a million years," writes Ratey.

To restore and maintain energy, we have to heed our very nature, and that means work up a sweat.

YOUR BRAIN'S OWN BUILT-IN ENERGY MAKER

Exercise increases blood volume in the brain, and that creates an optimal environment to grow new cells, strengthen neurons, and produce a potpourri of beneficial molecules, including a little protein with a long complicated name—*brain-derived neurotrophic factor* (or BDNF for short). Now you have my permission to forget its name, but do pay attention to what it does, because it can have a profound effect on your energy levels, not to mention depression, anxiety, addiction, and the aging process. It also helps keep your hormones and blood sugar in balance.

BDNF is the star of a class of what Ratey calls "master molecules." Researchers have found that if you sprinkle some BDNF neurons into a cell-filled petri dish, the cells automatically sprout new branches, called *dendrites*. That effect led Ratey to affectionately label BDNF "Miracle-Gro for the brain." Guess what increases the production of BDNF? You got it—*exercise*, in particular, cardio-vascular exercise.

"BDNF is the critical biological link between thought, emotions, and movement," Ratey told me when I interviewed him on the radio. Its actions are crucial for understanding why movement can profoundly impact your energy.

But wait, there's more.

When BDNF levels are elevated, the part of the brain that shows the most activity is the *hippocampus*, an area involved in memory and learning. "Without Miracle-Gro," said Ratey, "the brain closes itself off to the world." Just as giving your car a good wax job protects the paint from the elements, exercise—by initiating the production of BDNF—provides a buffer so the stress of daily life doesn't wear you down and drain your energy.

STRESS TURNS OFF THE ENERGY SPIGOT

By the way, if you're still skeptical about the interconnection of stress, thoughts, emotions, movement, and energy, consider this little biochemistry factoid (feel free to drop it into cocktail conversation; it will dazzle your friends): The major stress hormone in the body—cortisol—actually *shuts down* the BDNF factories in the cells. The more stress you're under, the more unrelenting it is, the less BDNF you make. That translates, ultimately, to a "closing off" to the world.

Mice with decreased levels of BDNF can't find their way out of a paper bag, either because they can't think well or because they don't have the energy to explore. Exercise—because it beefs up the BDNF factories—improves the infrastructure for learning, thinking, and relating to our environment.

Mice with decreased levels of BDNF can't find their way out of a paper bag, either because they can't think well or because they don't have the energy to explore.

"Exercise improves learning on three levels," Ratey explained. "First, it optimizes your mindset to improve alertness, attention, and motivation. Second, it prepares and encourages nerve cells to bind to one another, which is the cellular basis for logging in new information. Third, it spurs the development of new nerve cells from stem cells in the hippocampus." If that sounds a little heavy, allow me to break it down to the essentials: Exercise invigorates you mentally and physically. It increases your energy.

What's the obvious conclusion? Seems to me—and to other observers—that going for a ten-minute run might be the best thing you could do before tackling a mentally challenging task. It will not only energize your body, but it will also stimulate your brain.

#59
Practice the Power of Positive Exercise

Patricia Moreno is six feet tall (183 cm) and gorgeous.

When I first started as a personal trainer in 1990, Patricia was the most sought-after aerobics teacher in New York City. Aerobic instructors were the stars of the booming fitness industry of the 80s, which made Patricia a true superstar among stars. (We're talking about an era when "no pain, no gain" was the mantra, low-fat diets were all the rage, and "step" was a noun.)

Whenever and wherever her classes were held, the hallways would be packed with spandex-clad aerobicizers jockeying for a place in the class. Other teachers would typically have fifteen to twenty-five people in attendance. Patricia would have 100 (or whatever the legal capacity of the room was). She was, as they say in Hollywood, "a big draw."

She was that good. Still is.

And she had more energy than any human on the face of the earth.

ALIGN WITH A HIGHER ENERGY

She's no longer teaching aerobics, but her packed intenSati classes—part cardiovascular exercise, part yoga, part life coaching—are taught throughout the country and offer movement with a message of self-awareness and empowerment.

She's still six feet tall and gorgeous, has a "real woman" (i.e., curvy, not model-thin) body with minimum fat and a scary amount of muscular strength.

And she *still* has more energy than any human on the face of the earth.

Patricia—like me—is an optimist. She believes our natural state is one of energy, peace, and happiness, and even if we can't achieve it all the time, it can always be the bull's-eye we aim for.

"What depresses our whole energy and happiness is the way we're thinking," she told me.

Like many intuitive healers, Patricia believes energy exists on a vibrational continuum, with emotions such as anger, guilt, resentment, and fear on the lower end, while joy, peace, spirituality, generosity, and personal power exist on the higher end. When you're out of sync, feeling depressed, pessimistic, and uncertain, it's a good bet you're hanging on the low end of the continuum.

When you're in alignment with that higher energy, you know it. You feel fully alive, whole, and—well, *energized*.

So how do you get on the high side of the energy continuum?

CHANGE ENERGY-DRAINING THOUGHTS

In Patricia's classes, students shout positive, energetic affirmations while performing movements that express strength, power, and courage. "You may not be able to hold on to the thought 'I am strong,' for a full minute," Patricia told me, "but you sure can repeat it vocally for a full minute, and if you repeat it while doing a movement—such as the motion of a bow and arrow—it's enough to shift the belief or attitude that's causing you low energy into the direction of high energy and personal empowerment."

So, actions *and* words together pack a more powerful punch than thoughts do. In fact, used together in the way she recommends, they can *change* thoughts, especially the energy-draining kind.

You can try this at home, folks. Anything that gets you out and about in a quick, repetitive tempo can be the basis for reprogramming your brain and rebooting your energy circuits. First, get yourself in motion, and then, as you're doing it, repeat a word or an affirmation: "I'm feeling happier now" works well. So does "I'm feeling energetic!"

Even when the words don't describe how you actually feel, the mere act of *saying* the words as you move helps create the feeling of energy. You can dance, bike, walk, do jumping jacks, run—any repetitive motion that increases your heart rate will work. Speaking power phrases or affirmations, says Patricia, increases your oxygen uptake and helps program your brain, connecting the movement with the positive feeling.

REPEAT ONE ENERGETIC AFFIRMATION AT A TIME

Patricia suggests coupling the following energy-boosting affirmations with repetitive movement:

- All I need is within me now.
- All the energy I need is within me now.
- All the strength I need is within me now.
- All the love I need is within me now.
- All the courage I need is within me now.
- Every day in every way I'm better and better.
- Every day in every way I'm healthier and healthier.
- My body now restores itself to perfect weight and perfect health.

You may feel silly saying these out loud. I did, too. Doesn't matter—no one's listening. The point is, it works. And if the negative voices in your head are going on about how this couldn't possibly affect your energy, just ignore the little chatterboxes and do the exercise anyway.

"Building health and strength takes an attitude of courage," says Patricia.

Remember, you're aligning with your higher purpose. And who doesn't feel energetic and on fire doing that?

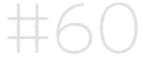

Start Your Day with the Sun Salutation

The exercise I'm about to describe to you is one of the beginning exercises in a yoga practice. It's called the Sun Salutation. I use it all the time, especially when I want to start my day with a nice little energy boost.

You don't have to practice yoga on a regular basis to get the energy boost of the Sun Salutation. Truth be told, I don't practice yoga, and I don't pretend to be anything like an expert on it. But I can tell you that the Sun Salutation is one of the best ways to start your day if you want to get your circulation going, get oxygen into your brain, stretch your muscles, and quicken your step. It's an energy bonanza, and it only takes a few minutes to perform.

The version I'm about to show to you comes courtesy of my friend Bernard Rosen, Ph.D., nutrition educator and consultant, and certified yoga teacher (www.brwellness.com).

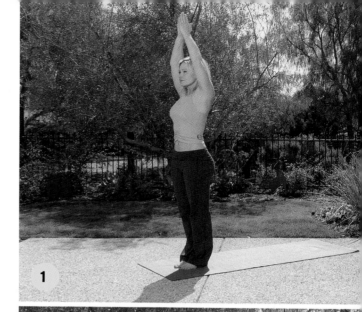

1. Stand with your feet parallel and hip-width apart (4 to 5 inches, or 10 to 13 cm) and your arms by your sides.

2. As you inhale, sweep your arms out to the side and overhead. Reach through the fingertips, keeping the arms straight—the palms come together and there is a slight back bend. (This is known in yoga as the Mountain Pose.)

3. As you exhale, fold forward from the hips as you bring your arms out to the sides and then your fingertips to the floor (forward bend). The idea here is to bend over straight from the waist and touch the floor with your legs straight, but few people will be able to do that. Don't worry about it. Go as far forward as you can go and, if you can reach them, grab your ankles. If you can't, grab your calves, or even your thighs. Pull your chest gently toward your legs as much as you can, while your chin is tucked under.

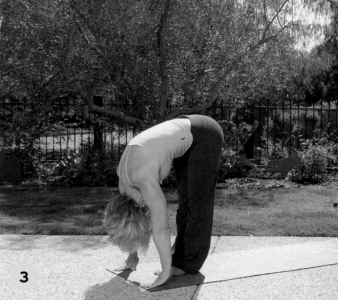

4. As you inhale, step your left foot back into a high lunge. The left leg is straight, the right leg remains forward, the right foot is even with the hands, the spine is long, and the hips are sinking. Tilt your head back as you look up.

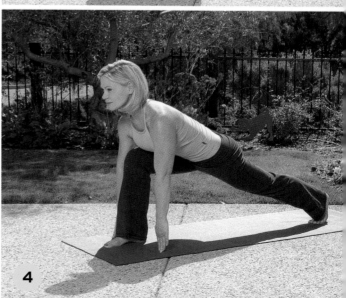

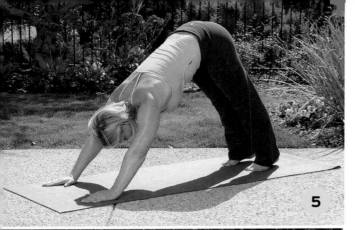

5

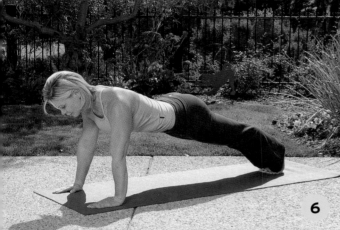

6

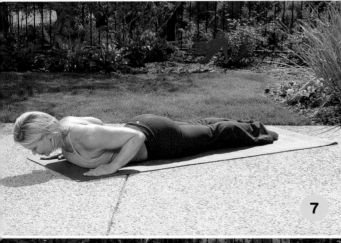

7

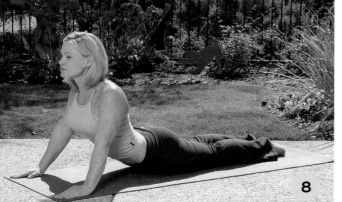

8

5. As you exhale, step your right foot back and move into an inverted "V" position (called the Downward Dog in yoga). Press into your hands and feet evenly, and relax your head and neck.

6. As you inhale, lower your hips as your body moves into a high push-up position (called the Plank in yoga). The hands are below the shoulders. Press into your hands, and press your heels toward the floor to lengthen your body.

7. As you exhale, lower your body to the floor.

8. As you inhale, lift the head and chest off the floor. Your hands are below your shoulders with your elbows in toward your body. Press the tops of the feet and the pelvis into the floor as you lift (called the Cobra Pose).

9. As you exhale, press into your hands, raise your hips, and return to the inverted "V" position (Downward Dog).

10. As you inhale, step your left foot forward into a high lunge. The right leg is straight, the left leg is forward and even with the hands, the spine is long, and the hips are sinking.

11. As you exhale, step your right foot forward to meet your left foot and fold into the standing forward bend.

12. As you inhale, sweep your arms out to the sides and come to standing with the arms overhead (Mountain Pose).

13. As you exhale, bring your arms down and press the hands together in front of the heart.

14. Repeat the steps above, but this time step the right foot back in step 4 and bring the right foot forward in step 10.

This is a basic version of the Sun Salutation (there are many!). It's a great way to start your day, and for little real physical effort, you get a very big energy bang for your buck. Try it!

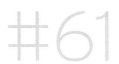

Work Smarter, Not Harder with Interval Training

Let me tell you why I'm not the biggest fan of long, slow cardio exercise and time-consuming workouts in the gym.

For one thing, I think most people waste far too much time in the gym. I don't know about you, but I'd like to be doing other things. Like playing tennis. Or writing books on energy. And I think a lot of what passes for "workouts" is actually pretty mindless activity that looks, frankly, kind of joyless to me. I see people on the treadmills at the gym running like rats, iPods in ears, staring at the TV monitors, and not looking all that happy.

LESS TIME, MORE RESULTS

I've been touting the benefits of shorter, more concentrated training for a long time. Coming from the gym culture, I've seen routines that took less than 12 minutes to perform that would leave the average steelworker collapsed in a puddle of his own sweat.

I'm not saying you should give up enjoyable long distance stuff such as hiking, biking, walking, or running, but I *am* saying that a lot of what passes for workouts is a waste of time. You can accomplish more with full-body circuit training and high-intensity interval training. That's what I do for energy and for exercise, and it's what I recommend.

The most efficient way to increase cardiovascular strength, brain health, and energy, is through interval training. There are different ways of doing interval training, but all include high-intensity bursts of exercise followed by lower intensity exercise (or in some cases rest). (Various examples follow; see pages 106–113.) High intensity generally refers to training between 70 and 85 percent of your maximum heart rate. (To calculate your maximum heart rate, subtract your age from 220.) Interval training is an especially effective method for burning fat and increasing VO_2 (aka oxygen uptake, which measures lung capacity and thus cardiovascular fitness).

Alternate your days of interval training with a longer, more steady state exercise that you enjoy, such as cycling or hiking. After just 10 minutes of interval training, you should have enough energy to blast through any day.

Putting Your Mind to the Muscle

I think exercise—like everything else—should have a quality of mindfulness (see page 101) to it.

Arnold Schwarzenegger, in his pre-*Terminator*, pre-Governator days, was fond of saying, "Put your mind into the muscle." Schwarzenegger claimed that it improved his results if he visualized his shoulders growing to the size of grapefruits while doing shoulder presses. In his mind's eye, he could actually "see" his deltoids expanding while he hoisted the weights.

Old-time bodybuilding gurus such as Vince Gironda (who was the owner of the legendary Vince's Gym in Southern California) didn't even allow music to be played in his facility, claiming it was too distracting. "You're here to lift, not to listen to music," he'd say.

Maybe you don't want to go that far, and you probably don't care about your deltoids looking like grapefruits, but there's more than a kernel of truth in the weight training philosophy of both Schwarzenegger and Gironda. Moral of the story: Don't multitask when you work out. Use it as a laboratory for practicing mindfulness and concentration. You'll get a lot more out of it, and you'll be able to accomplish much more in a lot less time.

#62
PACE Yourself

Al Sears, M.D., C.N.S., a friend and charter member of my Brain Trust,* has designed a form of interval training called Progressively Accelerating Cardiopulmonary Exertion, or PACE. He's a strong believer in the benefits of high-intensity exercise for improving health and increasing energy. So am I.

A brilliant doc, and a bit of a contrarian, Sears goes so far as to call traditional endurance exercise—steady, low-intensity aerobic exercise—a waste of time. "Heart attacks don't occur because of a lack of endurance. They occur when there is a sudden increase in cardiac demand that exceeds your heart's capacity," he says.

Sears says that interval training, with its short bursts of high-intensity exercise, not only trains the heart to withstand the greater stress, but it also creates a hormonal environment conducive to fat loss. And because it strengthens the heart, it increases energy.

HIGHS AND LOWS FOR ENERGY

The whole idea of PACE, and really, of any structured, well-designed interval training program, is to alternate periods of high-intensity exercise with what's called active rest. During active rest you don't stop moving, you just reduce the intensity so that you can recover and regroup. So, for example, if you just ran the steps of a stadium à la Rocky Balboa, active rest would be going back down at a very slow-paced jog. (It wouldn't be sitting down and catching your breath, which would be just plain old garden-variety "rest.") Get the picture?

*The experts on my speed-dial who I can count on to offer brilliant, cutting-edge information on almost any health-related topic.

When beginning the PACE program—or any program, for that matter—it's important to start out light and increase your effort over time. You can start PACE with an easy, 10-minute program. Warm up by walking at a brisk pace for 5 minutes (you can substitute biking, skating, or any other form of aerobic exercise for walking), then pick up the pace so you are jogging or running hard enough to break a sweat and really challenge your heart and lungs. Keep it up for 1 minute, and then lower the intensity for 1 minute to catch your breath and lower your heart rate. Repeat the cycle—1 minute of exertion followed by 1 minute of recovery—five times for a total workout time of 10 minutes.

After the warm-up, it looks like this:

Set 1: Exertion, 1 minute; Recovery, 1 minute
Set 2: Exertion, 1 minute; Recovery, 1 minute
Set 3: Exertion, 1 minute; Recovery, 1 minute
Set 4: Exertion, 1 minute; Recovery, 1 minute
Set 5: Exertion, 1 minute; Recovery, 1 minute

According to Sears, the speed and intensity of your exertion should be fast enough to break a sweat, but not so fast that you have trouble finishing the 10-minute program. If you're a gym member, this is the easiest thing in the world to do on a treadmill or stepper; just change the level from minute to minute. If you're accustomed to walking comfortably at a level of, say, 4 (on a scale of 1 to 10), go to 6 on your exertion phase and back down to 4 (or 3) on your recovery. Sears says that this allow you to train your ability to recover from exertion and stress, which, when you think about it, is one of the definitions of having more energy!

In Sears's book *PACE: Rediscover Your Native Fitness* (available at www.alsearsmd.com), he outlines all kinds of variations for accelerating your energy-promoting interval routines using the PACE program, with intervals ranging from 40 seconds to 10 minutes for the exertion phase and 2 minutes to 6 minutes for the recovery phase. Point is, this is a great way to do a structured interval training program without any machinery, especially if you prefer to exercise outdoors and like to walk or run.

Make the PACE workout part of your personal routine and you'll have more energy than ever.

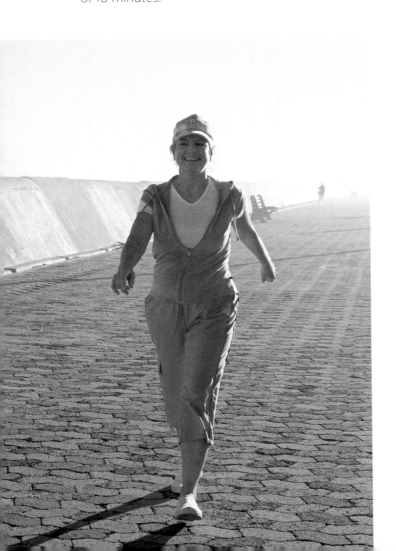

#63

Energize and Exercise with the Time-Saving X-iser

Is squeezing even 10 minutes for exercise out of your busy schedule too hard to manage? Well, guess what? I have just the program for you! With a mere 4 minutes a day, you can get a jolt of energy while burning fat, increasing endurance, improving balance, lowering blood pressure, stabilizing your core, and strengthening your muscles. Sound too good to be true?

I sure thought it was. (Remember, I come from the gym culture, where guys the size of barn doors spent entire mornings just doing "lats.") So convincing me you could get anything done at all in 4 minutes was, let's say, a bit of a stretch.

And then I tried burst training.

WHEN LESS CAN BE MORE

Burst training is 1 minute of high-intensity exercise, performed four times a day, three times a week, using an amazing, multitasking piece of machinery invented by exercise physiologist Mark J. Smith, Ph.D. It's called the X-iser, and it's a small, compact, incredibly well-designed and sturdy machine that looks like a miniature version of a stair-climber without the handles.

Stepping on the X-iser is kind of like doing multiple one-legged squats on both legs at the same time. This creates a great demand on the muscles because there is no rest period for the muscles during stepping, which means you're simultaneously challenging your aerobic and anaerobic systems. That's why the X-iser produces such incredible benefits in as little as 12 minutes per week and is safe and effective for everybody. I use the machine regularly, and I can tell you it's

without question one of the hardest and most effective workouts you can do. It gives a whole new meaning to energy efficiency.

Now I know you're probably skeptical. What can 1 minute of exercise, even if you do it four times a day, possibly accomplish? Well, think about it. You know that iconic scene in the first *Rocky* movie where Sylvester Stallone runs the steps of the stadium in Philadelphia? Suppose you did that exhausting, mind-numbingly difficult run every single day? Think you'd get better at it? Think you'd improve your aerobic fitness? Your endurance? Your energy? Let me save you the thinking time: The answer is "yes." In spades.

In fact, running up stairs is one of the best ways to burn calories, improve cardio conditioning and coordination, and increase energy. In the olden days, when I was a musical director living in the famous artists' complex in New York City called Manhattan Plaza (where my neighbors included Tennessee Williams, Larry David of *Seinfeld* fame, and the "real" Kramer, the one the *Seinfeld* character was based on), I used to run the forty-five flights of stairs from the bottom floor to the top floor a few times a week. It took less than 6 minutes and was one of the most intense, energizing exercises I ever did. Stair running is the bomb. Problem is, most of us don't live in forty-five-story buildings or near the *Rocky* stadium in Philadelphia. The X-iser gives you the ability to essentially do the same thing in your living room.

And it doesn't stop there. Burst training, which is really just a series of short bursts of very high-intensity exercise, is one of the most effective ways to exercise for weight loss, health, performance, endurance, and energy. The research backs me up on this. One study in a 2005 issue of the *Journal of Applied Physiology* found that a mere two weeks of as little as 8 minutes a week of burst training doubled the endurance and energy of participants. A study at Colorado State showed that 4 minutes on the X-iser burned the same number of calories as 20 minutes of traditional aerobic exercise. Burst training also burns fat for twenty-four hours after exercise. It basically teaches the body to burn fat more efficiently.

The X-iser allows you to do a number of other exercises besides the standard (and brutal) burst of 1 minute of stair climbing. You can hold weights in your hands. You can do push-ups on the steps. You can do all sorts of things, all of which basically come under the heading of interval training, which I now believe is the most effective way to get in shape, lose fat, and increase energy. Whether you use the PACE program (see page 106), the X-iser, or an interval program of your own devising (or one of the many I've suggested on pages 106–113), it's something you should definitely check out if you're serious about increasing your energy.

The only downside? You'll have to say good-bye to a lot of excuses that revolve around time.

To find out more about the X-iser, go to www.jonnybowden.com, and click on "exercise" under "shopping."

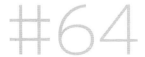

Do the Tabata Protocol

Back in the mid-1990s, Izumi Tabata, Ph.D., then a researcher at the National Institute of Fitness and Sports in Tokyo, studied an interval program designed by the head coach of Japan's speed-skating team. The routine consisted of 4-minute sessions alternating between 20 seconds of maximum effort with 10 seconds of recovery.

After comparing it to programs with varying degrees of intensity and duration, he found that the skaters' program was far more effective in increasing aerobic and anaerobic fitness (conventional wisdom at the time said high-intensity programs could increase one or the other, not both).

The routine was dubbed the Tabata Protocol. After following it for six weeks, five days a week, athletes increased their VO_2 max by 14 percent and their anaerobic ability by 38 percent. (Unless you're an exercise physiologist, those figures probably won't mean anything to you, but suffice to say those are two ways that scientists measure exercise capacity, and both measures improved significantly.)

HOW YOU CAN USE THE TABATA PROTOCOL FOR ENERGY

Why do I bring up a grueling routine designed for Olympic–medal winning skaters, you ask? Because you can follow the principle of the protocol while bringing the routine down to the level of a normal human.

To do that, you change the ratio of effort to rest from 2:1 to 2:3 or even 1:3, and you can dial down the intensity from all-out effort to between 70 to 85 percent of max. In plain English, that means you work out hard for 1 to 2 minutes and do "active rest" for 3 minutes, a far more doable option. (Active rest just means you're still moving, but not really working hard. So if you've just sprinted for 30 seconds, you might slow down to a walk for your "active rest" component. Make sense?)

For instance, after a 5-minute warm-up, sprint for 20 seconds, then rest for 30, and repeat up to eight times. (If that's too difficult to manage, start with 10 seconds of all-out effort, followed by 30 seconds of rest.) As you increase your fitness level, you can move closer to the Tabata Protocol ratio of 2:1 (20 seconds of exertion, 10 seconds of rest).

If this is sounding familiar because you've been carefully taking notes throughout the entire exercise section, it's because it *is* familiar—it's simply a clever variation on Al Sears's PACE program (see page 106) and Mark Smith's Burst Training for the X-iser (see page 108). All are well-designed interval training programs that can be summed up like this:

Work out hard. Rest. Repeat as needed.

What these interval programs have in common is that for a limited investment of time, you get the cortisol-lowering, BDNF-flowing (see page 100), dopamine-rushing results that translate to a boost in mood and energy (and it comes with a side of fat-burning, too).

Don't despair if all this sounds too hard. Even someone who walks for 20 minutes a day can do interval training. Let's say on a scale of 1 to 10, you walk at an exertion level of 5. Fine. For 20 to 30 seconds, move it up to a 7. Then go back down to walking at that comfortable 5 (called "active rest" or "recovery") while you catch your breath. You've just done an "interval." How hard was that? The rest is just details, different ways to up the stakes. The 7s become 8s, you do more frequent intervals, and you take shorter "active rest" periods. And you're on your way to a huge boost in energy!

#65-68

Try One of These 10-minute Energy-Boosting Workouts

The biggest obstacle to the 10-minute workout lives in your mind. It's the idea that if you do only 10 minutes, it doesn't count. It does.

Although it's true that you can get a lot of benefits out of longer workouts, it's equally true that 10 minutes counts and that it all adds up at the end of the day. If you've only got 10 minutes or so on a given day, here are four effective examples of what you can do. The possibilities are limited only by your imagination.

#65

The Low-Intensity (at Home, No Equipment Required)

1. **March in place:** 1 to 2 minutes.

2. **Wall push-up:** Stand about arm's length away from a wall. Extend both arms out and place both hands on the wall, shoulder-width apart. Elbows are shoulder level. Now lean in toward the wall, bending the elbows as you come forward, and straightening the elbows as you push back to the starting position. Do 10 reps.

3. **Squats to a chair:** Stand 8 to 12 inches away from a chair, facing away from the seat. Now bend your legs, push your butt out, and bend forward until you are seated on the chair. Beginners can rest for a second, then put your hands on your thighs, push off using your legs, and stand. Repeat for 10 reps. For non-beginners, let your butt touch the seat of the chair and come right back up, keeping tension on your muscles throughout the movement.

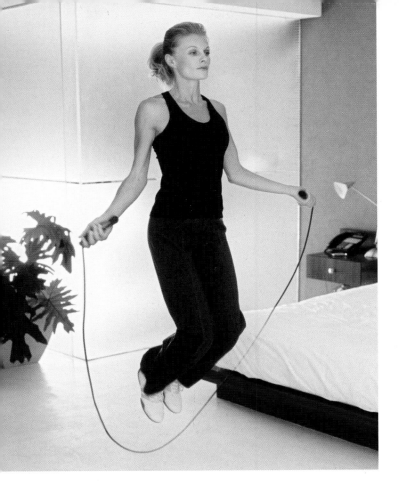

#66

The High-Intensity (at Home, No Equipment Required)

1. **Walk in place or do light calisthenics (such as jumping jacks):** 1 minute.

2. **Jump rope:** 1 minute.

3. **Push-ups:** As many as you can do in 1 minute.

4. **Crunches:** As many as you can do in 1 minute.

5. **Jump rope:** 2 minutes.

6. **Push-ups:** As many as you can do in 1 minute.

7. **Crunches:** As many as you can do in 1 minute.

8. **Jump rope:** 1 minute.

9. **Relax and breathe:** 1 minute.

4. **Wall push-up:** Repeat one set of 10 reps.

5. **Squats to a chair:** Repeat one set of 10 reps.

6. **Free dance:** 3 to 4 minutes. This can be anything you want it to be. You can sway to soft music or you can pretend to be Britney Spears. Think Tom Cruise in *Risky Business*. No one's watching. Have fun.

7. **Cool down, lie down, stretch, and breathe:** 1 to 2 minutes.

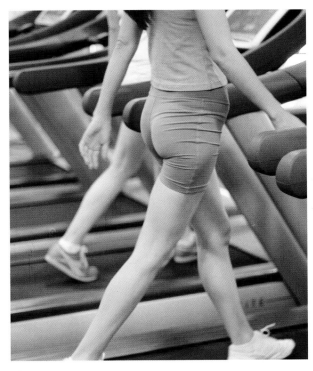

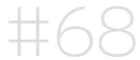

#67

The Moderate-Intensity Cardio Workout (Outdoors or on a Treadmill)

Tip: You can turn this into a high-intensity workout by just picking up the pace on the runs, and you can lower it a bit by changing the "run" intervals into "fast walks."

1. **Walk:** 1 ½ minutes, gradually picking up the pace.

2. **Run:** 30 seconds.

3. **Walk:** 1 ½ minutes.

4. **Run:** 30 seconds.

5. **Walk:** 1 ½ minutes.

6. **Run:** 30 seconds.

7. **Walk:** 1 ½ minutes.

8. **Run:** 30 seconds.

9. **Walk (gradually slowing down):** 2 minutes.

#68

The Moderate-Intensity Weight Training Workout (Gym-Based)

1. **Light calisthenics such as jumping jacks or pedaling on a stationary bike:** 1 minute.

2. **Chest press:** One set of 12 to 20 reps.

3. **Seated row:** One set of 12 to 20 reps.

4. **Shoulder press:** One set of 10 to 15 reps.

5. **Biceps curl:** One set of 10 to 15 reps.

6. **Triceps press-down:** One set of 10 to 15 reps.

7. **Leg extension:** One set of 12 to 20 reps.

8. **Hamstring curls:** One set of 12 to 20 reps.

9. **Crunches:** One set of 15 to 25 reps.

10. **Relax and breathe:** 1 to 2 minutes.

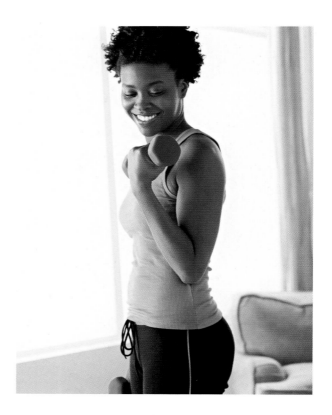

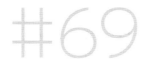

Practice the "No-Frills-No-Excuses-Anytime-Anywhere" Workout

We all know exercise helps with energy. The trouble is, not everyone has time for exercise. So I offer my own personal solution to the time demon—my own "no excuses" workout. I like it because I can do it in as little as 15 or 20 minutes, but can easily expand it to 30 or 40 minutes. Both beginners and advanced exercisers can do this routine. All are welcome!

You can do it anywhere; a gym with a treadmill is nice, but not necessary. A park or a city block in combination with four feet of space in a living room will do just as well. A little twiddling will let you customize it to virtually any combination of time slot and fitness level.

Here 'tis:

1. Run a mile.
2. Do some squats.
3. Do some push-ups.
4. Do some crunches.

THE DETAILS

If you're just starting, you might have to walk the mile, or jog-walk, and you might only be able to do a few repetitions of each of the three exercises. No problem. Do as few or as many of each as you can. But finish the circuit and you will have done a very effective mini routine.

Now, want to ratchet it up a notch or two? Run the mile faster. See whether you can do it in ten minutes or less. Do a set of serious squats—twenty reps, maybe with dumbbells or water bottles for added resistance. Don't rest. Go right to the push-ups. Try for fifteen. Do the crunches. Twenty-five, in perfect form.

You can stop right there or expand it even further by simply repeating the last three 2-cises: squats, push-ups, and crunches. Heck, if you're truly a sucker for punishment, add another mile run when you're done with your last crunch.

With a little imagination, you can easily see how hard this workout can be (or how easy). It's simple, elegant, and very effective. Get in the habit of doing this and your energy will go through the roof.

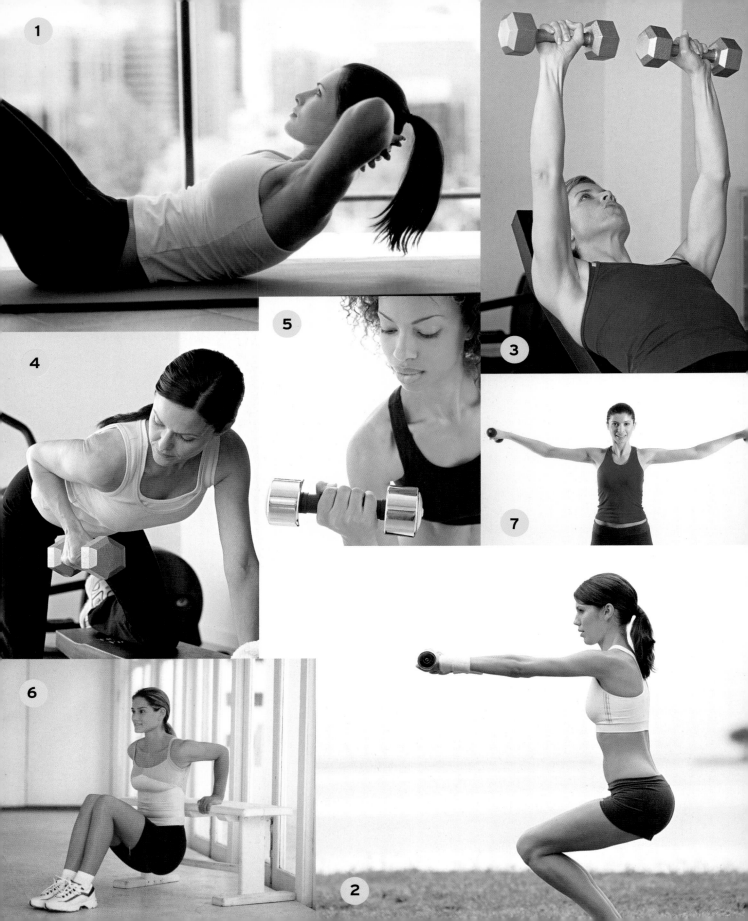

#70

Go Through Basic Training

For energy building, not to mention overall health, I recommend strength training two or three days a week.

Here's why: If your muscles are weak, your body takes more energy to perform daily tasks than it needs to, and that leaves less energy for you. (If your muscles are tired, *you* are tired.) Although most people think of muscle tone as something that looks great at the beach (which it does), it's actually about a lot more than that. People with strong, capable muscles sail through life a lot more easily than those who have muscles that are easily tired and fatigued.

Think about it. Picture a strong, muscularly fit person, who, for some reason, needs to jump up from his chair, run up the stairs to fetch something, and come back down. (Hey, just go along with me here for a minute and picture it, even if you don't find yourself routinely running up stairs.) If you're in shape, your leg muscles perform well for you, your heart rate goes up while you bound up the stairs, but it comes right back down a moment later. Your legs barely notice that they've just done the equivalent of a set of squats. You're good to go.

Now imagine a weak, untrained person doing the same thing. His heart will beat for half an hour after bounding up the stairs (I know this for a fact, because that person was me twenty or so years ago). His legs will have some lactic acid buildup because he doesn't metabolize the by-products of exercise quickly, so he'll feel sore and less energetic. Overall, a few short episodes like this will leave him fatigued for the rest of the day, whereas someone with conditioned, trained muscles wouldn't even notice the effort.

Get the picture?

Want another example? Think of a car that will go 200 miles an hour. You may never need to floor it, but think of how easily it sails down the highway at a mere 60. Compare that to a junker whose top speed is 60 if the wind is behind it. They may both do the same thing, but there's a light-year of difference in the ride (and effort).

You want to be like the car that can go 200. That's a car with a lot of energy. And to be in top form, energetically, you need conditioned muscles. Period.

SEVEN WAYS TO BUILD MUSCLE—AND ENERGY

Fortunately, it doesn't take all that much to train your muscles. I've put together seven basic exercises that will do the trick. Do the complete circuit, moving from one exercise to the next with minimum rest in between, about three times a week. (Of course, you can do more: two sets per exercise, or the whole circuit twice. Hey, go for broke and do it three times. What the heck.)

Side benefit: You'll also like how you look at the beach. And you'll actually have enough energy to get yourself there!

Here are my seven basic exercises for boosting energy.

1 Crunches—for the Ultimate Six-Pack

I constantly hear from people that they are doing hundreds of crunches. The minute I hear this, I know they're doing them wrong. (I also know there's a good chance they're using momentum and are setting themselves up for a lower back injury.) If you do a crunch properly, it's hard. Most people don't do them correctly. The good news is that when you do them correctly, you don't have to do nearly as many to get results.

Here's how: Lie on the floor with your legs bent, feet flat on the floor, and hands clasped behind your head with your elbows touching the ground. Your head should be in position with your body so that you could hold an apple between your chest and your chin.

Imagine Velcro-ing your lower back to the floor. You may feel like you're doing a small pelvic thrust slightly forward to accomplish this. Keep your lower back nice and stable in this position.

Curl your upper body forward and up holding the highest position for a full second before lowering your upper body back to the ground. Don't pull on your neck when you come up.

When you lower your upper torso back to the ground, don't return all the way to the relaxed position where your weight is supported by the ground, but rather to a point where your upper body is just above the ground and your abs are still contracted.

Remember to keep your elbows all the way back while doing the motion. Repeat for as many reps as you can manage in good form. The goal is to try for 10 to 20 reps.

Beginners: Remember that if you can do only one or two, that's fine. You'll work up to more, you can bet on it. Don't dwell on what you *can't* do, and just concentrate on what you *can* do.

Muscles worked: Abdominal muscles (the "six pack")

2 Squats—for a Bodacious Back View

Stand with your arms at your sides. Keep your feet shoulder-width apart and your head up. Slightly arch your lower back. Slowly bend your knees while pushing your rear out, until your thighs are about parallel to the ground. Squeeze your thighs and glutes for added contraction. At the same time as you bend, bring your arms up straight in front of

you for balance until they're extended straight out at shoulder height, palms facing each other.

Now come up until you're standing again, dropping your arms back to your sides as you come up, and repeat for 10 to 15 reps. Don't lock your knees when you return to a standing position. Adjust your foot stance until it feels comfortable.

You're going to perform one set, from 8 to 15 reps. (Remember that if you can only do a few repetitions to start, that's fine, too. This will be your personal starting point. You'll work up to where you can do 8 to 15. Note: this exercise can be done with or without weights.

Muscles worked: Thighs and glutes (butt)

3 Chest Presses—for Perfect Pecs

For this exercise you'll need a pair of dumbbells or filled water bottles.* For all exercises requiring weight, start with a weight you can comfortably do for 8 to 12 reps. If that weight is light enough for you to do more than 12 reps, increase it. If it's too heavy to perform 8 reps, decrease it. (For more information, see the sidebar on page 118.) Lie down on a bench, with your feet resting comfortably on the floor. (If you don't have a bench, you can use a step or even the floor.) Extend your arms overhead, shoulder-width apart, palms facing out, so that the dumbbells are positioned directly over your shoulders.

Bend your elbows about 90 degrees, gradually lowering the weights until they are above and a little beyond your shoulders. Now push the dumbbells up with an arcing motion until they're back in the starting position.

Muscles worked: Pectoralis (chest), deltoids (shoulders), and triceps (backs of arms)

The beauty of using water bottles is that you can fill them to whatever level you choose to provide just enough resistance to make the exercise difficult but doable. You can then fill to a higher level as you get stronger.

4 **One-Arm Rows—for Sexy Rhomboids**

You will need a single dumbbell or filled water bottle for this exercise. Bend over and rest your left hand on a bench or stool about 2 ½ feet (76 cm) high. Extend your right leg behind you so that you're far enough away from the bench that your back is flat; make sure you don't round your back and instead keep it as flat as possible (you may actually have to arch it a little to keep it in this position). Your back should be like a tabletop in this position. Your right arm will be hanging down straight.

Take a dumbbell in your right hand and bring it straight up toward your hip by bending your elbow and bringing it up behind you toward the ceiling. It should be almost like starting a lawnmower in slow motion. When the weight is about at hip level, lower it back down until your arm hangs straight down. That's one rep. After you complete 8 to 12 reps with your right arm, reverse everything and do the same number of reps with your left arm.

Muscles worked: Rhomboids (muscles in the back)

5 **Biceps Curls—for Firm Arms, Part I**

Stand with a pair of dumbbells (or filled water bottles) in your hands, palms facing out and feet shoulder-width apart.

Keeping your elbows close to your torso, curl the dumbbells toward your shoulders, and then bring them slowly back down. Repeat for 8 to 12 reps.

Muscles worked: Biceps (front of arms)

6 **Triceps Dips—for Firm Arms, Part II**

Sit on the edge of a bench or step, with your hands on the edge of the bench and your fingers facing forward. Lift your butt off the bench and lower it toward the floor by bending your arms at the elbows. Make sure you stay perpendicular to the ground, with your back straight. Don't push your hips forward. Lift yourself back up by straightening your arms, but don't reset your butt back on the bench until you're done. Repeat for 8 to 12 reps.

Muscles worked: Triceps (backs of arms)

7 **Lateral Raises—for Shapely Shoulders**

Take a dumbbell (or filled water bottle) in each hand and hold them at the sides of your body, palms facing inward. Stand with your feet shoulder-width apart, knees slightly bent. Don't lean backward.

Raise your arms up and out to the sides until they are parallel to the ground, then lower back down. Repeat for 8 to 12 reps.

Muscles worked: Medial deltoids (shoulders)

Jonny's Energy Exercise Plan for You

The following is a very basic workout that should set your energy on fire if you do it regularly. The seven exercises hit all the major muscle groups, as described in this entry. You can do one set of each, or if you're feeling perky, try for two.

Note, though, that recent research from one of the foremost exercise physiologists in America, Wayne Wescott, Ph.D., has shown that most people will get plenty of benefit from doing only one set of each exercise at about 75 percent of maximum weight, 8 to 12 reps per set. What that means is, if you're able to lift 100 pounds once for a movement, use 75 pounds for 8 to 12 reps. Obviously, the amount of weight you can lift will be different for each exercise (the legs are stronger than the arms), but this should give you a good idea.

If 8 reps are too hard, lower the weight (or pour some water out of that jug). If 12 reps are too easy, add some more weight (or water or sand). Don't drive yourself crazy trying to be exact, just go for the spirit of the workout—training all your muscles just enough to get them pumping and fire up your energy. It'll work! I promise.

If you're interested in more workout alternatives, you can find them in my Diet Boot Camp Program (www.jonnybowden.com) or on exercise videos or any of dozens of excellent books (I particularly like *Weight Training for Dummies* by my friend Liz Neporent, M.S., C.S.C.S.).

JONNY BOWDEN'S BASIC TRAINING FOR ENERGY WORKOUT

Home Version	Gym Version
10-15 minutes of cardio	10-15 minutes of cardio
Squats (1-2 sets)	Push-ups (1 set)
One-arm rows (1-2 sets)	Squats (1-2 sets)
Push-ups (1 set)	One-arm rows (1-2 sets)
Leg presses (1-2 sets)	Chest presses, regular or incline (1-2 sets)
Lateral pull-downs (1-2 sets)	Leg presses (1-2 sets)
Chest presses, regular or incline (1-2 sets)	Lateral pull-downs (1-2 sets)
Crunches (1-2 sets)	Crunches (1-2 sets)
Stretch and cool down	Stretch and cool down

71

Exercise En Masse

In a book on energy, exercise is important enough to get an entire section—and it has—but there's one thing you can do that qualifies as an easy energy tip: Take an exercise class.

There are a lot of reasons why taking a class gets special mention, even beyond the benefits of exercise itself. First and foremost, there is the collective energy of the group. Don't underestimate the power of being in a room with like-minded people all sweating to the same beat, moving to the same rhythm, breathing together, working together, intensely focused on the same goal—fitness, strength, beauty, and energy. It's powerful!

I don't really run (jog) anymore, having supplanted it with other cardio exercises, including hiking and tennis, but I can tell you this—when I *did* run, nothing was more energizing to me than running around the lake in Central Park, where you were constantly surrounded by other people doing the same thing.

Whether it's dancing, spinning, step classes, or kickboxing, one hour in an exercise class will give you an energy boost that can last for the whole day. And although I can't prove it scientifically, I can tell you that there's a boost in mood and energy that comes from working out in a group that you just can't get from exercising solo. If you're stuck in a rut when it comes to exercise, a class setting may be just the energy boost you're looking for.

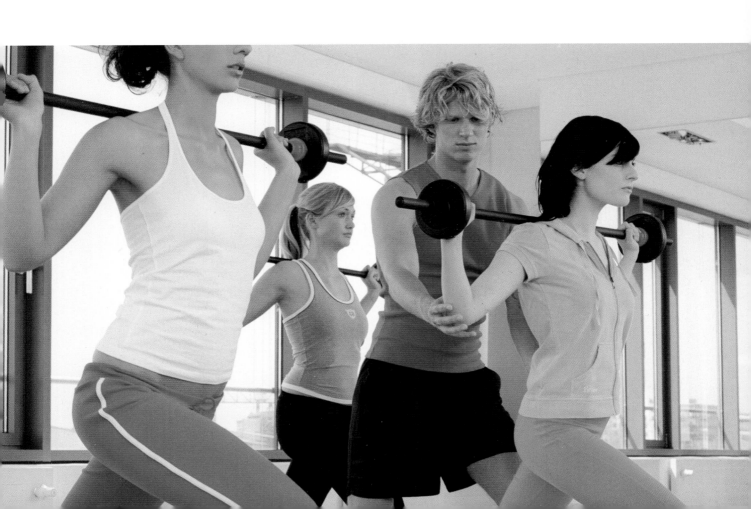

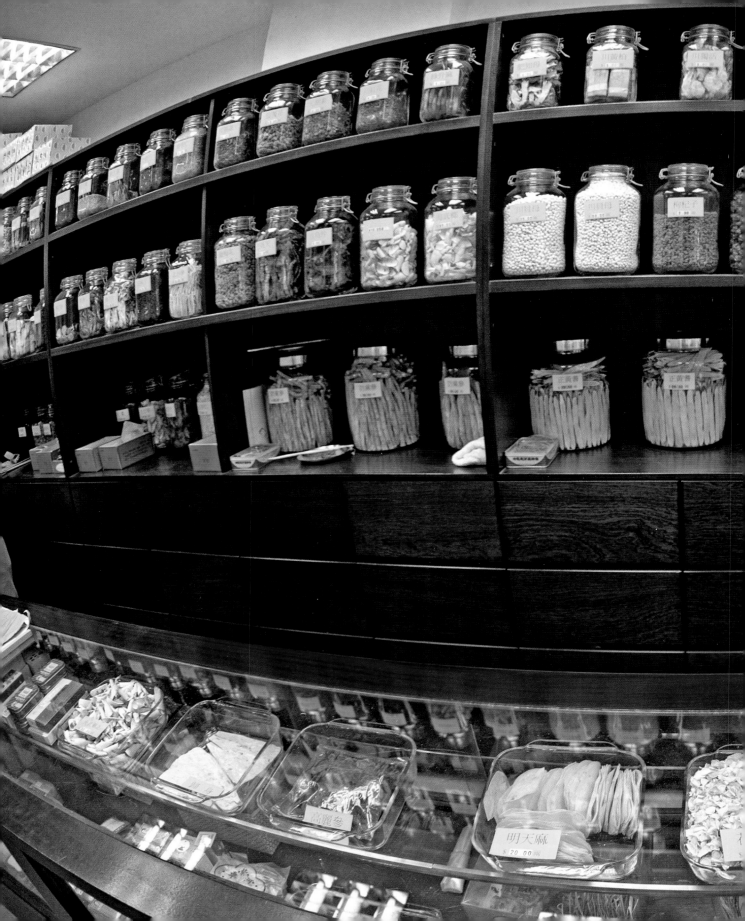

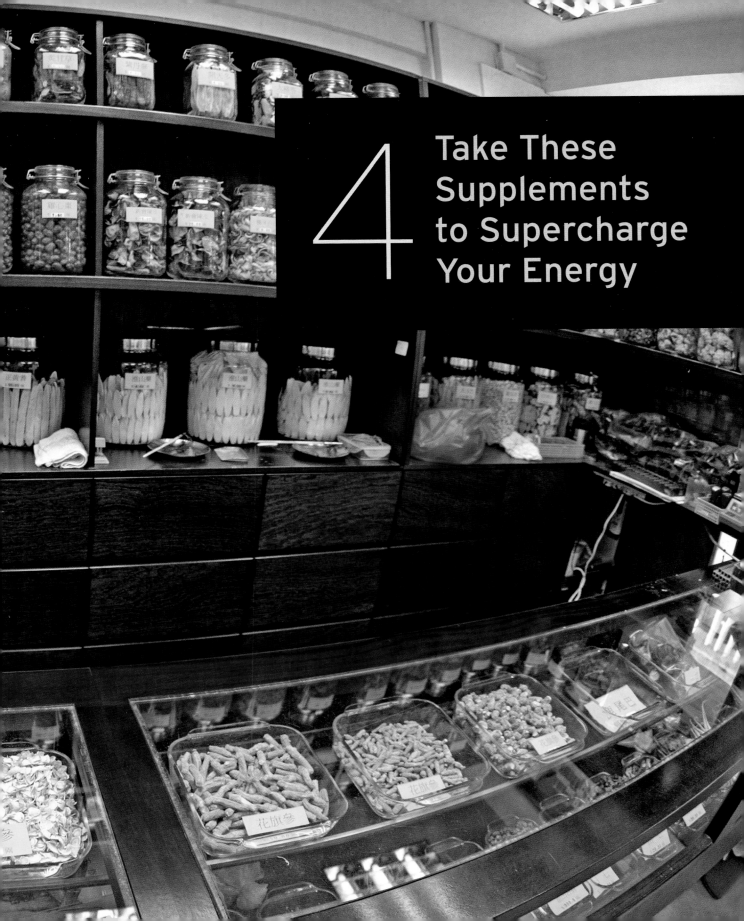

4

Take These Supplements to Supercharge Your Energy

Just so you know from the outset, I'm a big believer in supplements. I probably take a couple dozen of them a day. (At one point I probably took 100, which I suspect puts me in some all-time record-holding category, either for health fanaticism or sheer craziness, depending on your point of view.)

So please take what I'm about to tell you in the spirit in which it is intended. It is not—repeat, *not*—a slam on taking supplements, for energy or for anything else. Remember, I'm hardly anti-supplement. I wrote an entire book, *The Most Effective Natural Cures on Earth,* that is mostly devoted to how you can use nutritional supplements to improve a huge range of health conditions. So clearly, I think nutritional supplements (what we now call "nutraceuticals," a term that more fully captures their potential use as illness-fighting, health-promoting compounds) are the best thing since sliced whole grain bread. (Much better, actually, but that's another discussion.)

But—as you may have suspected—there's a "but."

THE "WHOLE" TRUTH AND NOTHING BUT THE TRUTH

I think the full value of taking supplements for energy is only realized when you're also doing a lot of *other* healthy things. Adding a few supplements to your program—even the best ones— won't compensate for a lifestyle of inadequate sleep, too much stress, a bad diet, and no exercise. Against energy drains like those, even a fantastic program of the best "energy" supplements would be outmatched. It would be like trying to bail out the Titanic with a bucket.

That said, even a great diet can be lacking in important nutrients. And you're unlikely to get certain nutrients and herbs from your diet no matter how good that diet is. Vegetarians will hardly ever get enough carnitine, and will almost never get enough B_{12}, despite what you may have heard. (Plant sources of B_{12} are simply not as good as animal sources are, despite what our vegan friends believe.)

Some nutrients, such as alpha-lipoic acid, are only found in tiny amounts in food. Other important nutrients are found only in foods we rarely eat (such as sweetbreads and organ meats). To get therapeutic amounts of still others, including vitamin E, selenium, and chromium, would require eating tons more foods than you're likely to consume no matter how healthfully you eat. Finally, some vitamins are literally eaten up by stress (the B vitamins and vitamin C). So no matter how you slice it, supplements can really add to your ability to get through your day with vigor and enthusiasm—*provided* you take the right ones *and* you take them for the right reasons. Let me explain.

A PILL FOR ENERGY?

There really aren't any supplements that will "give" you energy, although some herbs, such as ginseng and rhodiola, come close. But many supplements can help us indirectly. I spoke earlier in the book about how a swimmer can swim faster not just by getting a more high-tech-material Speedo, but also by dropping the weights that might be attached to his feet. In much the same way, many health or metabolic conditions could be draining your energy like the weights attached to the feet of our proverbial swimmer. Supplements can most definitely help remove those weights and, by helping with the conditions that are slowing you down and by making your metabolism run smoother, can thus increase your energy indirectly.

It's like getting a much needed oil change and tune-up for your car. It doesn't necessarily increase the top speed on the speedometer, but it makes it a lot more likely that, whatever the top speed happens to be, you'll be able to reach it effortlessly.

So what are some of the reasons for lack of energy that can be helped by supplements? Let's start with stress. Or high blood sugar. Bad digestion. Mild depression. And of course, a lack of key nutrients never makes anyone feel their best.

So when I say supplements should be taken the right way and for the right reasons, what I mean is this: *Don't take them expecting a quick fix, and don't expect them to work like a pharmaceutical stimulant.* Expect instead that these nutrients can plug important holes in your metabolic machinery. Many of these supplements are vitally important nutrients *whose absence can contribute mightily to fatigue.*

Ever go to the ear doctor as a child and have the wax removed from your ears? You walk out hearing absolutely everything, and feeling like someone just put an amplifier in your ear canal. Actually, your hearing didn't improve—it's just that a major obstacle was removed so that your ears could perform as they were meant to in the first place.

Supplements are a lot like that. In some cases, once you add these supplements to your program, you're going to feel a whole lot better. You may well feel that the supplement is giving you energy, but more likely it's helping to fix something that might have been, metaphorically speaking, broken, or at least not performing up to snuff. Some of the supplements in this chapter can help protect your brain, your cardiovascular system, your liver, and your heart, as well as provide the metabolic tools to "burn" fat, build muscle, and build important biochemicals that *are* involved in energy production.

You probably don't need to be like me and take all of them, but I strongly suggest you take at least some of them. For energy, I'd start with L-carnitine and CoQ10, an "energy cocktail" if there ever was one. For the occasional pick-me-up, I'd try ENADA. And, although they're not discussed in this section, I'd always start with a foundation of a multivitamin and at least 1 gram a day of fish oil. Beyond that, you can experiment with any of the other excellent supplements discussed in this section. I recommend giving any that interests you a trial of at least a couple of weeks at the recommended dosage. If you're willing to experiment, you'll soon come up with the program that's right for you. And you'll wonder why you didn't start sooner!

Some of the supplements in this chapter can help protect your brain, your cardiovascular system, your liver, and your heart, as well as provide the metabolic tools to "burn" fat, build muscle, and build important biochemicals that *are* involved in energy production.

#72

Take Coenzyme Q10, the Ubiquitous Energizer

Coenzyme Q10 just might be the most important energy nutrient you've never heard of. It's not a vitamin and not a mineral, but it's found in every cell in your body. It was first discovered in 1957 by two different researchers working in completely different parts of the world—Frederick Crane, Ph.D., of Wisconsin, who isolated the substance from the heart tissue of beef, and professor R. A. Morton, Ph.D., of England, who found an identical compound in the liver of rats. Morton, in fact, gave coenzyme Q10 its alternate name, *ubiquitone*, which he considered a catchy condensation of "ubiquitous quinone" (*ubiquitous* because it's found everywhere in the body and *quinone* because it has the same molecular structure as quinine. It appears that lab biologists are easily amused.).

So what's a coenzyme anyway, and why is this one so important for energy and overall health? You may remember from biology 101 that an enzyme is something that speeds the rate at which certain chemical processes can take place. You use enzymes in the laundry machine—they speed the chemical process by which the dirt on your teenager's jeans can be dissolved. Your body uses enzymes for hundreds of metabolic processes, including digestion, the conversion of food into nutrients, and the creation of energy in cells. Without enzymes, life as we know it would simply cease.

Well, a coenzyme is a substance that *enhances* the action of an enzyme. A coenzyme is necessary for an enzyme to work, much like a spark plug is to a piston. Many vitamins (such as B_1, B_2, and B_6) function as coenzymes. Coenzyme Q10 is the MacDaddy of coenzymes. It charges up the energy-production factories in the cells, improves the function of the little power stations in every cell called *mitochondria* (where energy is actually produced), and, as a bonus, helps protect cells from nasty little molecules called free radicals that can damage cells and their DNA and contribute to degenerative diseases (and sap your energy in the process).

The highest amounts of CoQ10 in the body are found in the heart (where Crane first found it) and the liver (where Morton found it) as well as the kidneys and pancreas. Because the heart especially relies upon CoQ10 to produce energy and to function efficiently, CoQ10 is absolutely essential to a healthy heart. In fact, CoQ10 is an accepted treatment in Europe and Japan for congestive heart failure.

But I digress.

NECESSARY FOR ENERGY, BUT HARD TO FIND

Coenzyme Q10 is a great supplement to take for many reasons. Although the body can actually make it (and does), it does so through a complicated seventeen-step process that requires at the very least seven different vitamins (vitamins B_2, B_3,

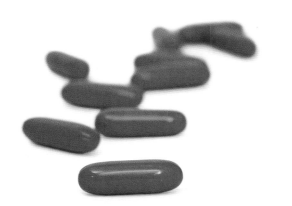

B$_6$, B$_{12}$, and C, folic acid, and pantothenic acid) plus a whole bunch of trace elements. Because plenty of people aren't getting optimal levels of those vitamins to begin with, there's likely to be less than optimal production of CoQ10—after all, if a factory isn't getting enough raw materials, its output suffers.

If you add to that the fact that coenzyme Q10 production slows down with age, and that many commonly prescribed medications block CoQ10 production (more on that in a moment), it starts to make a lot of sense to supplement with CoQ10. In fact, CoQ10 should be high on the list of supplements any high-energy person is going to want to take on a regular basis.

And no, you're not going to get optimal amounts from food. CoQ10 is found mainly in organ meats such as the heart, liver, and kidney—not popular dishes for most people—as well as beef, soy oil, peanuts, and sardines. But you'd need 1 pound (455 g) of sardines, 2 pounds (905 g) of beef, or 2½ pounds (1.13 kg) of peanuts to provide your body with a measly 30 mg of CoQ10, the absolute minimum dose to take for healthy folks looking for general protection. For people who are energy compromised, the recommended dose is much higher.

HEART HELPER

So how exactly does CoQ10 work? The body strips foods of *electrons*, tiny subatomic particles that carry a negative electric charge, which surround the nuclei of atoms. Our body then transports these electrons to an electron "receptor," which happens to be oxygen. (To get any energy from food we have to breathe oxygen!) This whole transportation system—not surprisingly called the *electron transport system*—is the final step

in converting intermediate energy carriers with weird names such as *nicotine adenine dinucleotide* (NAD) and *flavin mononucleotide* (FMN)—don't bother to remember them—into molecules of *adenosine triphosphate* (ATP). ATP is the famous "energy molecule" that functions like a battery, storing energy that's used to power anything from dozens of cellular processes you'd never notice to doing biceps curls at the gym. (Without enough ATP, you run out of steam really quickly. Lack of immediate ATP is one of the reasons your muscles "fail" after a certain amount of repetitions of bench presses or biceps curls.)

CoQ10 has the ability to increase ATP production. It's one of the electron carriers in the electron transport system, so it basically helps the cells use oxygen and create more energy.

Understanding this, it becomes easy to see why CoQ10 is so important for a healthy ticker. The average human heart beats more than 100,000 times a day. That's a lot of energy and a lot of work. No wonder the heart cells produce more energy than any other organ; they have to keep working even while you're sleeping. Being your heart (or mine) is a full-time job. It never gets to take a vacation.

SOLVING THE ENERGY SLOWDOWN

As we age, for a variety of reasons, the ability of our bodies to produce that energy starts to slow down. And without enough oxygen and vital nutrients, guess what? You start to feel rundown and tired. It's hardly surprising that there are low levels of CoQ10 associated with numerous diseases. Karl Folkers, Ph.D., an early coenzyme Q10 researcher, noted that a reduction of coenzyme Q10 levels in the body by just 25 percent (to 75 percent of optimal) may cause illness, and falling by 75 percent (25 percent of optimal levels) could cause death.

There are many reasons why CoQ10 production in the body could be compromised—aging, lack of optimal vitamin and mineral intake, stress, and medications are a few examples. (The statin drugs used to bring down cholesterol are among the biggest offenders; if you're on one of those, you should definitely supplement with CoQ10!)

—————— **WORTH KNOWING** ——————

Nearly all CoQ10 is manufactured in Japan and is marketed by a number of companies in capsules, powder-based capsules, and oil-based gelcaps. It's a fat-soluble nutrient, so I strongly recommend the oil-based gelcaps. If you take another form, it's best to take it with some fat for best absorption (such as a fish oil capsule, or a salad with olive oil). According to CoQ10 expert Peter H. Langsjoen, M.D., there can be big individual differences in absorption rates, with some people attaining fine blood levels on 100 mg a day and others requiring a good deal more. For the average person, 30 to 60 mg a day is a nice maintenance dose, but I'd recommend higher doses for those on statin meds or those with energy issues (100 mg or even higher).

#73

Catch a Ride on the Energy Shuttle Bus with Carnitine

I live in Los Angeles, so I hope you'll forgive a very local, LA analogy for what L-carnitine does in the body.

One of LA's most famous residents is Hugh Heffner, the octogenarian founder and editor in chief of *Playboy* magazine who famously lives in the eponymous Playboy Mansion in an elegant and exclusive section of town. Hef, as you may have heard, is known for his parties, but what you may *not* know is that invited guests can't just drive up to the Mansion. Instead, they drive to a large parking area not too far away. There, they board a bus that then takes them to the premises.

Well, in your body, carnitine acts like that shuttle bus to the Mansion. Except, instead of taking guests to the party, it takes fatty acids into the part of the cell where they can be burned for energy. Carnitine is literally the transport mechanism—the shuttle bus—by which fat gets escorted into little energy factories inside the cell called *mitochondria*, where all the action, including fat burning and energy production, takes place. No shuttle bus, no guests at the party. No carnitine, no energy production.

We can learn a lot about the role of carnitine in energy production by looking at what happens in the bodies of people with energy deficiency syndromes such as fibromyalgia and chronic fatigue syndrome. Low levels of a carnitine compound called *acetyl L-carnitine* (more about this in a moment) have been found in the blood or muscles of people with fibromyalgia and chronic fatigue in two different research centers. Carnitine prevents a substance called acetyl-CoA from building up and shutting down two critical energy production cycles in the body, the Kreb's cycle and the electron transport chain. Quite simply, if you want your body's energy production factories to work seamlessly and optimally, you need carnitine.

So what is carnitine anyway, and where do we get it?

FATIGUE FIGHTER

Although carnitine is often referred to in popular magazines as an amino acid, technically it's not. But it *is* an amino-acid-like *substance*. (In case you ever find yourself in one of those heated dinner party discussions about the amino acid status of carnitine, simply point out that an amino acid by definition needs an atom of nitrogen, which carnitine doesn't have, and you will immediately be declared the winner of the argument, and men and women will worship at your feet.)

Carnitine (also known as L-carnitine or levo-carnitine) is made in the body, mainly in the liver and kidneys, and most of it is found in the muscles. It's actually biosynthesized from the amino acids lysine and methionine, with help from vitamins C, B_6, and B_3, and iron. Because it's made in the body, conventional docs and dietitians tend to pooh-pooh the need for carnitine supplements, claiming we get all we need from the diet and the body makes the rest. Theoretically, this is true, but the key word is *theoretically*.

Carnitine is only found in any appreciable degree in animal products. Strict vegetarians or vegans may ingest as little as 1 mg a day. There's also speculation that during pregnancy, breast-feeding, or growth, the need for carnitine is greater than the amount the body naturally produces. And in conditions when fatigue and low energy are issues, supplemental carnitine may help a lot.

L-carnitine is a tremendous nutrient for the heart; it is part of what Stephen Sinatra, M.D., dubbed "the awesome foursome" for heart disease: L-carnitine, coenzyme Q10, D-ribose, and magnesium. One reason it's so important for the heart has to do with—guess what?—energy. Remember that the heart is a muscle and beats 100,000 times or so a day. It uses an *enormous* amount of energy, most of it from the fuel it gets from "burning" fatty acids. If the system by which fatty acids get forklifted over to the cell's mitochondria is compromised, then so is energy production, and the heart can't work as well.

"Carnitine fuels the cardiac engine," says my friend, nutritionist Robert Crayhon, M.S., C.N., author of *The Carnitine Miracle*. The exercise endurance of cardiac patients goes up remarkably on 900 mg of carnitine a day.

I mentioned in the beginning that L-carnitine performed the valuable function of escorting important fatty acids into the mitochondria of the cell, where they can be burned for energy. But L-carnitine has another mission as well. On its way back from dropping off that payload, it carries away extra fatty acids and waste products,

Quite simply, if you want your body's energy production factories to work seamlessly and optimally, you need carnitine.

or toxins, out of the fat-burning part of the cell for eventual elimination in the urine. If these wastes are not removed, they will clog the area, and this will ultimately affect the production of energy.

The thing of it is, we don't have much trouble producing all this cellular energy when we're young (did you ever see a six-year-old complain of fatigue?). But as we get older, our enzymatic systems start to get sluggish, and the heart may begin to get less of the essential nutrients it's come to depend on.

Next thing you know, you're in your 40s (or 50s or 60s or beyond), and your poor heart is virtually starving for energy. Like the plant in *Little Shop of Horrors* it's crying out, "Feed me! Feed me!" Your heart is soon struggling to deliver enough oxygen and vital nutrients to the organs, tissues, and every part of the body. And without enough oxygen and vital nutrients, there's simply less energy production in the cells to keep the body going. The result? You're rundown, tired, and fatigued.

Remember that you need energy not just to fight off fatigue, but also to build, repair, and renew cell membranes and other cellular structures; create immune components that help fight infection; and support the functioning of vital organs, such as the heart, liver, kidneys, and lungs. A shortage of energy translates into impaired functions that can lead straight to disease, ill health, and most certainly an impaired sense of well-being.

Some research has also shown additional benefits to L-carnitine supplementation beyond the boost in energy seen in many people. Studies show that L-carnitine elevates "good" HDL cholesterol, reduces triglycerides, and lowers blood pressure in hypertension. "I have never seen people feel such an improved state of overall wellness

and a natural increase in energy as they have when they increase their intake of carnitine," says Crayhon.

Most people get about 50 mg of L-carnitine in their diet, but many professionals think the optimal level is closer to 200 to 2,000 mg. You'll need at least 500 mg daily of an L-carnitine supplement to feel any difference, and that's the minimum. Most health professionals recommend between 1 and 3 grams, or even 4 grams a day if you're using the supplement for a specific purpose (such as increasing cellular energy).*

──────── **WORTH KNOWING** ────────

Carnitine works best with a low-carbohydrate diet, as high carbohydrates (especially the junky, processed, high-sugar kind) interfere with its action by boosting insulin. And it's worth taking some omega-3s (supplements or cold water fish) at the same time.

Some health professionals, including Mark Moyad, M.D., director of Preventive and Alternative Medicine at the University of Michigan Medical Center, believe that even as little as 500 mg of L-carnitine a day will give you an all-day energy boost. Personally, I think that's a low recommendation—I'd start with 1,000 mg (500 mg twice a day).

#74

Burn Calories and Get an Energy Edge with EGCG

I'm a huge fan of tea for both its health properties and as an energy drink in general. Although all tea is great, one particular compound in green tea, called *epigallocatechin gallate,* or EGCG for short, has been isolated and is available as a supplement. I think it's great for energy, even more so if you're not drinking tea on a regular basis.

EGCG is a member of a family of substances found in tea called *catechins*, which are in turn a member of a larger class of plant chemicals called *polyphenols*. These polyphenols are thought to be responsible for a large measure of the health benefits of tea, but EGCG in particular is of special interest to those of us looking to get an energy edge.

EGCG sparks a process in the body known as *thermogenesis*, or heat production (thermo means "heat," and genesis means "making new"). You may know the process of thermogenesis by its more common term, "fat burning." And sure enough, EGCG has been found to be of great interest to those on a weight management program for the same reason that it may help you with your energy.

AN ANCIENT ENERGIZER

Here's what we do know: Green tea consumption leads to a significant increase in calorie burning, a decrease in body weight, and a decrease in waist circumference, all while producing no real change in heart rate or blood pressure.

Researchers suspect that one of the ways it accomplishes this is by possibly prolonging the effects of norepinephrine, one of the stimulating chemicals in the body. Traditional Chinese medicine has long recommended green tea for all sorts of ailments and conditions, including headaches, body aches and pains, digestion, depression, immune enhancement, detoxification, and . . . as an *energizer*!

Makes sense. In one study, which appeared in the December 1999 *American Journal of Clinical Nutrition*, researchers measured energy expenditure (calories burned) in ten healthy young men who were randomly given either a standard green tea extract (375 mg of catechins and 150 mg of caffeine), 150 mg of caffeine by itself, or an inert placebo. Believe it or not, the caffeine was no better than a placebo at speeding metabolism, but the men receiving the green tea extract burned an average of 78 calories more a day. Another study, this one published in the September 2005 *British Journal of Nutrition*, found the increased calorie burn was a little higher—about 178 calories a day for a combination of 200 mg of caffeine with any dose of EGCG tested, from 90 to 400 mg.

Although that amount of calories per day isn't enormous, it's still significant, and those calories do add up. Considering all the other health benefits besides "metabolism boosting," and that there were zero negative side effects (e.g., no increase in heart rate), and *also* that green tea tends to stimulate not just calorie burning but fat burning as well, it's hard to argue that green tea extract—EGCG—wouldn't be a great addition to a supplement program for energy enhancement.

#75

Take Off with a Little Biological Rocket Fuel

For the almost twenty years I've known him, Oz Garcia, Ph.D., my close friend (and superstar nutritionist to the stars), has sworn by a little-known supplement named ENADA, calling it the ultimate energy supplement.

"It's one of the most rehabilitating supplements I've ever come across," he told me.

ENADA has actually changed names and is now known as Co-E1 NADH. It's an unwieldy name, but a terrific product. People who love it have called it "biological rocket fuel." A number of studies have shown that it can significantly improve at least four recognized symptoms of chronic fatigue syndrome, including unexplained tiredness, difficulty thinking, sleep disturbances, and headaches or sore throats. Researchers at the Sleep-Wake Disorders Center, Weill Cornell Medical College, found that it significantly improved measures of cognitive performance following a night of total sleep deprivation. Athletes use Co-E1 NADH to increase muscular energy supply. My friend Oz uses it all the time before he goes running.

So what is this stuff, anyway? NADH is the reduced form of NAD (*nicotinamide adenine dinucleotide*), a coenzyme that plays a key role in the energy production of cells, particularly in the brain and central nervous system. The more NADH a cell has available, the more energy it can produce.

NADH participates in the cellular processes that generate ATP (*adenosine triphosphate*) from glucose (sugar). ATP is known as the "energy molecule" because it's cellular fuel for your muscles. Co-E1 NADH may help people with chronic fatigue syndrome by triggering energy production through the generation of ATP. Some studies indicate it may improve mental and physical endurance, as well as cognitive performance, possibly by stimulating the cellular production of neurotransmitters.

Co-E1 NADH is available as a lozenge (I have a link on my website www.jonnybowden.com, under shopping/vitamins). Oz recommends starting with 2.5 mg upon waking, and increasing in increments of 2.5 mg to 5 mg, 7.5 mg, or 10 mg upon waking. You can also use it at different times of the day. "Always start low and work up," he advises.

You can also pop one in your mouth 30 minutes or so before athletic activity, or any time you need a little boost in mental energy.

#76

Take the Fatigue Fighter, D-Ribose

I first heard about D-Ribose as an energy nutrient in a gym in Los Angeles and promptly dismissed it. Why? Probably prejudice on my part. Most of what you hear around the gym regarding supplements is nonsense, and the guy who was touting this one claimed to have gotten it from a medical researcher who swore that it was the missing link in energy production, and if you just drank this product with D-Ribose in it you'd be benching 250 in no time, and running marathons in your spare time.

So, naturally, I paid no attention.

Several years later, my friend Stephen Sinatra, M.D., a cardiologist and nutritionist for whom I have great respect, wrote a book on metabolic cardiology that had an introduction by another physician, James Roberts, M.D.. Sinatra, a huge fan of D-Ribose, said that he had discovered the supplement through Roberts. Here's what he wrote in his book, *The Sinatra Solution: Metabolic Cardiology:*

"Before trying ribose on his patients, Dr. Roberts decided to use himself as a guinea pig. As a marathon runner, Dr. Roberts knew the importance of energy recovery on maintaining the physiological health of his muscles. He also knew the pain, soreness, stiffness and fatigue he felt following long distance training runs. Dr. Roberts soon found that taking ribose before and after a run eliminated the problems associated with training. After a long run his muscles felt good and his legs were no longer 'spongy.' The muscle pain and soreness he generally had for a couple of days after training were gone. And, he was no longer fatigued in the days following a strenuous workout. Dr. Roberts was convinced!"

Okay, that got my attention.

A VITAL SUGAR

So here's the deal. D-Ribose is actually a five-carbon sugar that is used by every living cell. It was discovered way back in 1905, and has long been known to be a component of RNA, which, you may remember from high school biology, is a nucleic acid that helps translate genetic information from DNA into proteins. In other words, it's vital. Because D-Ribose (ribose for short) is an essential part of RNA, it's *also* essential for all living things. And if that weren't enough to make its resume impressive, ribose is also a component of ATP (adenosine triphosphate), the "energy" molecule in the cell. Bottom line: It's critical for metabolism.

Between 1997 and 2004, a company called Bioenergy, Inc. amassed no fewer than twenty-four patents (issued or pending) relating to the use of ribose for increasing energy in tissues, and also for the treatment of cardiovascular diseases.

The primary dietary source of D-Ribose is veal and other red meat, but, as Sinatra points out, the amount you might get from your diet isn't enough to provide any meaningful support for anyone with low energy caused by heart disease, vascular disease, or even high intensity exercise recovery. The body makes ribose, and because of that, it's not considered an "essential" nutrient (meaning you have to get one from the diet). That's why technically there are no "D-ribose deficiencies." Deficiencies technically are defined as concentrations of nutrients that fall below normal levels, and because the body doesn't store ribose in the conventional sense, a ribose deficiency can't exist. But that doesn't mean you couldn't use more of it.

Cells basically produce ribose on demand, much like the barista at Starbucks—they don't make a bunch of it and leave it on the counter waiting to be used. But certain tissues, including the heart and the brain, can only make the amount of ribose they need when the cells *aren't* under stress. On top of that, ribose manufacturing is a slow process.

As a result, the tissues of the heart and muscles are unable to quickly replace energy pools once they've been depleted by either exercise or disease. This is a particular concern i n heart disease, when oxygen or blood flow is chronically impaired, but as we saw with Roberts' experience running marathons, it could also be the case with regular folks under certain conditions.

"Studies have shown that any amount of ribose you give to energy-starved cells will give the cells an energy boost," Sinatra told me.

PROMISING STUDIES

Will ribose supplementation help people with low energy? Truth be told, we don't know for absolute sure, but there's good reason to connect the dots from certain research with energy-depleted conditions, such as fibromyalgia and chronic fatigue syndrome. Both of these conditions are related to a shortage of cellular energy.

In a 2006 pilot study in the *Journal of Alternative and Complementary Medicine*, forty-one patients with chronic fatigue syndrome, fibromyalgia, or both were given 5 grams of D-Ribose three times a day over the course of about twenty-five days. By the end of the study, the participants reported significant improvements in sleep patterns, mental clarity, energy, and feelings of well-being. The average energy increase was 45 percent; about two-thirds of the people reported feeling "somewhat better to much better" while taking the D-Ribose supplements.

A study on young, healthy males also yielded promising results. Male recreational bodybuilders between the ages of eighteen and thirty-five were divided into two groups; one group was given ribose supplementation (10 grams per day), and the other group was given a placebo. The ribose-supplemented group had a significant increase in the total work performed in their workout as well as a significant increase in their one-repetition maximum-strength bench press. Sure, it was a small study, but it adds to the evidence that ribose may be effective in increasing energy.

The evidence for ribose supplementation in people whose energy is compromised because of heart issues is even more compelling. A number of studies have shown great value in using ribose (often along with other great heart nutrients, such as coenzyme Q10 and carnitine) for heart patients.

One of many peer-reviewed journal articles (in a 2003 issue of the *European Journal of Heart Failure*) showed that D-Ribose improved diastolic function and quality of life in patients with congestive heart failure, a condition in which energy is highly compromised.

It's more than possible that D-Ribose may help you with general fatigue, whether or not you are an athlete. I recommend starting with 5 to 10 grams a day (1 slightly rounded tablespoon of powder), in two divided doses (½ to 1 tablespoon each).

#77

Feed Your Brain for Energy

Ever hear the expression "the spirit is willing but the flesh is weak"? Well, biblical meanings aside, the concept has a lot to tell us about energy.

I can't actually think of a time when my mind has been alive, energetic, and enthusiastic, but my body's been too tired to do something. But there are plenty of times that the reverse is true: your body is perfectly able to perform, but you're mentally exhausted. Take-home point—energy starts (and frequently ends) in the brain.

That's why keeping your brain active, keeping the circuits firing on all cylinders, protecting your neurons from the damage known as oxidation (see sidebar below), and generally making sure that everything up there is working fine is probably the best overall strategy on the planet for maintaining terrific reserves of energy.**

**There's no one on the planet more anti-drug than I am, but consider this: Back in previous wars, when the military had physically exhausted troops on its hands, it would routinely provide the soldiers with amphetamines so they could complete their missions. The soldiers' physical energy wouldn't

change, but because amphetamines work on the brain, the drugged-out troops were able to perform as if they'd just woken up from nine hours of restful sleep, even though they were physically spent. Moral of the story: If your brain is energized, you are energized. But don't try this at home, folks.

That's why, no matter what else I may forget to take, I never forget to take my daily "brain supplements." The basic brain energy formula I recommend has three important ingredients: acetyl-l-carnitine, phosphatidylserine (PS), and glycerophosphocholine (GPC). In addition, I strongly recommend taking ginkgo, alpha-lipoic acid, and fish oil for a whole bunch of reasons, not the least of which is that they help support the brain (as well as a host of other organs and functions).

A PRESCRIPTION FOR MENTAL PRECISION

So what are all these ingredients, and why do they have such unpronounceable names?

I can't explain the esoteric names in a way that wouldn't put you to sleep, but I *can* tell you what they do and why they help with brain energy. In a nutshell, acetyl-l-carnitine helps energize the brain; phosphatidylserine, or PS, is great for memory; and GPC helps enhance mental focus. Together, they make a winning combination.

Neurologist David Perlmutter, M.D., author of *The Better Brain Book*, describes acetyl-l-carnitine as a neuronal energizer. He points out that it helps remove waste products from the little energy production factories in the cells (called *mitochondria*), enabling those energy-draining (and health-robbing) toxins to be eliminated from the body. Neurosurgeon Russell Blaylock, M.D., says acetyl-l-carnitine improves the function of those mitochondria, "returning them to the way they were when you were twenty."

PS is a member of a class of biochemicals called *phospholipids*, and has been available as a supplement for decades. It's been shown in many well-documented studies to restore brain function and help improve learning and concentration. My good friend, biochemist and nutritional supplement expert Parris Kidd, Ph.D., says, "Dietary supplementation with PS can alleviate, ameliorate, and sometimes reverse age-related decline of memory, learning, concentration, word skills, and mood."

Finally, GPC has been extensively researched for its effect on mental performance, attention, and concentration, and the results have been impressive indeed. (It's actually found in large quantities in breast milk, which ought to say something about its importance in human health!)

"I continue to be fascinated by GPC's capacities to sharpen mental performance, even in people who are healthy, and to give new vitality to the aging brain," says Kidd, who is one of the country's leading experts on GPC (www.dockidd.com).

I also recommend alpha-lipoic acid, a supplement with a huge resume of beneficial effects on the body and brain. Alpha-lipoic acid was combined with acetyl-l-carnitine in a series of animal experiments performed in 2002 by the legendary researcher Bruce Ames, Ph.D., at the University of California.

The appearance of the animal brains' improved and the animals showed significant increases in energy, Ames reported. "With these two supplements together, these old rats got up and did the Macarena."

Finally, don't underestimate the old standby for brain health, ginkgo biloba. It's a powerful antioxidant and neuro-protector. My friend Daniel Amen, M.D., who has looked at more than 10,000 SPECT scans (pictures of brains), says that from a health and function point of view, the healthiest looking brains he has seen are those on ginkgo.

So how do you take all these things? Well, let me count the ways. There are dozens of supplements sold that combine them in various formulas marketed for brain health, brain energy, memory enhancement, and the like. These vary widely in quality, and you should look for meaningful doses of the important ingredients (at least 100 mg of PS, 450 mg of GPC, and 300 mg of acetyl-l-carnitine). The formulas I like the best I list on my website, www.jonnybowden.com, under "shopping/vitamins" and "supplements/brain power."

I also recommend 100 mg a day of alpha-lipoic acid for general protection (and antiaging assistance!) and 120 to 240 mg of ginkgo.

Remember, too, that fish oil has many benefits for the brain, and although it won't directly "give" you energy, it will sure help protect the circuits in the brain that will!

─────── **WORTH KNOWING** ───────

Two other ingredients are often used in brain formulas, largely because both are precursors of that exciting, stimulating, energizing neurotransmitter dopamine. They are DL-phenylalanine and L-tyrosine, both amino acids. One formula, designed by Eric Braverman, M.D., combines both in a product aptly called Brain Energy. Brain Energy is also in the vitamin supplements section of my website, www.jonnybowden.com, under "brain power."

Oxidation and Your Brain

Here's the thing about oxygen: You can't live without it. But it can also do some nasty damage.

You may remember from high school biology that all molecules have something called *electrons* that orbit around the core of the molecule in matched pairs. Once in a while, one of these electrons gets loose from its pair bond, and goes on a bit of a rampage while it tries to find a mate. That rampage causes what's known as *oxidative damage,* or *oxidation.* (You can see the visible effects of this by watching what happens to apple slices left out in the air on the kitchen counter overnight.)

These rogue, unpaired electrons are known as *free radicals*. Each time one of these free radicals "hits" on an intact molecule looking to steal a mate for itself, it damages your cells and DNA. When this happens in the brain, the results are . . . well, not good. Antioxidants (including vitamin C, vitamin E, selenium, zinc, ginkgo, and plant compounds such as flavonoids) actually work by "donating" an electron to the rogue fellow, helping to prevent further damage.

Bottom line: Oxidative damage: bad. Protection against oxidative damage: priceless.

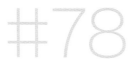

Take a B-Complex Vitamin

We have to work backward a bit to uncover the connection between taking B-vitamin supplements and improved energy, but you don't have to be Columbo to do it—it's pretty easy to uncover the relationship.

Consider, for openers, vitamin B_{12}. Clinical symptoms of B_{12} deficiency take many years to appear. And one of the biggest symptoms is fatigue.

Despite what our vegan and vegetarian friends may believe, B_{12} is only found in animal source foods. This isn't just my opinion; it's also the opinion of the U.S. Department of Agriculture, and it is stated as clearly as possible in the exhaustive *Encyclopedia of Dietary Supplements,* edited by Paul Coates, the director of the Office of Dietary Supplements for the National Institutes of Health. So let's stop with the "we can get all the B_{12} we need from plants" arguments. We can't.

Now why does that matter? Because B_{12} deficiency is far more prevalent than previously assumed, and vegetarians, even those who consume dairy products, are at risk. Because a lot of health-minded people shun meat these days (not because meat per se is bad, but because the meat we tend to buy is so horrible), this is a big concern.

Another problem is that B vitamins are eaten up alive during stress, and if you're reading this book, chances are that you and stress are not exactly strangers. That's an important reason why many people feel so much better supplementing with a B-complex vitamin (more on that below). Even the popular media seem to have caught on to this. An article in a 2003 issue of *Psychology Today* was appropriately titled "Vitamin B: A Key to Energy" and subtitled "To Fight Fatigue, Irritability, and Poor Concentration, Power Up with B Vitamins."

Not for nothing were the "Dr. Feelgoods" of the 1950s and 60s known for dispensing shots of vitamin B_{12}. It does make a lot of people feel better, especially if you're low in this vitamin to begin with. And as we get older, we lose a lot of our ability to absorb it from food.

THE B FAMILY: AN ENERGY ORCHESTRA

But it's not just B_{12} that's critical for energy. Vitamin B_6 is needed for the manufacturing of all kinds of brain chemicals and enzymes, and it is critical for making serotonin, the feel-good neurotransmitter in the brain. (That's one reason why, in *The Most Effective Natural Cures on Earth*, I recommended B_6 as a vital ingredient in my "PMS Cocktail." Serotonin levels frequently drop before and during menstruation, a fact that didn't escape the pharmaceutical manufacturer Eli Lilly, who recently repackaged its famous serotonin drug Prozac as Serafem, which is now prescribed for PMS. Vitamin B_6 seems to help the body replenish this important neurochemical naturally.)

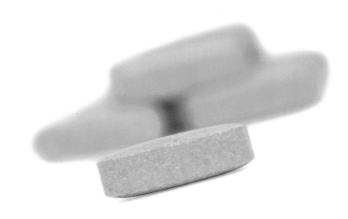

B_6, together with B_{12} and folic acid (another member of the B family), works to bring down a nasty inflammatory compound in the blood called *homocysteine*, which can increase your risk for heart disease, stroke, and Alzheimer's. Plus, B_6, together with B_{12}, contributes to the myelin sheath that covers nerve cells and is necessary for signals to travel through the brain at warp speed. Without enough B_{12} or folic acid, your poor blood cells can't carry enough oxygen to the brain. And that would sap anyone's energy.

All the B vitamins have important functions in the body, and some, such as thiamin (B_1) and riboflavin (B_2), are critical for normal energy production in human cells. In one 1997 study done in Wales, healthy women who took B_1 supplements had faster reaction times and reported feeling more clear-headed and energetic.

Although there are occasions where specific B vitamins can be useful (such as B_2 for headaches, the occasional shot of B_{12} for any number of things, and the aforementioned B_6 for moods and carpal tunnel syndrome), the B vitamins actually perform quite like an orchestra; if you really want that rich sound that the orchestra is capable of, you need all its members to play together. That's why most health professionals recommend taking a B-complex vitamin, even if you think you're low on one specific B.

If you do want to take one of the B family for a specific health reason, no problem. Just remember to also take a B complex, preferably at a different time during the day for maximum absorption. According to my friend, nutritionist extraordinaire Linda Lizotte, R.D., a high level of one of the B vitamins can cause an imbalance or deficiency in some of the others, which is not a problem if you're also supplementing with B complex.

#79

Zap Energy-Draining Organisms with Probiotics

I first got to thinking about the connection between energy and probiotics—those "good bugs" with weird-sounding names such as *lactobacillus* that are found in yogurt—when I was interviewed about energy for a national magazine. The writer wanted to know whether taking probiotics might help people increase their energy.

Frankly, at first I was surprised by the question, because the relationship between energy and probiotics isn't obvious at first glance. But when I thought about it, it seemed clear that there is indeed a logical connection. Probiotics support and increase immunity. Lowered immune defenses increase your likelihood of being sidelined by microbes, viruses, bacteria, and infections, all of which are known energy-drainers. Hence, giving

Without enough B_{12} or folic acid, your poor blood cells can't carry enough oxygen to the brain. And that would sap anyone's energy.

your immune system a nice little turbo charge makes plenty of sense if you want your energy to be at its highest.

Enter probiotics.

DIETARY DEFENSIVE SYSTEM

Like many things, the health benefits of these live bugs were discovered by accident. First scientists noticed that people in the mountains of Bulgaria were remarkably free of degenerative diseases. (They tended to be strong, energetic people who hardly ever got sick.) So researchers investigated their diet.

Fast forward through a number of studies, and voilà, the likely suspect was identified. These rugged mountaineers were eating a ton of yogurt that was very rich in a particular bacteria called *bulgaricus*, and bulgaricus has antiviral, antibacterial, and antifungal properties, as well as many other health benefits.

Bulgaricus—also known as *B. bifidum* or bifidobacteria—is part of a class of bacteria called *probiotics*, the most famous of which is lactobacillis. Your gut is populated by a huge amount of bacteria, some of it "good," as with lactobacillis, and some of it not so good, including candida, *E. coli,* and salmonella.

We all have both good and bad bacteria in our gut, but it's a turf issue, like flowers and weeds in the same garden. You need to keep the good ones in the majority and the bad ones at a minimum. The live cultures in real yogurt help do that, and they provide many health benefits.

HOW YOGURT HELPS

Many health professionals believe that absolutely everyone should supplement with probiotics, unless they're eating plenty of yogurt with live cultures. "By maintaining good gut flora, you'll prevent all kinds of different diseases, especially chronic ones," says my friend, naturopathic physician Sonja Pettersen, N.M.D. "Probiotics help control inflammation, which is a central feature of so many degenerative diseases, including heart disease. Probiotics, like the bulgaris found in the yogurt in Bulgaria, help increase NK cells (a powerful immune system weapon). They increase antibodies when we have infections. They improve digestion. They have anticancer properties."

And they clearly boost immunity. Probiotics basically work by colonizing the small intestine and edging out the disease-causing organisms. They stimulate the body's immune system. Probiotics may also have a positive effect on blood sugar. An article in the August 2007 *Journal of the American College of Nutrition* reported that daily ingestions of tablets containing powdered fermented milk (yogurt) with lactobacillus reduced elevated blood pressure in mildly hypertensive patients without any adverse side effects whatsoever.

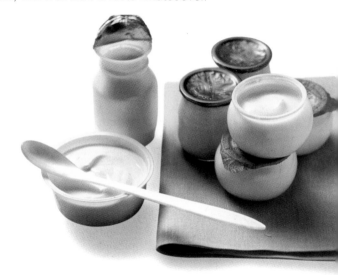

THE ACID TEST

You can give your immunity a boost and increase your energy by either taking probiotics as a daily supplement or by eating plenty of real yogurt. Remember, yogurt is just milk that was left out to sour, so it's a naturally fermented food that's allowed to develop its own bacteria (just like sauerkraut or any other fermented food). "The more acidic the yogurt is, the more likely there's good bacteria in it," Pettersen says. "The product has to actually contain live cultures."

The National Yogurt Association (NYA) has developed a "Live and Active Cultures" (LAC) seal for the yogurt label to identify yogurt that contains significant levels of live and active cultures. Be aware that a label stating "made with active cultures" does not mean the same as the LAC label. The LAC label means that the yogurt contains at least 100 million cultures per gram of yogurt at the time of manufacture and after pasteurization.

In addition to boosting your energy by helping your immune system do its job more effectively, probiotics may actually have an unexpected side benefit. Just as this book was going to press, a study in the May 2, 2008, *Journal of Psychiatric Research* found that probiotics may have an anti-depressant activity. Although the study was done on rats, the evidence was compelling. To my mind, anything that improves mood boosts energy. Probiotics might wind up boosting your energy in more ways than one.

#80-82
Adapt to Energy with These Three Supplements

If your house or apartment has ever been too cold or too hot, you've probably fiddled with the thermostat. If you can understand how a thermostat works, you can understand what an adaptagen is, and how it can help with energy.

The key to the whole thing is adjustment; adaptagens act as a counterbalance to whatever is out of whack in your body. Let's say you set the temperature on your thermostat to a nice comfortable 72ºF (22ºC). If the temperature in the room is currently too *cold*, the adjustment mechanism in the thermostat will bring it *up* (to 72ºF, or 22ºC), but if it's too *hot*, it will bring it *down* (to 72ºF, or 22ºC). The thermostat behaves exactly the way an adaptagenic herb behaves in your body—it smoothes things out, increasing energy when you're feeling fatigue, and relaxing you when you're feeling too stimulated. It "looks" at the existing situation and helps you adapt, doing whatever's needed to bring you into balance—hence the name adaptagen.

The three herbs in this section are all known as adaptagens, though they have many other (and sometimes wide-reaching) effects and uses. For our purposes, however, we'll concentrate on their ability to reduce stress, lower fatigue, or generally make you feel better and more alert, especially if you're feeling overstressed or fatigued to begin with.

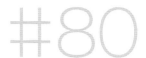

Ashwagadha, the Antistress Agent

Ashwagandha (*Withania somnifera*) is an herb commonly used in the traditional medical system of India called Ayurvedic medicine. In Ayurvedic medicine, it's considered a *rasayana* herb, which is an herb that works to increase longevity and health. The herb is a biologically rich brew of active chemicals, including all sorts of unpronounceable names such as alkaloids, steroidal lactones, saponins, and withanolides. Many of ashwagandha's benefits are probably due to these compounds, though—as in much of natural and herbal medicine—it's not entirely clear exactly which constituents of the plant are responsible for its observed benefits. The plant is also a rich source of iron.

Ashwagandha has been used in traditional herbal medicine for more than 2,000 years, mainly as a "vitalizer" or "energizer" of the body. It seems to have a noticeable antistress effect. In a number of animal studies, it increases the length of time animals are able to exercise and reduces atrophy of the adrenal glands, which produce stress hormones. In one review, the authors speculate that if their results could be reproduced in humans, they would support the use of ashwagandha to treat nervous exhaustion due to stress. Its mildly "taming" effects on the central nervous system of a number of different species (dogs, cats, and monkeys) make sense, considering so many people use ashwagandha for relaxation.

According to my friends at the American Botanical Council, some research suggests that ashwagandha may enhance brain functions such as memory and cognition. That's probably because the root of the herb contains *choline*, which is an essential part of *acetylcholine*, an important neurotransmitter that's critical for both memory and learning. Ashwagandha seems to decrease the activity of an enzyme called *acetylcholinesterase*, which breaks down acetylcholine, thus leaving more of it around in your brain to make you think better. (That's actually how Aricept, an Alzheimer's medication, works.)

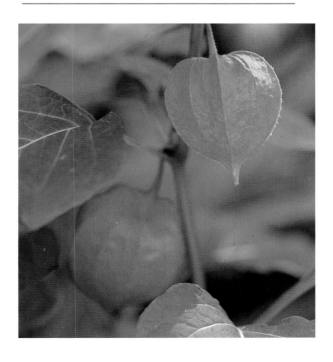

#81

Panax Ginseng, for Cognitive Performance Improvement

If the first thing you think of when you think about "herbs for energy" is ginseng, you're hardly alone. Panax ginseng (which includes both the American ginseng [*Panax quinquefolius*], and the Asian ginseng [*Panax ginseng*]) is probably one of the most investigated plants in the world for its medicinal uses. The term Panax actually means "all-heal" in Greek. (Note: "Siberian ginseng" [*Eleutherococcus senticosus*] is actually not ginseng at all, but a different adaptagen with entirely different active ingredients.)

In Eastern medicine, ginseng roots are prized for their ability to treat tiredness and fatigue. In fact, a common side effect is the inability to sleep, which should tell you something! A 2005 study in the *Journal of Psychopharmacology* is just one of many showing that Panax ginseng can improve cognitive performance in healthy volunteers, though the exact mechanism by which it works isn't known. The researchers of this study concluded that "Panax ginseng can improve performance and subjective feelings of mental fatigue during sustained mental activity."

To be truthful, not every study produced the same positive results, but enough have that the prestigious (and conservative) *Encyclopedia of Dietary Supplements*, edited by Paul Coates, the director of the Office of Dietary Supplements of the National Institutes for Health, states, "The indications of Panax ginseng root and standardized extracts supported by clinical data are for the *enhancement of mental and physical capacities*, and increased resistance against infections, in cases of weakness, exhaustion, tiredness, loss of concentration, and during convalescence" (italics mine).

The active ingredients in ginseng are a class of phytochemicals (plant compounds) called *ginsenosides*; interestingly, sometimes when you increase the dose of these ginsenosides beyond certain limits, the positive results are reversed. That may account for why some research studies haven't produced positive results (though plenty have).

The Chinese have used ginseng since ancient times to fight off weakness and fatigue. One study of rats using tests of learning and memory found that both improved after an oral dose of 20 mg of the extract per kg of body weight, but remained the same or even decreased after 100 mg of extract per kg of body weight, showing again that the dose is very important.

There are plenty of studies on humans as well. One study found a small but consistent antifatigue effect among night-shift nurses, as well as a benefit in mood. Another showed a favorable effect in attention and mental processing among healthy male volunteers given 100 mg of ginseng extract twice a day for twelve weeks, and yet another study demonstrated significant improvements in endurance among forty-three top triathletes receiving 200 mg of a standardized ginseng extract per day for ten weeks. Positive effects on cognition have also been observed using a combination of Panax ginseng and ginkgo biloba.

If you want to try this herb, 1 to 2 grams a day of the ginseng root, or 200 to 400 mg of the standardized extract (supplied in capsules) is a good place to start, though some research indicates a higher dose might be better. A recent study at the Mayo Clinic found that taking 1,000 to 2,000 mg a day of the herb can give you an all-day energy boost.

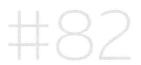

Rhodiola—for Fighting Depression and Fatigue

Rhodiola is another herb with a pretty strong resume of published research documenting its ability to fight fatigue, improve reaction time, improve attention, and reduce stress. It's a plant (also known as golden root and roseroot) that grows in cold and mountainous places, including the Arctic, the Central Asian and Rocky Mountains, the Alps, the Pyrenees, Scandinavia, Iceland, and other regions. In fact, in Russia it has been used for hundreds of years specifically to help cope with the harsh Siberian climate, and it is said to have been used by the Vikings as well.

Rhodiola is a valuable adaptagen. In one study, published in the *International Journal of Sport Nutrition and Exercise Metabolism*, rhodiola improved endurance exercise capacity. In another study, published in the *Nordic Journal of Psychiatry*, Armenian researchers found that patients from eighteen to seventy years of age with mild to moderate depression improved significantly on measures of overall depression, insomnia, and emotional instability following doses of either 340 mg a day or 680 mg a day.

Other studies have shown pronounced anti-fatigue effects for the supplement. One particularly well-known study (from the Department of Neurology at Yerevan State Medical University in Armenia) investigated the effect of low-dose treatment with rhodiola on fatigue in young, healthy physicians working night duty. One group received a placebo and one group was given a standardized extract of rhodiola. The researchers wanted to see whether rhodiola supplementation would have any effect on total mental performance, so they used a measure calculated as the Fatigue Index,

consisting of five different standardized tests for perception and cognitive function (such as short-term memory and ability to concentrate). Sure enough, they found a statistically significant improvement in the Fatigue Index for the rhodiola group, with no improvement shown in the group given the placebo. The Fatigue Index was also significantly improved in a group of 161 healthy cadets ages nineteen to twenty-one after a single dose of rhodiola was administered.

Want more? A 2000 double-blind, placebo-controlled, randomized study—considered the gold standard in research designs—investigated the effect of rhodiola supplementation on forty foreign students during a stressful exam period. Russian researchers divided the students into two groups, and gave one group rhodiola and the other a placebo. The rhodiola group demonstrated significantly improved scores in physical fitness and mental fatigue. The rhodiola group also had significantly higher scores in a self-assessment of general well-being.

Rhodiola has low toxicity and extremely low occurrences of side effects. According to the *Physicians Desk Reference for Herbal Medicines*, most users find that it improves their mood, energy, and mental clarity. For that reason, you shouldn't take it at night, because it can easily disrupt sleep.

If you want to try this herb, a good place to start is with 50 to 200 mg a day. And remember not to take it at night.

--------- **WORTH KNOWING** ---------

Because rhodiola does have an antidepressant effect, people with bipolar disorder shouldn't use it. Like many other antidepressants, natural or pharmaceutical, rhodiola has the potential for inducing mania in people with bipolar disorder.

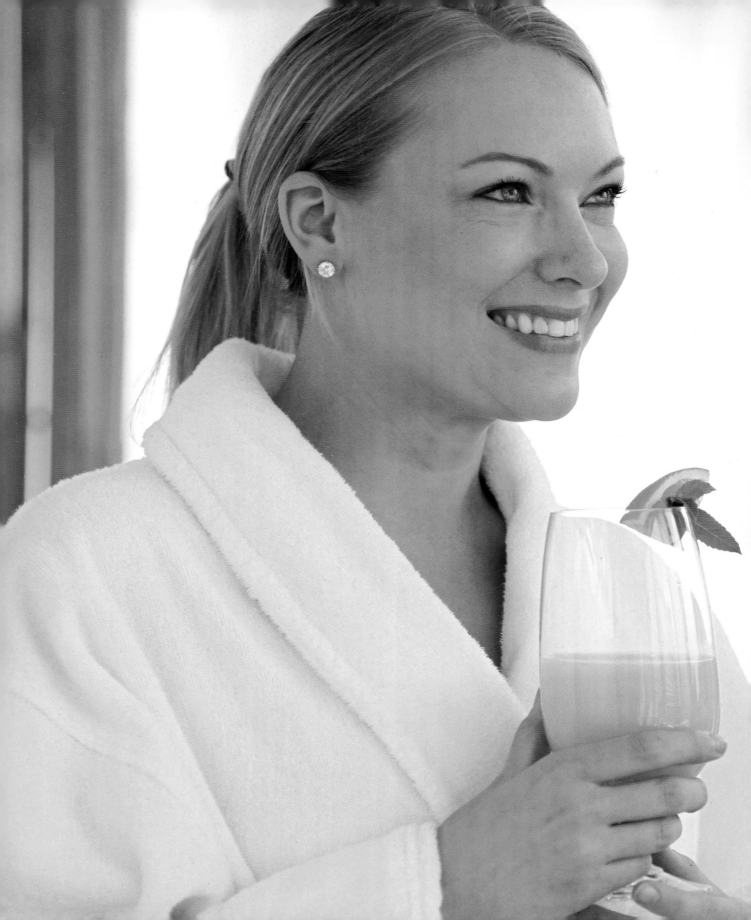

5 Detox from Energy Sappers

The term detoxification has been around forever, but it remains, in my opinion, one of the most misunderstood and misused terms in nutrition. It's been used to describe a staggeringly wide range of procedures, from total fasting to spiritual retreats to highly sophisticated nutritional regimens for the removal of specific toxins.

So to understand how best to do a detoxifying cleanse we first have to figure out what we're specifically trying to accomplish—exactly which toxins we're trying to cleanse the body of—and why. Then we can determine the best way to do it.

For our purposes, we're going to use detoxing as a means to an end, the end being a boost in our energy level. It's like rebooting a sluggish computer (or more accurately, like emptying the trash that's taking up a huge amount of memory).

TAKE OUT THE TRASH

There's no doubt in my mind that giving your body a rest is a good thing from an energy point of view. It takes a lot of energy to process bad food, not to mention the effect that food has on hormones, neurotransmitters, blood sugar, and all the other energy controllers in your body.

A low level of exposure to chemicals and toxins, whether they come from the outside environment, from inside the home, or from products you use on a daily basis—all of which I address in this chapter—may sap energy in small insidious ways that you don't notice at first, but which cumulatively add up, preventing you from being your energetic best.

My advice: Get rid of them.

OVERPRICED AND UNNECESSARY "SOLUTIONS"

Walk into any health food store and you're likely to find an entire shelf full of products specifically aimed at the person who wants to do a detox. You'll see teas, vitamin supplements, laxatives masquerading as cleanses, kits, instruction books, and even "medical foods" all meant to help you perform a cleanse.

So let's get one thing out of the way right off the bat: You don't need any of them. I think you can get the same benefits—maybe more—by using some of the detox techniques found right in this chapter.

I think detoxing can be done without spending any money on special cleansing kits or products, and that you can do just as good a job with a low-tech approach. (Don't get me wrong—such products may *help*, especially the fiber products, but they're not *necessary*, and many are just overpriced laxatives.)

JUMP-START YOUR ENERGY THROUGH DETOX

I think detoxification is a great idea, but I won't lie to you: The term itself is highly controversial. On one side there are those who claim we can't even measure or identify all the toxic chemicals in our environment or our bodies, so how do we even know we're getting rid of them?

Tests on blood, hair, and urine don't even exist for half the stuff we're exposed to on a regular basis, and even when they do, measuring levels after a detox have shown disappointing results. (My friend Mehmet Oz, M.D., once put a group of women in a house and fed half of them their "regular" fast food diet while the other half ate smoothies and vegetables. At the end of the week there was no measurable difference in their blood tests.)

On the other hand, there are those who claim that such tests aren't the best way to measure the kinds of changes that can begin to take place in the body when you go on a detox. In any case, a week may not be enough to show what's happening. The idea that changing your diet from all fast food to all fruits and vegetables accomplishes nothing just doesn't pass the "smell" test. If nothing else, a week or two of "clean" food, clean air, clean water, and a reduction of exposure to outside chemicals can be invigorating and can give the digestive system and the liver a much needed rest from its usual overload—ask anyone who's been to a spa!

A GENTLE AND EASY WAY TO START

The tips in this section all address ways that you can begin to eliminate energy-draining toxins either from food or from your environment. You can try a gentle program such as Elson Haas's SNACC program (see page 146), a more rigorous one like the Master Cleanse, or even a program of your own devising that's somewhere in the middle. And why not clean up your environment at the same time, eliminating even more possible causes of fatigue and low energy?

Remember, most energy drains are like a slow leak in your tire. The cause isn't always immediate and obvious, but the result is the same; it just takes longer to manifest. By lightening the body's load, you'll be giving your digestive system and your liver a much needed break, and your energy will get a much needed boost at the same time.

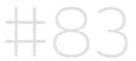

Eliminate Fatigue with Dr. Haas's Detox Program

Maybe you think of detox as a time-out for badly behaving celebrities. A retreat from the public, a $1,000-a-day haven where they can work on their addictions and their image. Often, it is.

But this isn't about celebrities and their addictions; it's about *you*. Specifically, it's about how you can cleanse your body and mind of the toxic agents that drain your energy one drip at a time.

It starts with your diet. Proponents claim a detox fast can speed along the elimination of toxins; give your digestive system a rest; make you look better, feel better, and sleep better; improve your mood; and leave you energized.

"Detoxification is the missing link in Western nutrition," says my friend, Elson Haas, M.D., the Detox Doc, and author of *The New Detox Diet* (www.elsonhaas.com). Haas has run detox programs as part of his medical practice for more than thirty years.

"Fasting is the single greatest natural healing therapy I know, and when applied to the right people, it helps reduce many problems and helps with greater energy and vitality," he told me

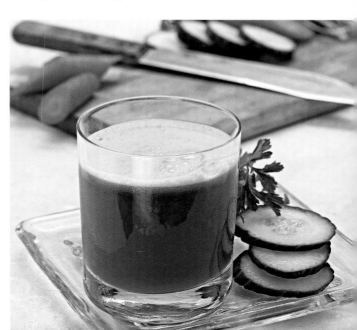

recently. "People need to take a break from their substances (SNACCs—sugar, nicotine, alcohol, caffeine, and chemicals). A detox fast can give the body a rest so it can rebalance."

By fast he doesn't mean a diet of water. "A more common and liberal definition of fasting would include the juices of fresh fruit and vegetables as well as herbal teas," Haas explained. "Fresh juices are easily assimilated, require minimum digestion, and still supply many nutrients. They also stimulate our body to clear wastes. Juice fasting is safer than water fasting since it supports the body nutritionally while cleansing and maintains your energy level."

THE BASIC FORMULA: THE SNACC PROGRAM

Haas starts all his patients on what he calls the SNACC program—simply eliminating sugar, nicotine, alcohol, caffeine, and chemicals. (Most people can get a huge benefit from just this stage, even if they don't go on to the next.) He then puts them on a simple, clean daily diet consisting of one piece of fruit, one bowl of cooked whole grains (millet, brown rice, amaranth, quinoa, or oatmeal), and two to four heaping bowls of steamed vegetables throughout the day. "For any who feel fatigued, or feel they just need protein, 3 to 4 ounces of fish, poultry, or beans can be added," he told me. Typically, people stay on this program for a week or even two, and then slowly begin to add back more of their typical daily foods.

But there are cautions as well. Naturopathic physician Sonja Pettersen, N.M.D., told me that people who have been exposed to extremely toxic chemicals (agent orange or chemotherapy, for example) should never go on a stringent detox without supervision. "Those toxins are stored in your fat," she explained, "and you don't want someone releasing all that stuff without supervision."

Detoxification, whether defined as an absence of the "bad stuff" (sugar, chemicals, nicotine); a mild restriction of your normal daily calories; a few days or a week of vegetables, juices, and fruit smoothies; or a complete juice fast, can be beneficial for many people. But it can be difficult. Best advice: If you want to give it a try, start with a one- or two-day fast and work up to a longer period. Excellent menu plans, as well as smoothie recipes and suggestions for beginning and ending the program, can be found in Haas's book, *The New Detox Diet*.

Here's a basic program, courtesy of Haas.

DETOX DETAILS

One week before fasting, eliminate:
    Sugar
    Nicotine
    Alcohol
    Caffeine

One or two days before fasting, eliminate:
    Red meats
    Milk products
    Eggs
    Wheat and baked goods

DR. ELSON HAAS'S DETOX SAMPLE MENU PLAN

Upon Rising
Drink two glasses of filtered water, one glass with half a lemon squeezed into it.

Breakfast
Eat one piece of fresh fruit (at room temperature), such as an apple, a pear, a banana, a citrus fruit, or some grapes. Chew well.

Fifteen to Thirty Minutes Later

Consume one bowl of cooked whole grains—millet, brown rice, amaranth, or quinoa. You can try oatmeal, but note that it contains gluten for those who are glutensensitive. For sweetness, use 2 tablespoons of fruit juice. For more savory flavoring, add 1 tablespoon (14 g) of Better Butter (see below) and a little sea salt or tamari.

Lunch

Eat one or two medium bowls of steamed vegetables (save the water). Use a variety, including roots, stems, and greens. For example, use potatoes or yams, green beans, broccoli or cauliflower, carrots or beets, asparagus, kale or chard, and cabbage. Flavor with 1 to 2 teaspoons (5 to 9 g) of Better Butter.

Dinner

Eat the same as you did for lunch. If you feel fatigued or as though you need protein, add 3 to 4 ounces (85 to 115 g) of fish, poultry, or beans to this meal (or have the protein between lunch and dinner).

Special Drinks (late morning to mid-afternoon)

Drink the water collected from steaming vegetables. Add a bit of garlic salt or veggie salt.

Better Butter Recipe

Makes 32 servings

1 cup (240 ml) extra-virgin olive oil (preferably organic)
1 cup (2 sticks, 225 g) organic butter

In a glass bowl, combine the olive oil and butter until well mixed. Cover and store in the refrigerator for up to two weeks.

From The New Detox Diet *by Elson M. Haas, M.D. Reprinted with permission.*

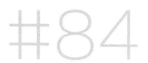

#84

Try the Master Cleanse

It's impossible to talk to people who have done the "Master Cleanse" without hearing them talk about the effect it had on their energy.

So what is the Master Cleanse, anyway? It's a controversial program that was first developed in the 1970s by a man named Stanley Burroughs, whose only claim to eternal fame is that he published a little booklet about it—*The Master Cleanser*—that is still sold in health food stores everywhere.

Although many conservative dietitians dismiss the Master Cleanse as hogwash, the fact is that it's been used for decades with great results by many people, including some that I have great respect and regard for, including Elson Haas, M.D. Don't let its periodic appearance in celebrity magazines as the "secret" behind some star's weight loss and newfound energy blind you to its value for some people some times. I'm including it in this book, not because I recommend it for everyone, but because so many people swear by it that I thought you should at least know what it is and how to do it, should you want to try it.

GROUND ZERO FOR THE MASTER CLEANSE

One of the best-known proponents of the Master Cleanse is a man named Peter Glickman, who has devoted his life to teaching people how to incorporate the Master Cleanse into their lives as part of a program of healing and renewal. When I interviewed him for this book, he explained how he developed this passion.

"Around 2002, food had become my enemy," he explained. "I was feeling exhausted. I had no energy. My wife had gotten into the whole raw vegan diet thing, and for two months I watched as she got skinnier and healthier. Her eyes sparkled. Meanwhile, I just felt more tired. Finally, I decided to give raw vegan eating a try for six months."

Glickman lost 42 pounds. Not surprisingly, his energy went through the roof. When I asked him what prompted him to try the Master Cleanse, he was refreshingly frank. "I just woke up one morning and felt like I needed a cleanse." He's been a convert—and a proponent—ever since.

RECIPE FOR REVIVING ENERGY

Many people use the Master Cleanse as an energy tonic, and more than a few have used it for weight loss, though like all juice fasts, that shouldn't be the main reason you do it. The Master Cleanse, also known as the Lemonade Diet, is basically a fast in which you take in nothing but the following drink all day long, as wanted, for a period of time ranging from one to ten days.

Here's the recipe for a single serving:

2 tablespoons (30 ml) organic lemon juice (about ½ lemon)

2 tablespoons (40 g) organic Grade B maple syrup (not the commercial kind used on pancakes)

¹/₁₀ teaspoon cayenne pepper

8 to 10 ounces (235 to 285 ml) filtered water, boiled or heated to the temperature at which you'd make a cup of tea

Combine all the ingredients in a glass and drink.

There's some good tradition behind the ingredients in the drink. Lemon juice and hot water is a drink of choice for singers, and in Indian (Ayruvedic) and traditional Chinese medicine, lemon is thought to cause the liver to excrete more bile. Because bile

salts are one of the ways that the body detoxifies itself, prompting the secretion of bile is thought to be a good thing. Lemon is also a diuretic, and it contains a number of antioxidants to boot. (My friend, Ann Louise Gittleman, Ph.D., has used the hot water and lemon drink as a component of her very popular "fat flush diet" for years.) The cayenne pepper is thought to stimulate metabolism. And Grade B maple syrup is less filtered and processed than the more common Grade A, and therefore believed to contain more minerals and enzymes than the latter.

Whether you can go for a day—or ten—on just that drink is a personal matter. Since the Master Cleanse is really just a slight variation on a water fast (with lemon and maple syrup adding a few nutrients), it's possible you might not feel really perky during the first day or so as your body starts dumping whatever it's holding on to in the fat cells. That said, I'd be lying if I told you that it doesn't work for certain folks. After just a few days on the program, some people report that they feel more energetic than they have in years. Also, some people find that even drinking it throughout the morning and afternoon and then having one small, "clean" meal in the late afternoon or early evening (not technically a Master Cleanse, since on the Master Cleanse the drink would be all you'd have) can still produce some energy benefits. But this is one detox program where I'd truly recommend checking with a health professional familiar with detoxification diets before starting it. There may be other ways to get the same result that aren't as challenging.

If you want to find out more, check out Glickman's video introduction to the program on his website, www.therawfoodsite.com/master-cleanse.htm. It's probably the best resource for all things Master Cleanse.

Fasting Through the Ages for Energy, Penance, and Clarity

Fasting as a strategy for enhancing health and attaining spiritual enlightenment has been around since the beginning of recorded history. The Greek philosophers Plato and Socrates were said to have fasted for mental clarity and physical discipline. Hippocrates appreciated the therapeutic benefits of fasting.

Throughout both the Old and the New Testaments there are stories of people fasting, including the forty days and forty nights that Christ was said to have abstained from food. It has been used (and is still being used) by many religious sects—including Christians, Jews, Muslims, and Buddhists—as penance or for purification. Fasting has been a tool of political prisoners and disciples of civil disobedience. From Mohandas Gandhi to guests at high-end spas, from religious awakening to simple rejuvenation, fasting has served many people and purposes throughout the ages.

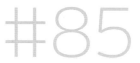

Energize by Brushing and Bathing Away Toxins

I first heard about dry skin brushing from my friend Ann Louise Gittleman, Ph.D., who highly recommends the practice as part of her famous "fat flush" program. I've since become a convert.

Think about it. The skin is the body's largest organ, eliminating about a pound of waste a day through the pores. If you're trying to rid your body of energy-depleting substances, helping the skin perform its natural functions makes a lot of sense. Detox experts believe dry skin brushing stimulates the lymphatic system, helping to promote the body's natural detoxification process.

If you want to give this a try, use a natural-bristle brush—soft, but stiff enough to cause some friction—with a long handle for those hard-to-reach parts of the body. Before you begin, make sure the room is warm and you have plenty of towels and a comfortable place to sit. (Note: It's a good idea to make sure you won't be disturbed so you can do this quietly without interruption.)

Using firm, rhythmic strokes, brush the sole of your right foot, then move to the top of your foot and ankle. Brush your shin and calf, then your knee to the top of your thigh, covering the area several times. Next, brush your buttocks. Always brush in an upward direction, and cover the whole surface. Repeat on the left side of your body, again starting with the sole.

The skin is the body's largest organ, eliminating about a pound of waste a day through the pores.

Brush your back from the waist to the shoulders and neck, covering the whole surface several times. Now brush your right arm. Begin with the palm of your hand, then the back of your hand, and brush from your wrist to your elbow in an upward direction. Make sure you brush your entire forearm. Next, brush from your elbow to your shoulder, in upward strokes, covering the surface of your upper arm. Repeat the procedure on your left arm.

Lightly brush your abdomen in a circular, counterclockwise motion, to follow the flow of your intestines. Brush lightly around and over your breasts, avoiding your nipples. Because the skin on your neck is very sensitive, either avoid brushing it or brush very lightly.

Either with a softer brush or a dry flannel, carefully brush your face. Take a warm shower or bath. You may want to end with contrast showers—3 minutes of warm water, followed by 1 minute of cold water. You can repeat the cycle, but be sure to end with the cold rinse.

----------- **WORTH KNOWING** -----------

You can accelerate the detoxification process by soaking away toxins in an Epsom salts bath, which many people find both relaxing and energizing. Epsom salts are nothing more than magnesium sulfate, and magnesium is one of the most relaxing nutrients on the planet. It's absorbed into the skin and may help flush toxins and heavy metals from the body.

Make sure your tub is very clean before filling it with the hottest water you can stand. Add 2 cups (96 g) of Epsom salts (you can build up to 4 cups, or 195 g) and soak for at least 15 minutes (or as long as half an hour). Then take a shower and dry off with a clean towel.

Dry skin brushing is a great accompaniment to your Far infrared sauna experience (see below). Try brushing before or after your sauna—it's a totally energizing experience that will relax and invigorate you at the same time.

#86

Banish Toxins and Boost Energy with an Infrared Sauna

One of my best friends in the world is the renowned nutritionist and antiaging expert Oz Garcia, Ph.D., who I've been pals and colleagues with since 1990, when we were both on staff at Equinox Fitness Clubs in New York City. I think he's one of the brightest people on the planet, and when he recommends something, I listen. He tends to be right an awful lot of the time.

It was Oz who first told me about the energy enhancement benefits, which he calls no less than miraculous, of infrared saunas. "They're one of the most healing, beneficial treatments I know for energy, detoxification, and vitality," he told me.

That we're exposed to a veritable cornucopia of toxic chemicals on a daily basis is a given. Less clear is their direct relationship to our daily life and energy level. Personally, I think the relationship is huge. Here's why: If your body uses its resources to defend itself against toxins, pollutants, medications, carcinogens, pesticides, and other chemical riffraff, then it's using up valuable energy and draining at least some of your vitality. Who wouldn't be tired from the sheer effort?

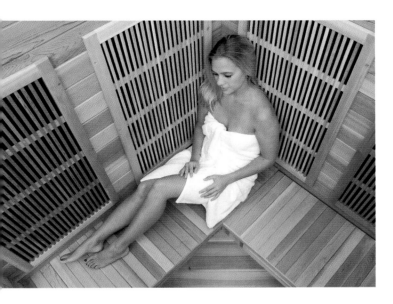

Establishment voices will scoff that these environmental toxins aren't harmful in small doses, that our bodies are perfectly able to get rid of them naturally, and that many of them haven't been "proven" to be harmful in the first place. These same folks will then reassure us that, in any case, the government keeps its eyes on this stuff anyway, so what's to worry about?

Well, if you believe that, I've got this lovely bridge you might be interested in buying . . . .

The truth is that no one knows the end effect of being exposed to the almost 80,000 chemicals that are now in the atmosphere, environment, and food supply; no one knows the "safe" dosage of many of them; and no one knows for sure how such constant exposure can ultimately affect our health and energy, especially given that, for many of us, our immune systems and detoxification pathways aren't performing optimally to begin with. I'd prefer to err on the side of caution, and do everything I can to support my body in getting rid of what shouldn't have been there in the first place.

Infrared saunas can help.

THIS ISN'T YOUR FATHER'S SAUNA

Now don't misunderstand me. There's a world of difference between the sauna in your gym and the infrared sauna I'm talking about here. Infrared radiation is electromagnetic radiation of a wavelength longer than that of visible light, but shorter than that of radio waves. This radiating energy penetrates the body and heats it directly and more efficiently. Because of the longer wavelength of far infrared, the skin is penetrated more deeply than with conventional saunas. The body slowly warms up while preserving vital electrolytes such as sodium, chloride, potassium, and magnesium.

"Since the heat is generated in the skin layers below the surface, the slow gentle warming is completely different, and invokes different physiological processes to get rid of the heat other than the evaporation of sweat from the skin's surface", Lewis Meltz, D.C., an expert in infrared saunas, told me. (A regular old garden-variety sauna simply works by placing very hot coals in a room and generating extremely hot air, which simply makes you sweat.)

"Infrared saunas are one of the most healing, beneficial treatments I know for energy, detoxification, and vitality."

—Oz Garcia, Ph.D., nutritional counselor and antiaging expert

"You need to think of the effects of far infrared photons of light like a process similar to the photosynthesis process in plants," Meltz explained. "Far infrared rays are converted by the body into electrochemical impulses and sent to the pineal and pituitary glands, which in turn produce healthy hormones that are sent through the central nervous system to all the cells of your body. Thus, light is essential to the functioning of our entire endocrine system."

Because photosynthesis is the process by which plants get their energy from the sun and convert it into the energy they need to live, the parallel is a good one. Far infrared rays help fine-tune our systems so that we can make our body's natural energy-producing mechanisms work at optimal efficiency.

Meltz shared with me the *Mayo Clinic Proceedings of 1999,* which report how superficial heat—or the inherent production of infrared energy—is naturally associated with a wide variety of healing responses. "As our ancestors knew instinctively," he told me, "there are times when the body needs a boost of infrared radiant heat energy to ensure optimum tissue repair and healing." Because our bodies are in a constant cycle of breakdown and repair (also known as "healing"), anything that contributes to or accelerates the latter is going to increase our energy.

Plus, let's be honest, it feels great. And anything that feels that good reduces stress, which increases energy. As my grandmother used to say, "What could be bad?"

WHERE TO SEEK THE HEAT

Of all the infrared saunas I've looked into, I'm most impressed with the home saunas made by Life Saunas International. They have some really cool features, such as incorporating color (which they call "chromo-therapy") to invoke the many different emotional and psychological benefits that color can provide.

These infrared saunas also have an oxygen ionizer to reduce free-radical damage and encourage that feeling of well-being that comes from negative ions (such as the ones near a waterfall, or that you experience right after a rainfall, when everything feels so peaceful and energizing).

I think some time in an infrared sauna such as the LifeFIT system makes a lot of sense as part of a detox program and as well as an overall program for increasing energy and general well-being. I've arranged for a link on my website (www.jonnybowden.com under "Shopping") that which goes directly to Life Saunas International, where you can read more about their home units. They're surprisingly affordable and will make a huge difference in your energy.

#87

Clean Up Your Air

What you don't see can affect your energy.

And that's especially true when it's in the air you breathe.

Here's the deal: Where there's smoke, there's combustion pollutants. And they can be—and frequently are—hidden energy drainers. That includes Uncle Harry's cigar, the cozy wood-burning stove, unvented kerosene and gas space heaters, and gas stoves.

Combustion gases and particles also come from tobacco smoke, chimneys and flues that are improperly installed or maintained, and cracked furnace heat exchangers. Pollutants from fireplaces and woodstoves with no dedicated outdoor air supply can be back-drafted from the chimney into the living space, particularly in weatherized homes. The major pollutants released are carbon monoxide, nitrogen dioxide, and particles. None is good for your energy or your overall health.

Some of the symptoms that even low concentrations of carbon monoxide (CO_2) can cause include headaches, dizziness, weakness, nausea, and fatigue, and that's just in healthy people. In people with chronic heart disease, it's even worse. And it's particularly insidious because you may experience these energy-draining symptoms without having any idea what's causing them. The symptoms of carbon monoxide poisoning, for example, are often confused with the flu or even with food poisoning. CO_2 is fatal at very high concentrations, so it makes sense that it's energy-draining at lower concentrations.

If you want your energy to be at its best all the time, you need to have clean food, clean water, sunlight, healthy relationships, and, yup, clean air. Don't overlook this important component of health and vitality.

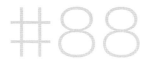

Engage in Biological Warfare and Detox Your Home

The biological contaminants in your home have a lot more to do with energy than you might think. Read on.

Biological contaminants range from the nearly invisible—dust mites—to the hard to ignore—your Great Dane. All of them can affect your energy in slow and subtle ways.

Get rid of them.

In addition to dust mites and animal dander, other biological contaminants include bacteria, mold, mildew, and viruses. After repeated exposure, some biological contaminants trigger allergic reactions that can affect the lungs, throat, nose, and eyes. These contaminants can (and do) also trigger some types of asthma. Infectious illnesses, such as influenza, measles, and chicken pox are transmitted through the air. Molds and mildews release disease-causing toxins. Other symptoms caused by biological pollutants include sneezing, watery eyes, coughing, shortness of breath, dizziness, lethargy, fever, and digestive problems.

Beginning to see the connection?

TAKE THESE STEPS TO BAN THE BIOLOGICALS

- Keep the humidity level below 50 percent (the humidity has to be at least 60 percent for mold to grow).
- Install and use fans vented to outdoors in kitchens and bathrooms, which can also reduce levels of organic pollutants that vaporize from hot water used in showers and dishwashers.

- Vent clothes dryers to the outdoors.

- To help prevent moisture buildup, ventilate the attic and crawl spaces.

- Clean cool mist and ultrasonic humidifiers in accordance with the manufacturer's instructions and refill with clean water daily. Be vigilant, because these machines can become breeding grounds for biological contaminants.

- Empty water trays in air conditioners, dehumidifiers, and refrigerators frequently.

- Thoroughly clean and dry (or remove) water-damaged carpets and building materials as soon as possible after damage. These can harbor mold and bacteria.

- Clean and disinfect the basement floor drain regularly. Before finishing a basement, patch all water leaks and be sure to have adequate heat and ventilation to prevent condensation. Keep the relative humidity levels between 30 and 50 percent (if necessary, use a dehumidifier).

- Keep the house clean to help reduce the amount of animal dander, pollen, dust mites, and other allergy-causing contaminants. If you suffer from allergies, use allergen-proof mattress encasements, wash bedding in hot (130°F or 54°C) water (to kill dust mites), and avoid dust-collecting furniture and knick-knacks, especially those that can't be washed in hot water. Because vacuuming can actually increase airborne levels of mite allergens and other biological contaminants, allergy sufferers should head outside while the house is being vacuumed. Using central vacuum systems that are vented to the outdoors or vacuums with high-efficiency filters may also help.

One grassroots organization that is working hard to help people—women especially—reduce everyday exposure to toxic chemicals in the home is Women's Voices for the Earth. You can find out more about toxins in cleaning and household products and what to do about them at the group's website, www.womenandenvironment.org.

HOME, TOXIC HOME

You probably think that keeping your home (and yourself) clean will help reduce toxins, right? To a certain extent that's true, the key term being "to a certain extent."

You scrub your toilet, scour the bathroom and kitchen tiles, clean the floors, polish the furniture, run the dishwasher, wash your clothes, shine your silver, spray some air freshener, pick up your dry cleaning, shampoo your hair, slather on body lotion, spritz some perfume, put on your makeup, and breathe easily. Not so fast.

If you aren't discriminating in the products you buy, every single task mentioned above introduces chemicals into your home and, in many cases, your body. They are called volatile organic compounds, or VOCs. (Organic in this case doesn't mean it came from Grandma's farm. Organic here means *carbon-based*, and because these substances exist as a vapor or gas, they are considered volatile.)

Many of these VOCs have short-term adverse effects, including eye, nose, and throat irritation; headaches; and fatigue. Long-term exposure can cause loss of coordination; nausea; and damage to the liver, kidneys, and central nervous system. Some organics can cause cancer in animals and are suspected of causing cancer in humans.

You may not be able to control the pollutants you are exposed to outside, but you can certainly limit the toxins in your immediate environment—your home. And you should: The

U.S. Environmental Protection Agency (EPA) has deemed indoor air pollution as one of the nation's top health concerns. That's because Americans spend about 90 percent of their time indoors and the air inside can be up to 100 times more contaminated than the air outside. In fact, according to a five-year study carried out by the EPA, peak concentrations of twenty toxic compounds, some linked to cancer and birth defects, were 200 to 500 times higher inside homes than outdoors.

In addition to VOCs, your home might contain combustion pollutants and biological pollutants. The best way to deal with these toxic intruders is to go to the source and eliminate or prevent* them, or bring the outdoors in, and ventilate.

MY CHEMICAL ROMANCE

Due to the chemicals in our homes and the products we put on our bodies, we have a veritable alphabet soup of chemicals brewing in our systems, such as PFCs, PBDEs, BPAs, and so on. (Don't even ask what those initials stand for; it's scarier than you can imagine.) Some of these chemicals are so ubiquitous that virtually all of us have them in our bloodstreams, according to the U.S. Centers for Disease Control and Prevention (CDC). That certainly can't be good for our health, much less our energy levels!

For instance, researchers measured levels of twelve different *perfluorochemicals* (PFCs)—a broad class of manufactured chemicals—in the blood of more than 3,600 subjects. They found three types of PFCs in an almost unbelievable

When I spent some time in Japan a few years ago, I was struck by the loveliness of their custom of leaving your shoes outside when you enter a home. I thought it the height of civility and assumed it was "just" a tradition, only learning later that the custom started because the Japanese are way more cognizant of the level of pollution and toxicity found on the bottoms of our shoes than Americans are.

98 percent of people tested. That's 3,528 out of 3,600 people walking around with a chemical soup inside them that shouldn't even be in their environment, let alone in their bloodstreams!

BLINDED BY SCIENCE

Where do these lovely chemicals come from? Everywhere. The culprits include a wide range of products, such as, but not limited to, stain-resistant carpets and fabrics, nonstick cookware, and some nail polishes, all of which have been known to contain PFCs. (PFCs are used in products to resist oil, stains, heat, water, and grease.)

The effect of these chemicals on humans is completely unknown, but animal studies aren't exactly reassuring. In animals, studies have shown that some PFCs can cause tumors, damage organs, and affect the reproductive system.

Then there are PBDEs (polybrominated diphenyl ethers—I told you not to ask). PBDEs are a whole other class of chemicals found in such things as flame retardants used in electronics, the back coatings of upholstery and drapes, and inside small appliances and other plastic or foam products. One particular type of PBDE, affectionately named BDE-47, was detected in the blood of almost all 2,040 folks tested by the CDC for the presence of this chemical.

Although animal studies have shown that high levels of PBDEs damage the thyroid and liver, researchers don't know the affect of the much lower levels found in humans. Maybe small amounts are safe. Maybe they aren't. Maybe they don't affect some people, but seriously affect others. The very theory of biochemical individuality (i.e., everybody's different) would seem to argue that at the very least there's likely to be a significant subset of the population for whom exposure to all this stuff is a real problem. (For the rest of us, it can't be good either.) Who really knows for sure?

A QUESTION OF SAFETY

Even if those small amounts are safe, that's just saying they won't kill us. Exposure certainly can't affect our health and our energy in a good way.

Based on its study that found bisphenol A (BPA) in 93 percent of the subjects tested, the CDC didn't have to go out on a limb to say that this indicated widespread exposure to BPA in the United States. That would fall under the category of "duh." BPA is used in polycarbonate plastics, which is everything from linings of food cans to plastic dinnerware and refillable beverage containers. In experiments where animals were given high doses of BPA, it had an estrogen-like effect on the uterus and prostate glands.

Once again, scientists don't know whether trace amounts could pose health risks to humans. The usual scientist pabulum—"more studies are needed"—seems like an inadequate way to deal with what is a big environmental and health concern for many people.

Researchers from the CDC also found *phthalates*—plasticizers used to soften plastic and vinyls and found in many shampoos, makeup, and lotions—in virtually every person tested. Ditto for chemical residue from pesticides. In fact, the average person had thirteen pesticides in his or her system.

Beginning to get the picture? What's polluting the environment is also polluting us, coursing through our own energy ecosystem.

TOXINS, TOXINS, WHO'S GOT THE TOXINS?

Even if it can't be proven in a court of law that a given toxin causes a disease, that doesn't mean it's a good thing for you to be exposed to. And that's for more reasons than you might think.

First, the damage from exposure to any given toxin in typical amounts may not be staggering, but it could be cumulative over time. Second, no one has studied the interaction of the thousands of chemicals, drugs, and other foreign compounds we're exposed to on a daily basis. Third, individuals vary so much biochemically that some of us just aren't that efficient at getting rid of toxins, so it's likely to affect some of us more than others.

This cumulative effect of the chemical potpourri we are exposed to is what clinical ecologists call the "body burden." Unfortunately, no one can tell us the effect of this burden. One thing's for sure—it can't be good. Regardless of what the tipping point is for disease and ill health, the less exposure you have to harsh chemicals, pollutants, and toxins, the better.

─────── **WORTH KNOWING** ───────

The Environmental Working Group (www.ewg.org) maintains a website that lists the ingredients of some 25,000 personal care products.

"Under federal law, companies can put virtually anything they wish into personal care products, and many of them do," says Jane Houlihan, vice president of research at EWG. "Mercury, lead, and placenta extract—all of these and many other hazardous materials are in products that millions of Americans, including children, use every day."

To find out what's in your products, log on to www.cosmeticsdatabase.com.

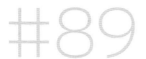

Clean Green and Breathe Easier

One of my favorite comic routines is an old bit by the great comedian Lenny Bruce. Bruce was making fun of a consumer how-to booklet given out to tourists in Florida, called *Do's and Don'ts for Swimmers in Shark-Infested Waters*.

"Okay, are you ready for the first 'Do'?" he asked the audience. "Get out of the water as soon as possible." Dramatic pause. Then, sarcastically, "Gee, doc, glad you thought of that!"

Well, at the risk of channeling my inner Lenny, the first "do" when it comes to removing energy-draining toxins from your environment is this: Don't put them there in the first place. That includes toxic cleaning products.

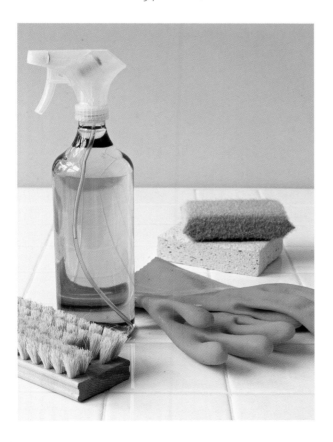

Remember, toxins can—and do—drain your energy. The body needs to devote a lot of resources to ridding itself of foreign invaders, and the diversion of those valuable resources can have a profound effect on your energy. Although building detoxification into your regular routine as part of an energy-saving regime is a great idea (see the rest of this section for ideas), preventing as many energy-draining toxins from contaminating your environment in the first place is even wiser.

THE GREEN REVOLUTION

There are many safe cleaning products on the market. Buy them. Look for products certified by Greenguard Environmental Institute (www.greenguard.org) or Green Seal (www.greenseal.org/findaproduct).

Read product labels (unfortunately, many of the products don't list their ingredients). But if there are warnings about usage (such as "eye irritant," "if swallowed, do not induce vomiting; call a physician," or "handle in a well-ventilated area"), then you can bet the ingredients are toxic. Do look for products that are petroleum-free, chlorine-free, ammonia-free, phosphate-free, alcohol-free, synthetic perfume- and dye-free, and fully biodegradable.

OUST THE ANTIBACTERIALS

And while you're at it, avoid antibacterial products. More and more soaps and cleaning products are antibacterial, which can be problematic for the following reasons:

1. These products kill good bacteria along with bad bacteria.

2. Many of them can irritate your skin.

3. Their use may help promote super-germs that are resistant to antibiotics.

4. Introducing antibacterial agents into the environment can upset the balance of good bacteria.

5. Most important, by eliminating any challenge to our own immune systems, we're making it a less powerful defender against all the things that can sap our energy. A little dirt can actually be a good thing, sometimes.

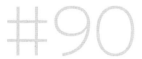

Fight Fatigue by Giving Your Liver Milk Thistle

You can help your liver do its job more effectively—and boost your energy in the bargain—by taking a daily dose of an herb called milk thistle.

I consider the liver the most misunderstood and underappreciated organ in the human body. It's the energy underdog, because when it's not working right, the first thing to suffer is your energy. (The most pronounced, immediate, and obvious symptom of hepatitis—a disease of the liver—is crushing fatigue.)

Unlike the heart, which gets sonnets composed in its honor, and the brain, which makes the cover of *Time*, or the skin, which has spawned a multibillion dollar industry devoted to keeping it young and smooth, the liver is the Rodney Dangerfield of the body—"It don't get no respect."

But it should.

The liver is the body's chemical refinery, processing center, storage facility, and waste treatment plant all rolled into one. Besides converting food into energy, it creates bile to aid in digestion and store glucose. In addition, it's a major detoxification center (see Neutralizing Energy Sappers on page 159).

A HEALTHY LIVER IS THE KEY TO MORE ENERGY

Giving the liver all the nutrients it needs to perform its daily tasks is one of the most important things you can do to boost your energy. In addition to all the terrific minerals, vitamins, and phytochemicals found in the plant kingdom (and in abundance in fresh vegetable juices), certain supplements can help.

At the top of the list is an herb called milk thistle. Milk thistle's active ingredient, silymarin, has been found to have a liver-protecting effect in a number of studies. Silymarin and its related

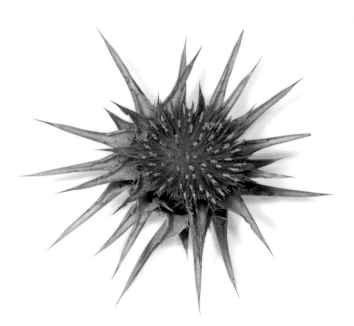

compounds seem to inhibit the entrance of toxins into the liver by somehow altering the outer membrane of the liver cells. Milk thistle is also a powerful anti-inflammatory and antioxidant.

I recommend a dose of between 400 and 900 mg a day (in divided doses), with the larger doses for those who suspect their energy has been compromised by toxins, including alcohol, acetaminophen (such as found in Tylenol), and other known liver toxins. (Make sure your milk thistle is "standardized" for 80 percent silymarin, the active ingredient. That means a 100 mg capsule of milk thistle delivers 80 mg of silymarin.) And for general energy maintenance, 200 to 400 mg of milk thistle (standardized to 80 percent silymarin) is a good idea.

Neutralizing Energy Sappers

The liver—and to a lesser degree, the lungs and skin—is responsible for neutralizing—or, in more popular terms, detoxifying—every chemical, pesticide, and medication that enters our bodies through any pathway (from the mouth to the skin to the hair), not to mention other intruders that we breathe, eat, drink, spray, and slather on our bodies.

If it's a toxin that doesn't belong in the body, it's the job of the liver to get rid of it. And most of those toxins can silently zap our energy. Some of these toxins are in and out of our system quickly, but others are persistent, lodging in fat cells, contributing to a feeling of malaise and, ultimately, a lack of energy.

When we have a good balance of nutrients and our system isn't overstressed, then the liver functions as a reliable waste treatment plant, excreting an arsenal of enzymes to transform fat-soluble toxins into water-soluble ones, and allowing them to be processed by the kidneys or bowels and then excreted.

If there aren't enough nutrients in the body to generate the enzymes or if the liver treatment plant is flooded with chemicals, then some of those toxins are stored in fat cells or transformed into *free radicals*. They then head back into the bloodstream, where they get recirculated and can damage the endocrine system, the nervous system, and the immune system. A great time is had by all.

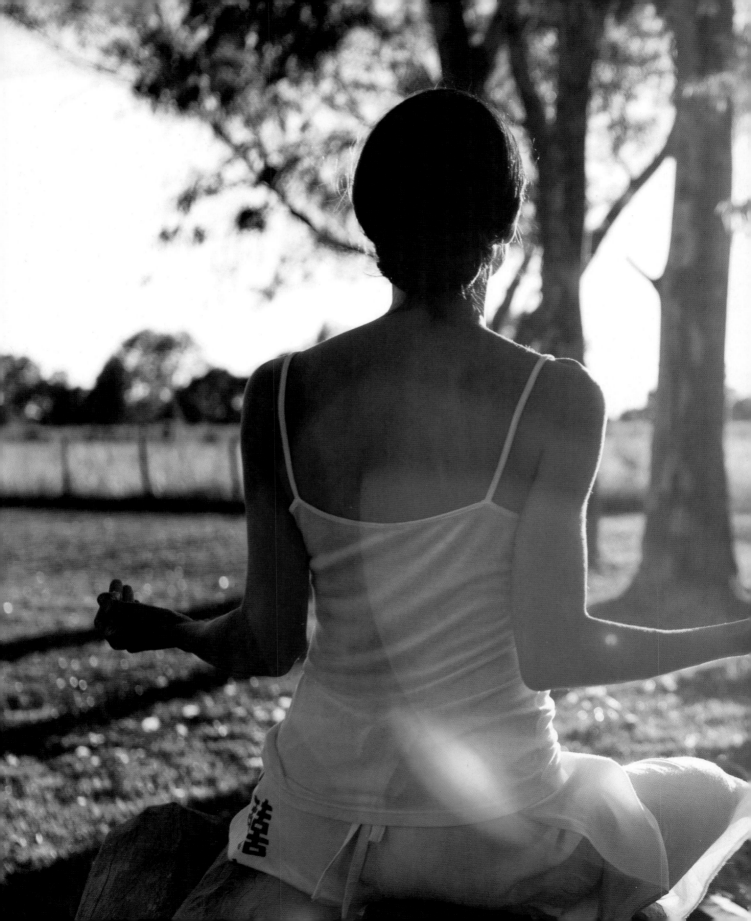

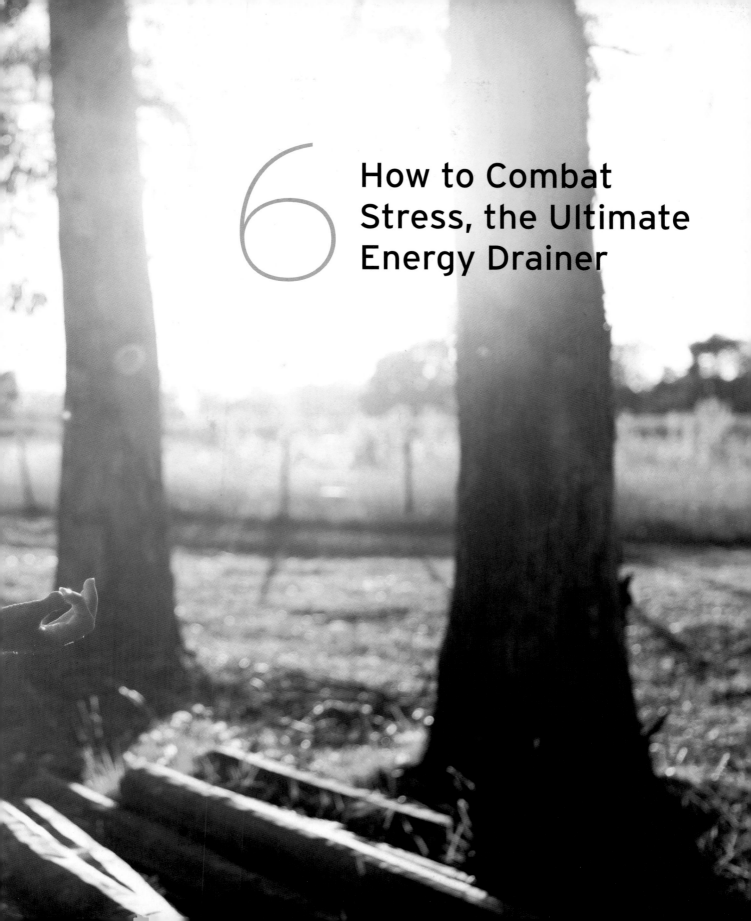

6
How to Combat Stress, the Ultimate Energy Drainer

Want a perfect recipe for sabotaging your energy reserves? No problem. Here it is in three easy steps:

Step 1: Get yourself some stress.

Step 2: Do everything you can to increase it.

Step 3: Do absolutely nothing to relieve it.

You'll be a walking zombie in no time. (Now if you feel like you're already on the way to the above-mentioned zombiehood, keep reading. There's a lot you can do to turn things around.)

Look, there's no two ways about it. Stress is a major energy killer. Maybe not in the short term—in fact, there are some people (we call them "adrenaline junkies") who seem to thrive on stress. But even the folks who eat stress for breakfast eventually wind up paying the price.

And that price almost always has to do with energy.

The term *stress* was actually coined by a Hungarian endocrinologist named Hans Selye back in 1936. Through a series of experiments and accidental discoveries involving some manhandled lab rodents (you don't want to know), he discovered the general adaptation syndrome, or GAS, which he called a universal response to stress. GAS comprises three stages. Stage one is alarm—it's when the zebra notices a lion about to charge and quickly figures out that it better run like the devil. (Hormones, including cortisol and adrenaline, kick in quickly to help him do this.)

Stage two is resistance. That's when we figure out that we better come up with a coping mechanism for any persistent stressor that won't go away (such as your boss or the traffic on the freeway).

Stage three is exhaustion. The body simply can't keep up with the long-term energetic demands of stress, and glands (such as the adrenals) or whole systems (including the immune system) become depleted and/or exhausted. Resources are used up as quickly as your savings account in a recession.

And your energy goes into the toilet.

Sound familiar?

REDUCE STRESS, GAIN ENERGY

I promised you there was hope, though, and there is. It's called stress reduction, and I consider it to be the unsung hero of just about every plan to regain health, maintain weight, and recapture (and increase) your energy. Why? Because stress has profound effects on all of these. High levels of stress hormones can shrink sections of the brain (such as the hippocampus), lower immunity, contribute to weight gain, and shorten your life. And high levels of stress hormones will eat your energy for breakfast.

The tips and suggestions in this section are some of the ways you can blow off some of that stress that, if left unattended, will build up like steam in a pressure cooker that has no escape valve. I can't emphasize how important these simple techniques are for increasing your energy (not to mention your lifespan!).

Most are really simple. Few cost any money. And all are effective.

Which should you do? Doesn't matter. Stress reduction is like exercise—the best techniques are the ones you actually use.

I'm not much for pat answers or slogans, but I'll make an exception here. When it comes to stress reduction—*just do it*!

#91

Breathe the Right Way for Better Energy

Right now, one of the hottest topics in nutrition and health is oxygen depletion. You can't have energy if you don't have enough oxygen, and you can't get enough oxygen if you don't breathe.

Breathe. Sounds simple. We all know how to do it, right? Well, maybe. Sure, we know how to breathe, but breathing the *right way*, well, that's a different matter.

As babies we did it naturally, inhaling from the stomach, pushing our little bellies way out, and then exhaling just as deeply, expelling as much "bad air" as we could.

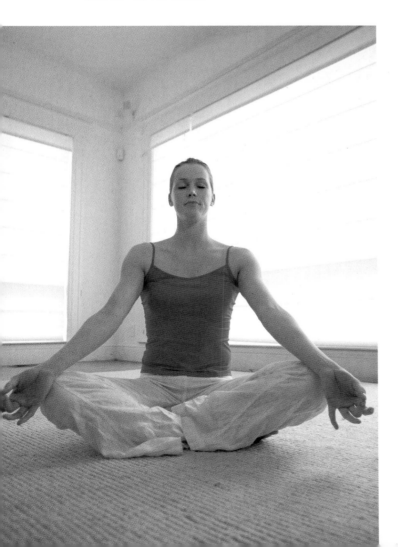

LET IT FLOW, LET IT FLOW, LET IT FLOW

Enter stress, anxiety, a harried lifestyle, and way too many hours hunched over the computer, and all of a sudden it's a different story. Your chest tightens—your whole upper body gets tense. To make breathing matters worse, we suck in our abs to look thinner, constricting our diaphragms and making it difficult to take slow, deep breaths—before you know it, we become *shallow breathers*. (I know, sounds like the premise of a *Seinfeld* episode. But it's no joke.)

When breathing emanates from the chest instead of deep down in the diaphragm, it restricts the amount of oxygen we inhale and the amount of carbon dioxide we exhale. Because oxygen is needed to fuel every cell and system in our body, over time fast, shallow breathing can lead to mental and physical fatigue and tension. The typical adult has a resting breathing rate of twelve to fifteen times per minute; the optimum rate is about six breaths per minute.

Inhaling through your nose and taking slow, deep breaths enables your lungs to fill with oxygen (as opposed to fast, shallow breathing, which fills only the top of the lungs with air), triggering the parasympathetic nervous system, which promotes relaxation (which in turn means less stress and way more energy).

We used to know how to do that naturally when we were babies. But then we grew up.

EXERCISES IN AWARENESS

Getting back to our natural breathing pattern starts, like a lot of things in this book, with awareness.

"Unlike any other function of the body, breathing can be entirely voluntary or entirely involuntary," says Andrew Weil, M.D. Because we have control over breathing, we can also influence such functions as heartbeat, circulation, digestion, and, yes, energy.

By doing a breathing check every few hours, and incorporating breathing exercises into your daily routine, you can slow your breathing rate and graduate from the ranks of shallow breathers to those of deep breathers.

For relaxation, try this deep breathing exercise:

Sit (or lie down) in a comfortable position, with your back straight and your body relaxed. With one hand on your abdomen and one hand on your chest, slowly inhale through your nose. Keep your abdomen relaxed as you feel it fully expand. Be sure to relax your face, mouth, tongue, and jaw. Hold your breath for 4 or 5 seconds, then purse your lips as though you were about to whistle, and slowly exhale through your mouth, retracting your abdomen completely. Concentrate on the air leaving your lungs. Pause, and then repeat this exercise four or five times.

Weil also suggests the following three exercises, any of which should have a huge effect on your energy levels.

EXERCISE 1: THE STIMULATING BREATH

The Stimulating Breath (also called Bellows Breath) is adapted from a yogic breathing technique. Its aim is to raise vital energy and increase alertness.

1. Sit with your back straight and place the tip of your tongue against the ridge of tissue behind your upper front teeth. Keep it there throughout the exercise. Inhale and exhale rapidly through your nose, keeping your mouth closed but relaxed.

Your breaths in and out should be equal in duration, but as short as possible. (Be forewarned: This is a noisy breathing exercise.)

2. Try for three in-and-out breath cycles per second. This produces a quick movement of the diaphragm, suggesting a bellows. You should feel muscular effort at the base of your neck above the collarbones and at the diaphragm. Breathe normally after each cycle.

3. Do not do this exercise for more than 15 seconds on your first try. Each time you practice the Stimulating Breath, you can increase your time by 5 seconds or so, until you reach a full minute.

If done properly, you should feel invigorated. According to Weil, it's a feeling comparable to the heightened awareness you feel after a good workout. Try this breathing exercise the next time you need an energy boost and feel yourself reaching for a cup of coffee.

EXERCISE 2: THE 4-7-8 (OR RELAXING BREATH) EXERCISE

This exercise is utterly simple, takes almost no time, requires no equipment, and can be done anywhere. Although you can do the exercise in any position, sit with your back straight while learning the exercise.

Place the tip of your tongue against the ridge of tissue just behind your upper front teeth, and keep it there throughout the entire exercise. You will exhale through your mouth around your tongue; try pursing your lips slightly if this seems awkward.

1. Exhale completely through your mouth, making a whoosh sound.

2. Close your mouth and inhale quietly through your nose to a mental count of four. Hold your breath for a count of seven.

3. Exhale completely through your mouth, making a whoosh sound to a count of eight.

4. This is one breath cycle. Now inhale again and repeat the cycle three more times for a total of four cycles.

Note that you always inhale quietly through your nose and exhale audibly through your mouth. The tip of your tongue stays in position the whole time. Exhalation takes twice as long as inhalation. The absolute time you spend on each phase is not important, but the ratio of 4:7:8 is important. If you have trouble holding your breath, speed up the exercise but keep to the ratio of 4:7:8 for the three phases. With practice, you can slow it all down and get used to inhaling and exhaling more and more deeply.

This exercise is a natural tranquilizer for the nervous system. Unlike tranquilizing drugs, which are often effective when you first take them but then lose their power over time, this exercise is subtle when you first try it but gains in power with repetition and practice. Do it at least twice a day. You cannot do it too frequently. Do not do more than four breaths at one time for the first month of practice. Later, if you wish, you can extend it to eight breaths. If you feel a little lightheaded when you first breathe this way, do not be concerned; it will pass. (If it doesn't, just discontinue the exercise. But it will.)

Once you develop this technique by practicing it every day, consider it a useful tool that you will always have with you. Use it immediately after anything upsetting happens—before you have time to react. Use it whenever you are aware of internal tension. Use it to help you fall asleep. I can't recommend this exercise highly enough—everyone can benefit from it.

EXERCISE 3: BREATH COUNTING

If you want to get a feel for this stress-relieving work, try breath counting, a deceptively simple technique used in Zen practice.

Sit in a comfortable position with your spine straight and your head inclined slightly forward. Gently close your eyes and take a few deep breaths. Then breathe naturally without trying to influence how you do it. Ideally, your breathing will be quiet and slow, but your depth and rhythm may vary.

1. To begin the exercise, count "one" to yourself as you exhale.

2. The next time you exhale, count "two," and so on, up to "five." Then begin a new cycle, counting "one" on the next exhalation.

3. Never count higher than "five," and count only when you exhale. You will know your attention has wandered when you find yourself up to "eight," "twelve," and even "nineteen."

4. Try to do 10 minutes of this form of meditation. For more information, visit www.drweil.com.

#92

Practice Qi Gong

Ever wonder why a cat grooms itself all day?

Well, clearly, it's not primping for a night out on the town. So there must be some other reason. And through some inventive research at Princeton University, we now understand exactly *why* cats like to groom. (I know, that question's never far from your mind.) Even if you're not a cat person, read on, because what I'm about to explain has some major implications for your well-being and energy.

Remember serotonin? It's one of your brain's "feel good" neurotransmitters. Because there are only about 200,000 serotonin neurons in your brain, and they have to service millions of cells, and because serotonin has a profound (although complicated and not completely understood) effect on well-being and mood, it's no wonder that as a society, we spend an awful lot of money to keep the serotonin flowing. In fact, there's a $130 billion industry (as of 2000) based on drugs that do just that (they're called selective serotonin reuptake inhibitors, or SSRIs).

Back to the cat.

Barry Jacobs, Ph.D., and his colleagues in the psychology labs at Princeton inserted electrodes into the brain stems of cats and then recorded what was happening over the course of each cat's day. Which was not much.

Until the cats started grooming themselves.

Once they started grooming, their serotonin activity increased fortyfold!

No wonder they do it all the time.

But here's the thing: What that (and other) research has taught us is that *concentrated, repetitive motion raises serotonin activity.* And that brings us to one of the best energy enhancers in the world—qi gong.

MIND-BODY ENERGY EXERCISE

Qi gong originated in China thousands of years ago. It's actually a family of mind-body exercises that share the following elements: regulation of the body, regulation of breathing, and regulation of the mind. If a practice doesn't include all three elements, and if all three don't occur simultaneously, then it's not a member of the qi gong family.

Three decades ago, Herbert Benson, M.D., the pioneering doctor who was among the first to introduce the concept of mind-body medicine to the United States, studied qi gong while he was researching what he termed "the relaxation response."* He concluded that to reach a state of deep relaxation all you have to do is control your body, breathing, and mind.

In qi gong, as in many meditative practices, you control your mind by simply concentrating on a single thought. It can be a word, a mantra, a sound, a letter. You regulate your breathing in some controlled way (such as breathing in for a slow count of four and breathing out for a slow count of four), and you add regular, specific movement to handle the body part of it. Those three components are the trifecta of increased serotonin activity (and with it, greater energy and well-being).

PRACTICE MAKES PERFECT (ENERGY)

At the University of Southern California, Irvine, Shin Lin, Ph.D., a visiting professor from Shanghai University, has been researching the measurable effects of qi gong and tai chi. Lin and his colleagues use an EEG to measure brain waves. They use an EKG to measure heart waves and the

*I wrote about the relaxation response in detail in my book The Most Effective Natural Cures on Earth.

sympathetic-parasympathetic nervous system balance. They measure blood pressure. They use a laser Doppler to measure peripheral blood flow. These guys are serious; they're performing rigorous, scientific investigation about what happens in the body and what happens to energy when you perform certain exercises.

And here's what they found: *significant, measurable, beneficial effects on the nervous system when subjects did qi gong and tai chi.*

We don't often think of energy as something you can measure, but Lin's lab is doing exactly that. Lin and his research associates don't stop with the EEG, the EKG, and the laser Doppler measurements, though. They also quantify the actual human energy field using infrared thermography to measure heat, counting photons to measure light, and measuring electrical fields with a highly complex system called gas discharge visualization.

What they've demonstrated is that when you practice certain movements, such as those in qi gong, your energy increases. You get enhanced blood flow, signaling more energetic activity. You actually raise all the markers for energy—heat, light, and gas. Your energy *objectively, measurably, and significantly* increases. Couple that with an increase in serotonin levels and you've got a great prescription for boosting your overall energy.

So why not just do regular exercise?

Well, actually, you should (see chapter 3). But the thing about tai chi and qi gong is that you get many of the blood-circulating effects of exercise without the increase in stress hormones that usually accompanies a strenuous workout. In Lin's lab, they have Bowflexes, stationary bikes, and weight training equipment. Although all these do great things, they also raise levels of cortisol (the stress hormone), and weight lifting actually temporarily constricts rather than dilates the blood vessels. Tai chi and qi gong are excellent complements to conventional Western exercise and allow you to reach a relaxed, calm state while at the same time increasing your energy.

Which means you've got one up on that grooming cat.

#93

Invigorate with Aromatherapy

I live in Los Angeles, which sometimes—okay, often—feels like a foreign country. But after closely observing the natives, one of the things I've learned is this: *Smells have energy.*

You can't walk into an upscale boutique or visit a spa without being struck by the wonderful, gentle aromas of carefully chosen oils that have the power to invigorate and energize you (just as they also have the power to calm and relax you). You can get the same effect yourself without the high price tag by channeling the energy-boosting power of aromatherapy.

When you practice certain movements, such as those in qi gong, your energy increases.

Aromatherapy is the practice of using essential oils distilled from the fragrant parts of different plants—flowers, bark, leaves, roots, or fruits—to promote physical and emotional health and well-being.

Essential oils are the highly concentrated essences of various flowers. And when I say highly concentrated, I'm not kidding. For example, you'd need 220 pounds (100 kg) of lavender flowers to make 1 pound (455 g) of essential oil! People who use aromatherapy to improve mood, well-being, and energy know that each type of essential oil has a different chemical structure, which in turn affects how it smells, how it's absorbed, and how it's used by the body. Because the oils are so concentrated, they're often diluted in water or vegetable oil. Some scents act as stimulants, others have a calming effect, and some can boost your energy through the roof.

THE POWER IS IN THE PATHWAYS

We don't know exactly how aromatherapy works, but one theory is that our smell receptors send chemical messages along nerve pathways to the brain's limbic system, which is ground zero for moods and emotions. (This is one reason why it's standard operating procedure to use potpourri and freshly baked cookies as "bait" when you're selling a house!)

Another slightly more granola-ish theory about why aromatherapy works suggests that because essential oils are extracted from plants, they have a life force that can affect the body in unique ways. Who knows? But you don't have to know exactly how it works to know that aromatherapy can boost your energy.*

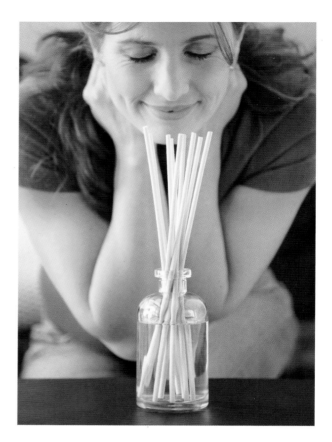

By measuring brain-wave activity, researchers have found that clove, basil, ylang-ylang, black pepper, and cinnamon oils act as stimulants. Other studies have shown peppermint, eucalyptus, jasmine, neroli, and rose oils are energizing, while lavender, chamomile, lemon, and sandalwood oils are relaxing.

Studies have also suggested that a little aromatherapy goes a long way toward making employees more alert and attentive. Workers in one Tokyo office building have a variety of aromas—lemon, rose, or cypress—wafting through their air-conditioning system. Another Japanese company fills the air with peppermint to fight fatigue.

If you doubt that smells can have a powerful effect on energy, just ask anyone who's ever passed out and then had smelling salts waved under his or her nose!

MIST, SPRITZ, OR DIFFUSE

There are several ways to reap the benefits of aromatherapy. With a few drops of essential oil, an aromatherapy diffuser will disperse a fine mist of scented steam throughout the room. (Diffusers range in price from $60 to $120.)

You can also add two or three drops of oil to a cold lightbulb ring (a ceramic or metal ring designed to be placed directly on lightbulbs) or to a handful of potpourri. Essential oil can turn a bath into an aromatherapy session (just add a drop or two).

For a great pick-me-up while housekeeping, add two to four drops of eucalyptus oil directly into the vacuum cleaner bag (you can also mix eucalyptus with lemon oil for a refreshing, clean smell). To make your own air freshener, add a few drops of oil to a spray bottle filled with water, then shake and spritz.

To add an air of energy to a room, try eucalyptus, peppermint, rosemary, jasmine, or cinnamon. For a calming effect—which helps reduce stress and thus ultimately boosts energy, though not in the short term—go for lavender, chamomile, sandalwood, or lemon (which also happens to be really refreshing). Because essential oils can elicit different responses in different people, experiment to find the scent that works best for you.

─────── **WORTH KNOWING** ───────

A word of caution: When working with undiluted essential oils, make sure you're in a well-ventilated room, and take frequent breaks. If the oil gets on your skin and irritates it, quickly dilute it with vegetable oil.

#94
Open the Door and Go Green!

Recently, I spent the weekend with my brother, Jeffrey, and his wife, Nancy, at their lakeside cabin in the mountains of Massachusetts. I arrived late Friday evening after four grueling days in Manhattan (if you've ever lived in New York, you'll know that's pretty much the norm).

The next morning, before anyone was up, I got into a kayak, paddled to the center of the lake, and stopped to catch my breath—not so much from the exercise, but from the spectacle of nature. Gazing at the gently rolling hills that framed the lake, watching the water sparkle as the sun climbed the sky, listening to a chorus of birds playing along with the water lapping against the kayak, I was transfixed. The stress I had carried with me from New York—an unsettled feeling of having to tie up loose ends and a looming deadline for this book—all seemed inconsequential.

I surveyed the pastoral scene, watched the hills turn from green to blue as the clouds rolled by, breathed in pine and fresh water and honeysuckle, and from my perspective, all was right with the world.

It struck me that at that moment there was no place on earth I would rather have been. That was the power of being totally in the present, and it was exhilarating. I paddled back to shore with my energy batteries fully recharged. It was so much like "therapy" that it got me wondering whether being outdoors has the same effect on other people.

STRESS REDUCTION AND FATIGUE RECOVERY

It turns out I wasn't the only one who wondered the same thing. A mental health organization in Britain called Mind recently coined the term *ecotherapy* to describe what it believes should be a frontline treatment modality for a number of mental health problems. In fact, research dating back to at least the 1980s demonstrates that exposure to the outdoors specifically can have a remarkable effect on variables ranging from depression to energy to concentration. The research is clear—green is golden.

One reason for the healing, energizing power of green is what's called the restorative effect. "There are actually two different restorative effects," said Stephen Kaplan, Ph.D., of the University of Michigan, and one of the leading researchers in the field. "One is the reduction of stress, which can be seen in measurably lower

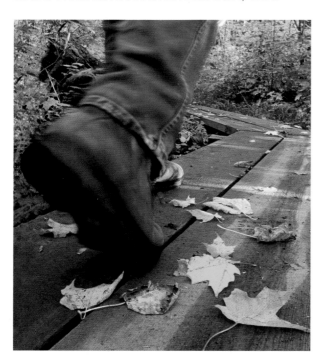

levels of stress hormones like cortisol. The other is recovery from mental fatigue." (See Shift Your Attention on page 250.)

After reading through this book, I hope I've convinced you by now that stress is one of the biggest energy robbers on the planet. But what to do about it? Sometimes the answer is as simple as opening the front door. At a time when our rural areas represent a smaller proportion of our environment than ever before, and prescription antidepressants represent a multibillion dollar industry, "green activities" may be the ultimate definition of a natural cure for low energy.

ECOTHERAPY: A NEW WAY TO RECHARGE YOUR BATTERIES

Enter ecotherapy—i.e., outdoor activities and exercise that can encompass anything from flying a kite to gardening to taking regular walks, but must take place in a natural setting, one where you can escape office buildings, traffic, and the concrete jungle of stress and responsibilities.

Mind, a nonprofit agency that dates back to the 1940s, has done a substantial amount of research on the connection between health, energy, and well-being on the one hand, and Mother Nature on the other. Their scientists believe, with quite a bit of research to back them up, that what they call "green exercise" (namely, outdoor activities) has profound mental health benefits.

One study compared a walk in a country park to a walk inside a shopping mall. By keeping the amount of walking and the level of intensity constant, researchers could identify whether simply being outdoors had any additional benefit to the exercisers, such as increasing their energy, sense of well-being, or overall mood. The results were dramatic. A whopping 71 percent of participants reported feeling better after the "green walk." Whereas half the mall walkers reported *increased* feelings of tension and 44 percent reported *lower* feelings of self-esteem, fully 90 percent of the outdoor exercisers reported *increased* self-esteem after their country walk, and 71 percent said they felt *less* tense.

In a second similar study, 94 percent of subjects reported that green activities had benefited their mental health, including lifting feelings of depression. Ninety percent felt it was the combination of exercise together with nature that was responsible for the effect. Typical comments included, "I feel better about myself and have a sense of achievement," and "I am more relaxed, have better focus of mind, greater coordination, and greater self-esteem."

The researchers didn't specifically ask the walkers whether they felt more energy after the outdoor walk, but on what planet would higher feelings of self-esteem and well-being together with improved mood *not* translate into higher energy?

Not the one I live on!

So escape to the outdoors. Get lost in nature. Spend some time in the moment, and come back energized.

#95

Listen to the Music

The people who run the clothing shops in the mall know what they're doing when it comes to raising energy levels.

I had to run an errand the other day to return some clothes I had bought for my girlfriend,

Anja (who has very picky taste, but don't get me started). To tell you the truth, my energy wasn't so high. (Three sets of singles tennis, plus five hours of writing, and it was only 4:00 in the afternoon!) I don't know about you, but when I'm fading and my energy is down, the last thing I feel like doing is shopping. I just wanted to get in, return the clothes, and get out, and even if the entire Hugo Boss men's collection at Nordstrom was on fire sale I wouldn't have noticed. (Okay, maybe I *would* have noticed, but I wouldn't have felt like doing anything about it.)

So in this low-energy state, I wandered into the mall.

And a funny thing happened.

I walked into the store, and this cool, trendy, Euro-hip club music was playing. Not loud enough to be annoying, but not so soft as to not be felt physically. It immediately put me in a different mood. I felt my energy perk up. Hey, that shirt *would* look good (and it's 50 percent off!). All of a sudden, the music switched to "Baby, You're Amazing." I thought, hey, you know, Anja would look so cool in that necklace! The music segued into the unmistakable funk of James Brown's "I Feel Good!" and all of a sudden I was bopping along (and parting with my credit card).

Tell me that's never happened to you!

WANTED: A GOOD ENERGY PLAYLIST

The healing and power of music is well known. New research by Claudius Conrad, M.D., a surgical resident at Harvard Medical School, shows that patients listening to music show a jump in pituitary growth hormone, which is known to be crucial to healing. It also lowers inflammatory compounds such as interleukin-6.

Other research has shown that music can change your heart rate, respiration, brain waves, and levels of an array of chemicals. It can dramatically reduce stress hormones, relieve anxiety, lower blood pressure, and ease pain. Pleasurable music activates the reward centers of the brain, sending a flood of dopamine, the "feel good" hormone, throughout the body.

Listening to music stimulates virtually every area of the brain, from the primitive regions—the brain stem—to the executive function—the frontal lobe. It can lull you to sleep or make you want to dance (in fact, even when you are perfectly still, listening to music activates the brain area responsible for movement). Just try to feel low energy while putting on a loud recording of Sly's "Dance to the Music" or Chic's "We Are Family." Go on. I dare you.

Music can elicit a kaleidoscope of emotions (listen to enough movie soundtracks and you get the idea). It has the power to tap deep into our reserve of memories, evoking vivid images of a time and place long forgotten.

"Throughout our lives, as we hear music, we create memory links between a particular set of notes and a particular place, time, or set of events," says Daniel Levitin, author of *This Is Your Brain on Music*. We all have a soundtrack to our lives. Want some instant energy? Listen to yours. (Highlights from mine include "Kind of Blue" by Miles Davis; the David Diamond 4th Symphony; any track anywhere on which the pianist Richard Tee played in the rhythm section; and the entire catalogs of James Taylor, Earth, Wind and Fire, and Michael McDonald.)

A CHORD OF ONE'S OWN

What type of music should you play? That depends on your taste and whether you want to be calmed or energized. Are you in the mood for instrumental music to accompany your work and get you into a state of flow, or are you hoping to get into a full-out groove and escape from the stresses of the day?

Generally, writes Levitin, music with major chords strikes us as happy, and songs that rely on minor chords sound "sad, or reflective, or even exotic. The most basic rock and country music songs use only major chords: 'Johnny B. Goode,' 'Blowin' in the Wind,' 'Honky Tonk Woman,' and 'Mammas Don't Let Your Babies Grow Up to Be Cowboys,' for example."

Music has such an enormous power to energize that a whole cottage industry has sprung up around the creation of workout tapes with specific metronome markings (120 beats per second will get anyone jumping!). Figure out what you respond to, and then put it on your playlist.

It's well known that surgeons operate better while listening to music. If music can boost the energy and focus of the person operating on a brain, it can boost yours.

Sometimes increasing energy is simply about changing focus, as when you have a strong case of "attentional fatigue" (see page 250) and simply need to focus somewhere else (such as when you're perfectly able to eat dessert even when you're stuffed after a meal). Taking a few minutes to plug into your MP3 player or iPod and "go somewhere else" can be energizing and mood changing all by itself. Believe me. It doesn't take more than the first few bars of Cheryl Lynn's "Got to Be Real" to do it for me! Ditto with Earth, Wind and Fire's "That's the Way of the World."

For heightened focus, try slower tempo, instrumental music. In one study, 58 percent of people said listening to the blues aided in concentration, while 39 percent said country or folk music helped them focus (golden oldies and world music each garnered about 9 percent). And consider a profession where high energy, focus, and concentration aren't just a luxury, but a necessity: surgery. Ever since the *Journal of the American Medical Association* published "The Phonograph in the Operating Room" in 1914, it's been well known that surgeons operate better while listening to music (just watch *Grey's Anatomy* or *Nip/Tuck* if you don't believe me!). If music can boost the energy and focus of the person operating on a brain, it can boost yours.

When you need energy to get out of a slump, or to help you through some mindless task or chore, go up-tempo. How can you not be energized listening to Aretha belt out "Respect" or James Brown singing "I Feel Good"? When you want to wind down after sitting in traffic for two hours or arguing with the boss, a song with a driving pulse is probably not going to ease your stress, but something slow tempo, with a beat lower than your heart rate (say under 60 or 70 beats per minute), should help soothe the soul. There's a ton of music available under the labels of "meditation" or "spa" that is soothing and stress reducing, and since stress eats up your energy reserves, anything that will help stop that energy drain is going to pay off in energy dividends down the road.

"We humans are a musical species. Our auditory systems, our nervous systems are indeed exquisitely tuned for music," writes the great neurologist, Oliver Sacks, M.D. So do what comes naturally: Listen to music. As you listen, pay attention to how different songs make you feel, and then create your own playlists for different moods and circumstances.

Music can be one of the greatest energizers on the planet. So rock on, listen to the music, and feel your energy dance.

#96

Practice Yoga for Yourself, Your Energy, and Your Life

Here's an energy tip that crosses the boundaries of many of the categories in this book: Practice yoga.

Yoga is good for overall *health* and well-being; it's an *exercise* that improves strength and flexibility; it can foster *personal* and *spiritual* development; it promotes *sleep*; it may aid in *detoxing* the body; and it is the ultimate example of mono-tasking, providing the kind of focus needed to better *organize* your thoughts, your priorities, and your life. And yes, it is a wonderful way to *manage stress*, promote relaxation, and increase energy.

You don't have to know your Ashtanga from your Vinyasa to be impressed with the myriad benefits you can derive from yoga. Research backs up what practitioners have known for centuries—yoga, with its precise moves and controlled breathing, can relieve anxiety, increase concentration, promote a meditative state, and improve mood and energy.

A recent study points to why yoga may be effective at improving mood. An hour of yoga produced a 27 percent surge in brain levels of GABA (gamma-aminobutyric acid), a neurotransmitter that's often low in people who are depressed or anxious. Yoga has also been shown to reduce fatigue in subjects with multiple sclerosis and relieve lower back pain in chronic sufferers. In yet another study, this one on subjects with chronic insomnia, researchers found significant improvements in sleep in those who practiced 30 to 45 minutes of Kundalini yoga once a day for eight weeks. Reduction in fatigue, pain, and anxiety translates into one thing everyone wants: more energy for living!

But wait, there's more. Yoga can also reduce heart rate and blood pressure, increase lung capacity, improve body composition, relax tense muscles, and improve overall physical fitness. Talk about an energy super-charge!

The practice of yoga began thousands of years ago as a way to attain spiritual enlightenment through physical and mental training. Today there are many yoga disciplines that vary in style and intensity, but all remain rooted in yogic tradition by incorporating various *asanas* (poses) and *pranayama* (breathing techniques). In yoga, breath signifies *prana*, or vital energy, and is the connection between the physical and the spiritual. Practicing yoga helps develop mind-body stamina. By focusing on the breath, you can clear the mind of distraction, as you ease the body into a pose.

Yoga practitioners often describe that increase in focus and clarity as feeling like the energy equivalent of a penetrating laser light.

In principle and practice, yoga promotes flexibility. Asanas can be adjusted to meet an individual's fitness level or to work around an injury. With thousands of poses and a wide variety of disciplines to choose from, yoga can be fashioned to suit a wide range of personalities, sensibilities, and goals. Done consistently, it can almost definitely send your energy into the stratosphere.

FIND YOUR FORM

The most common form of yoga in the United States and Europe is hatha yoga. It encompasses a variety of styles, both strenuous and gentle; some focus on the physical, others the meditative. Some forms of yoga are exacting in the number and sequence of asanas, and others are more free-flowing.

Lyenga yoga emphasizes precision and form, and employs belts, pillows, and other props to help students reach poses that would otherwise be beyond their limits. In Ashtanga yoga, on the other hand, asanas are performed one after another, quickly and continuously. Bikram yoga is a

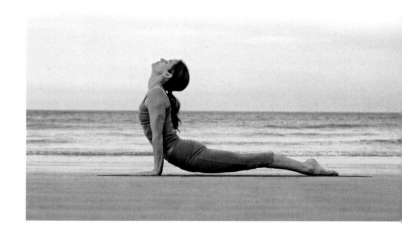

particular style developed in Los Angeles by Bikram Choudhury, a former Olympic gold medalist. It is practiced in a hot, humid room (typically from 95°F, or 35°C, to 115°F, or 46°C) and is rapidly gaining popularity around the world. Then there are the many hybrid classes, which mix and match yoga styles. Why not try a few, and pick the one that most suits you and gives you the greatest sense of well-being and increased energy?

Whether your ultimate goal is a lifetime of inner peace or just an hour of peace and quiet, by practicing yoga—clearing your mind, challenging your body, and controlling your breathing—you can attain a state of relaxation and invigoration.

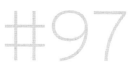

Try EFT for Emotional Energy

If you feel like you don't have any energy, here's something I can guarantee you: An enormous part of the problem can be traced to your habits—not only what you consistently do, but what you consistently *don't* do.

And one of the biggest habits we all have that ties into energy is suppressing our emotions. In fact, that's probably one of the biggest energy drains I know of.

Emotional Freedom Technique, or EFT, is a simple method to release emotions. In the process, it frees the energy that's suppressed along with your feelings.

I first wrote about EFT in my book *The Most Effective Natural Cures on Earth*. But quite honestly, I based what I wrote on the experience of others—people who reported feeling lighter, more energetic, and happier as a result of doing the technique. I was impressed enough with the reports I was hearing from my colleagues to feel it merited inclusion in my book. But since writing that book, I've tried EFT myself. I can now report from my own experience that EFT is one of the most energy-liberating techniques on the planet.

And it's free.

Interested?

"All of us have been taught to suppress our emotions from a very early age," says Glen Depke, N.D., a traditional naturopath and one of the country's leading practitioners of EFT. (Glen, one of my dearest friends, is currently the head nutritionist at the Mercola Optimal Wellness Center in Illinois, as well as the center's chief EFT practitioner.) "EFT is a simple energy technique to release those suppressed emotions that can be bringing down our energy," he told me.

TAPPING INTO ENERGY

Emotional Freedom Technique is a kind of non-invasive acupuncture, in which you use your fingers to tap specific energy meridians in the body for the purpose of releasing long-held beliefs and thoughts that can hold you back from fully expressing who you are.

"By helping us release those suppressed emotions, we create an open space where a person will be able to put in whatever patterns he or she chooses," Depke explains.

I'll give you a personal example. I've long had a block when it comes to my tennis playing. I'm a really good player during warm-up and practice, and a really terrible competitor (or at least I used to be, prior to EFT). Part of the reason was that I had a belief system based around the idea that when it comes to athletics, I'm a loser. That deeply held belief, embedded from a lifetime of childhood traumas around gym class (don't ask), actually caused me to tighten up my arms, breath shallowly when serving, and in general forget everything I knew about tennis strokes once the pressure was on. In athletic terms it's called "choking."

By tapping on the energetic meridian points while stating simple statements (such as "Even though I feel like a loser in tennis, I love and accept myself") I was able to loosen the hold these entrenched beliefs had on my psyche. After doing EFT for just a few sessions, I started winning matches. Not all the time, obviously—EFT doesn't give you a 140-mile-per-hour serve, unfortunately—but enough so that the energy I had around losing dissipated.

"If you're in a free-flowing energetic state and then you suppress your emotion, that will block energy. The blocked energy has a physical

location in your body. Wherever you block that energy it creates disharmony. The longer the emotion is suppressed, the greater the disharmony. Long-standing disharmony leads to dysfunction, and ultimately to a physical manifestation such as a disease state," says Depke. That disharmony also leads to a complete lack of energy.

For everyday, garden-variety fatigue, Depke suggests asking yourself the following questions:

- What are the typical negative emotions you experience on a regular basis?
- Are you frustrated with your spouse, your children, or your job?
- Are you angry?

"Typically the superficial challenges in our life are not the problem," Depke advised me. "They're a reflection of a deeper suppressed emotion. What you do with EFT is release the suppressed emotion to create harmony, function, and a high energetic state of natural health."

DO-IT-YOURSELF ENERGY

EFT is actually based on traditional Chinese medicine and acupressure points. You use your own hand to stimulate the flow of energy, tapping on these points (seven of them) while addressing your emotions as well as the situation that ties into it. "That's what allows the energy to flow freely and for a person to enjoy optimal health," says Depke.

The inventor of EFT is a Stanford University engineer named Gary Craig, who maintains a website where you can download a free manual on how to do the technique on yourself (www.emofree.com). EFT has been endorsed by some of the most impressive people in the field of energy medicine, including Deepak Chopra, M.D. ("EFT offers great healing benefits"), molecular biologist and star of the self-help film *The Secret* Candace Pert, Ph.D. ("EFT is at the forefront of the new healing movement"), life coach and frequent *Oprah* guest Cheryl Richardson, and many others. You can actually view videos of the technique on YouTube, as well as on Craig's website.

Depke suggests that a great way to start learning about how to use EFT to increase your own energy is by downloading the free manual. You may also find, as I did, that a few sessions with an experienced EFT therapist can produce unbelievable energy benefits. Depke himself even does highly effective phone consultations (www.depkewellness.com).

#98

Get a Massage

When he was in his twilight years, legendary comedian Bob Hope told his friend, Lee Iacocca, the former CEO of Chrysler, that the secret to living to be 100 boiled down to doing three things every day: Getting a massage, eating fruit, and having sex.

Iacocca thought for a second, and then said, "Hey, two out of three ain't bad."

Although I don't know how closely Bob Hope followed his own formula for longevity, I do know he lived to be 100.

Because this isn't a book about living to 100 (although following the principles of it may help you reach the century mark) and because I've already spoken about the health benefits of eating fruit and will talk about the upside to having sex later (see page 265), I'll focus on how massage can help protect your health and keep you energized.

KNEADED ENERGY

The term *massage therapy* actually covers more than eighty types of practices and techniques. In all, therapists press, rub, knead, and otherwise manipulate the muscles and other soft tissues of the body, often varying pressure and movement. Most often, they use their hands and fingers, but may also use their forearms, elbows, or feet. Massage relaxes the soft tissues, increases delivery of blood and oxygen to the massaged areas, warms them, and decreases pain. Usually, massage also reduces stress and enhances relaxation.

"When stored or blocked emotions are released through touch or other physical methods," writes Candace Pert, Ph.D., author of *Molecules of Emotion*, "there is a clearing of our internal pathways, which we experience as energy."

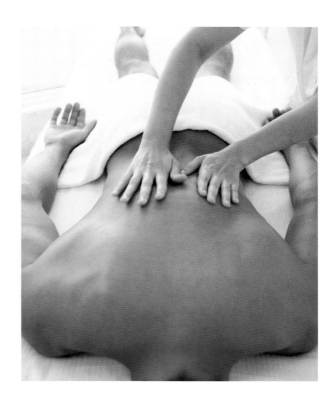

Like most forms of bodywork, massage does not lend itself to the gold standard of Western research, the double-blind clinical trial. (Just to show you how ridiculous it is to demand this kind of research for everything, consider what a double-blind, placebo-controlled trial would look like: You'd need a "placebo massage" and a "real massage." Let me know when you figure that one out. Oh, and the massage therapist would have to be "blind" to knowing whether or not she was administering the "real" massage or the "fake" massage.)

So, okay, no double-blind, placebo-controlled studies on massage. Big deal. But there has been published, peer-reviewed research that has shown massage can reduce pain, lower anxiety, improve circulation, decrease inflammation, enhance the immune system, and improve lung function in children with asthma. Like exercise, massage can reduce fatigue and enhance focus.

THE WAY MASSAGE WORKS

Although scientists continue to research the effects of massage, according to the National Center for Complementary and Alternative Medicine (NCCAM), they have come up with some theories as to how it works its magic.

- Massage might provide stimulation that helps block pain signals sent to the brain.
- It may shift the nervous system away from the sympathetic and toward the parasympathetic. When under stress, the sympathetic nervous system produces the fight-or-flight response (your heart rate and breathing rate go up, your blood vessels narrow, and your muscles tighten). The parasympathetic nervous system creates what some call the "rest and digest" response (your heart rate and breathing rate slow down, your blood vessels dilate, and activity increases in many parts of your digestive tract).

- Massage might stimulate the release of certain chemicals in the body, such as serotonin and endorphins, while inhibiting the stress hormone, cortisol.

- It might prevent fibrosis (the formation of scarlike tissue) and might help break up adhesions. It might also increase the flow of lymphatic fluid, helping to strengthen the immune system. And it may reduce lactic acid buildup.

- It appears to improve sleep, which can help control pain and aid the healing process.

- The mere interaction between therapist and patient might elicit some health benefits.

- There's another benefit to massage therapy that research can't measure—it provides a time and space to unplug all gadgets, disengage from the outside world, and focus inward. Plus you get to listen to all that cool, calming music, inhale that incense, and smell the almond oil being rubbed all over your body. Cost of massage: about $90. Ability to calm the body and quiet the mind: priceless.

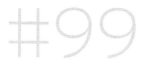

Dance to the Music

If you've never seen *Risky Business*, let me recommend that you watch it. And if you haven't seen it in a while, it might be worth revisiting. It's an iconic movie, in large part because of a dancing scene.

In it, Tom Cruise plays a teenager—alone at home and unobserved—who dances up a storm (dressed in a shirt, socks, and tighty-whities) and puts on the greatest air-guitar performance in movie history. The audience is completely and utterly his, in part because almost everyone can relate to the joy and energy of being *willing to do something that makes you look ridiculous as long as no one is watching.*

Kind of like a karaoke bar minus the audience and the alcohol.

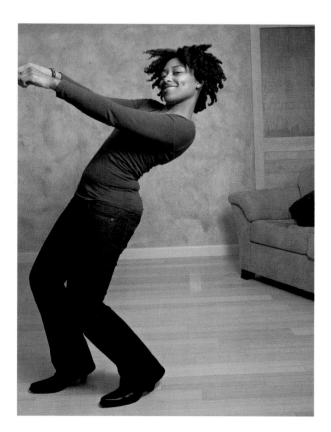

LET GO AND LET THE ENERGY FLOW

One of the biggest reasons we don't dance in public is because of inhibitions. Inhibitions *inhibit*. They act as a giant parental superego, telling you what to do and what not to do, and most of the time, that may be a good thing (for society, certainly, and maybe even for you). But sometimes the superego gets a little carried away and winds up putting the kibosh on our creative impulses. And when creative juices dry up, energy can wither away.

There's a saying among comics that to be really great on stage, you have to be willing to make a fool of yourself. Well, guess what? That's a truth that extends to a lot of areas of life. Dancing, for example. (Full disclosure—the fear of looking like a klutz and the desire to look cool has kept me off the dance floor on many an occasion.)

Here's the thing—you may never be able to fully let go and dance up a storm in public. But you can do it in private. And it will boost your energy like there's no tomorrow.

How do I know? I've done it. It's my own personal form of air guitar. Dancing—the wildest, most uninhibited, reckless, silly, crazy dancing you can imagine—does a number of things. It's a highly aerobic workout that'll get oxygen pumping throughout the body and brain, energizing you almost immediately. But more important, it's a chain-breaker. Even if no one sees you, the letting loose of inhibitions, the physical expression of what your body is holding on to, the giving in to the demands of the creative spirit to express itself physically is one of the greatest energy unleashers on the planet.

So go ahead. Put on your favorite music—Springsteen's "Born in the USA," Michael Jackson's "Thriller," Sly and the Family Stone's "Dance to the Music," Rick James's "Super Freak," Beyoncé, the Bee Gees—whatever gets you moving—and pretend to be a rock star. Try it for 5 minutes and throw caution to the wind. Throw your arms around, wiggle your hips, and don't worry about how you look (no one is watching); just close your eyes and dance.

Trust me on this—your energy will go through the roof.

P.S. If you're thinking to yourself, "He can't possibly mean me," then be assured that I *especially* mean you.

#100

Disconnect for a Day

Consider for the moment one of the great energy drainers of the twenty-first century: information overload.

Now think for a moment about what you might do about it.

The answer is quite a lot, actually. And it starts with a disconnect vacation.

These days we're deluged with information, coming at us from every possible angle. It's relentless: emails, RSS feeds, blogs, social networking sites, YouTube, television, magazines, newspapers, memos, DVDs, radio, fax machines, BlackBerries, satellite radio—it's exhausting just listing the sources, let alone reading or listening to them. And more will be invented tomorrow.

I sometimes think that if I had an X-ray photo of the average person's mind it would look like a personalized cable news channel, with breaking news crawling at the bottom, headline themes on top, and somewhere in between sports scores, weather reports, calendars, appointments, and people's names and titles flashing by in an instant.

THE ENERGY DRAIN OF INFORMATION SATURATION

Knowledge may be power; however, information overload is anything but. Information overload is just, well, noise.

When we gorge on media, it's about as satisfying as downing a vat of cotton candy, and in both cases, we eventually feel the aftereffects (either with an upset stomach or a throbbing headache). The age of information saturation has rewired our brains and given us all a mild case of ADD. More than that, it's left most of us feeling more than a little overwhelmed and exhausted.

The great philosopher, social critic, and historian Theodore Roszak once said, "A weekday edition of the *New York Times* contains more information than the average person was likely to come across in a lifetime in seventeenth-century England." Even if you don't read the *Times* on a daily basis, you can probably relate to the sentiment. And Roszak made that statement almost twenty years ago.

We spend countless hours trying to keep up, to the detriment of important things such as relationships, health, and energy.

TUNE OUT AND REV UP

So here's my suggestion for an immediate boost in energy: Have a media-free day. No Internet, no email, no television, no iPods, no radio, no newspapers, no magazines. And no BlackBerries (you know who you are!). For one day consider the possibility that there is nothing you need to know. Instead, spend that attention on your own experience, feeling your own energy accumulate rather than letting it dissipate as you attend to millions of distractions, most of which, when you really think about it, won't make much difference in the long run anyway.

Now you may have to do this on a weekend, but that's okay. With your free hours, enjoy leisurely meals with family or friends, have real conversations, take time to think, take a hike, take a swim, take a nap, and, at the end of your day off, take stock. Did the world as we know it end because you weren't plugged in?

Now let me be honest: No one is more guilty of being overly plugged in than I am. That's why I know the truth of what I'm saying. When you take a break (however temporarily) and disconnect, you will be amazed at the ultimate boost you'll get in your energy. Learning how to do so may actually make you a more discerning and discriminating consumer of information once you reconnect. You'll be amazed to find how much time you waste attending to things that really, ultimately, don't matter, at least not to you or anyone you care about.

If you end the day more relaxed, more satisfied, and more energized, consider limiting your media intake every day—perhaps do without television on Mondays, ban Web-surfing on Tuesdays, leave your BlackBerry in the office during lunch, and so on. You might find that a little less useless information makes you a lot more productive and energized.

#101
Relax and Recharge

You want the kind of sustained, invigorating energy that lasts a lifetime, that keeps you doing interesting and engaging things deep into your ninth decade and beyond, that fires you up with enthusiasm for every new project and every new day. Think Art Linkletter (see page 17). That's the kind of energy we're talking about.

To achieve that lasting, sustainable energy, you need to do some serious relaxing. It sounds like a paradox, but it's not. Think of relaxing as a temporary stop at the gas station that allows you to refuel your tank. You can put off that pit stop for just so long, but eventually, if you don't relax, you're going to run out of gas.

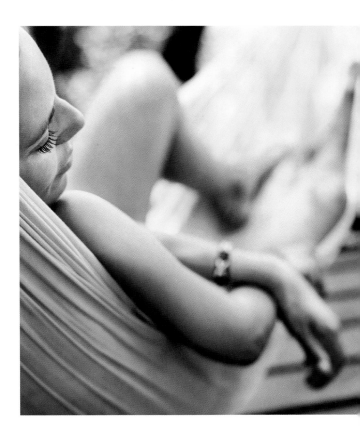

Relaxation is the key to replenishing your energy stores. It has to do with something called *homeostasis*. In medicine, the prefix *homeo* means "similar," "same," or "unchanging." *Stasis* means "stagnation," "inactivity," or "motionless." Get the picture?

Homeostasis is also the maintenance of a stable internal environment in the body despite changes in the external environment. It's what keeps you in balance. It's the inherent tendency of any living organism toward physiological and psychological stability and equilibrium. When one side of the seesaw goes up, the other side goes down. When both are equal distance from the ground, the seesaw is perfectly balanced, or in homeostasis. From your body's point of view, this is a desirable state.

HOMEOSTASIS: YOUR BODY IS LAZY!

Truth be told, your body is a bit like a slacker teenager. It actually *likes* to lie around on the couch and resist change or activity. While *you* might feel like doing jumping jacks, running a marathon, or writing the novel of the century, your body will always try to "recover" from that activity and bring you back to its ideal balanced state—the body's version of lying around on the couch and relaxing.

That's balance. Nothing too much going out, nothing too much going in. No muss, no fuss, no stress. Input equals output. Perfect . . . well, homeostasis.

Here's why: The part of your nervous system that acts as a control system, maintaining balance—or homeostasis—in the body is the autonomic nervous system, and it contains two major parts: the sympathetic and the parasympathetic nervous systems. They typically function in opposition to one another.

The sympathetic nervous system is the one that's aroused when you're running around, burning through your day, writing reports, shooting archery, playing soccer, doing laundry, hunting big game, whatever. It's the sympathetic nervous system that elevates your heart rate and gets sugar into the bloodstream when you need to run from a predator. It's the sympathetic nervous system that's responsible for your primitive fight-or-flight response, whether that means fighting a woolly mammoth in prehistoric times, or fighting the traffic on the Los Angeles freeway.

But, aha, it's the parasympathetic nervous system that calms you and restocks your body with the chemicals you used up running around playing Master of the Universe. While the sympathetic nervous system is responsible for fight or flight, the parasympathetic nervous system is responsible for

Constant whirlwind activity needs to stop for a refueling. That's where relaxation comes in.

rest and digest. You can't have that ideal state of balance, of homeostasis, without the two nervous systems cooperating.

THE ELEPHANT ON THE SEESAW

Here's what happens if you don't give the parasympathetic nervous system equal time. The sympathetic nervous system becomes like an elephant sitting on that seesaw. When it finally decides it needs to take a rest and dismount, the seesaw goes crashing to the ground and splinters into a thousand pieces. Why? Because there's been nothing on the other side to *balance* it.

Relaxation is the other side of the energy coin. Constant whirlwind activity needs to stop for a refueling. That's where relaxation comes in. I've seen so many people in my travels who consider relaxation "time wasted." "It's sitting around doing nothing," they claim. Not even close to the truth.

Relaxation is your body balancing the seesaw, activating the critical parasympathetic nervous system, acting as a corrective to that elephant of an overactive sympathetic nervous system, and creating the kind of balance and harmony your body craves—homeostasis.

I've never studied martial arts, but friends of mine tell me that their most powerful strokes come from a position of balance. As an avid tennis player, and I can tell you that's certainly true in tennis. I suspect it's true in most sports and indeed in most areas of life in general.

You just can't perform at full strength with full power if you're not in a balanced state, and without allowing time for the body to recuperate, balance will always elude you. Without balance, you'll always be withdrawing from your body's energy bank account, and eventually your stash will run out. For optimal energy, you need to balance those withdrawals with deposits in the form of relaxation.

If you don't make time to relax, you ultimately won't have time for anything else. Relaxation is a critical part of your energy prescription. You can rest assured that all those movers and shakers that you see burning through their day with boundless energy have spent plenty of time behind the scenes replenishing, restoring, and refurbishing their energy signature with some serious downtime.

You should, too.

So recharge your batteries. Regularly. Religiously. Without fail.

It's critical to your health, and essential to your energy.

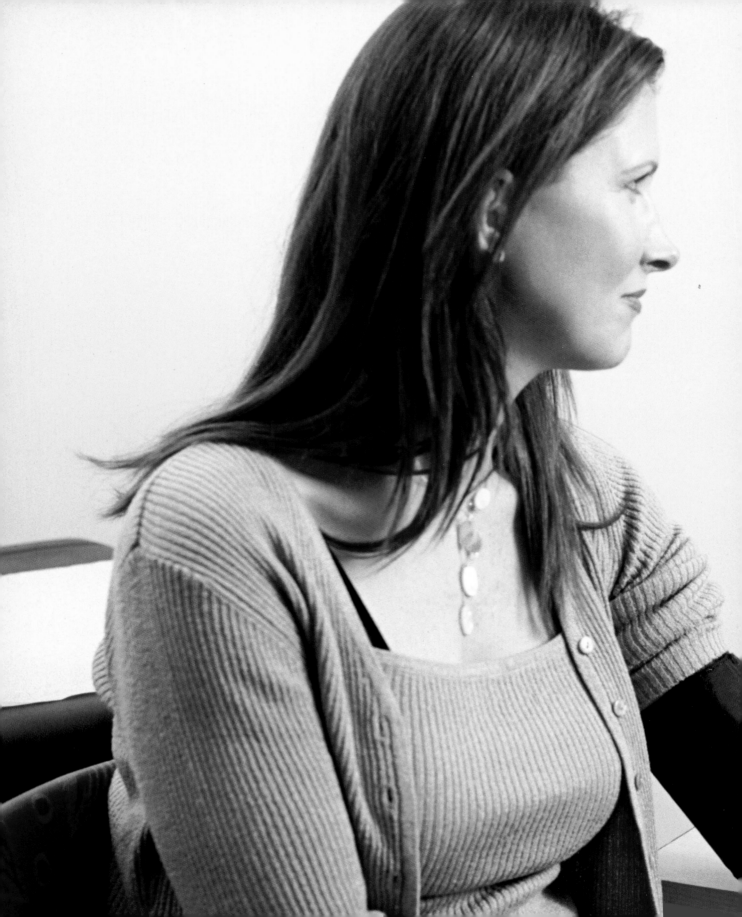

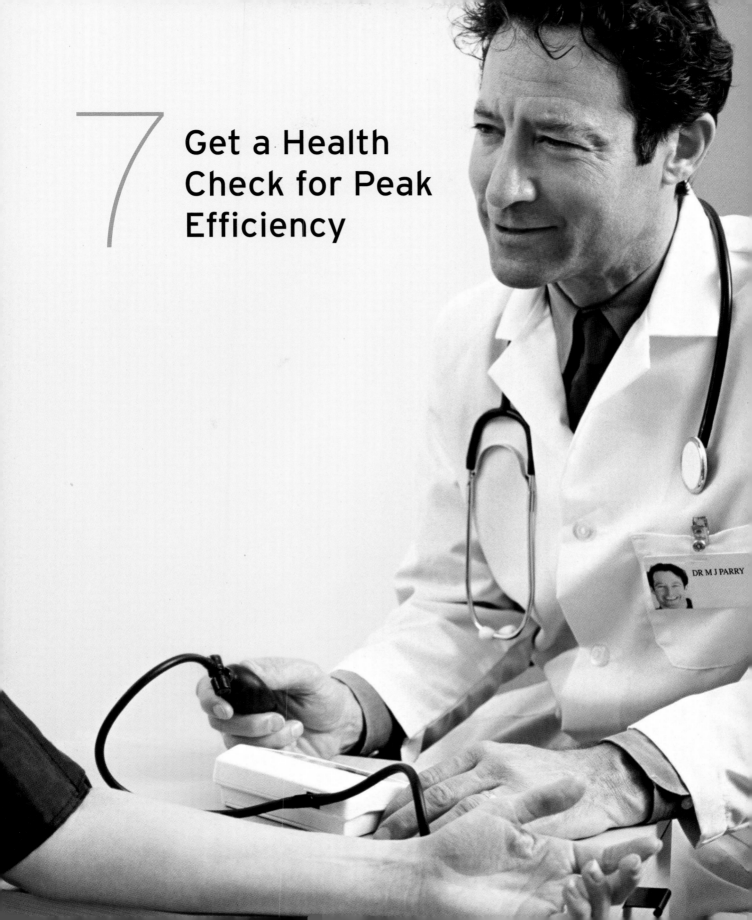

7

Get a Health Check for Peak Efficiency

By now, I hope it's becoming clear that the central theory of this book is that your energy is a by-product of the way you live your life. Great energy is, after all, a side effect (albeit a really desirable one) of the way you eat and exercise, multiplied by the way you think, feel, produce, and organize, as well as how you experience your life. Remember the mantra: Everything's related to everything.

So it shouldn't be much of a surprise that the things you do to take care of your overall health have a profound effect on your energy. It's pretty hard to conceive of someone in terrible health who isn't tired most of the time. Now that doesn't necessarily mean that if you're tired all the time you're in terrible health, but chances are something's going on that could be improved. And if you're truly in great health and have all your ducks in a row—emotionally, physically, and spiritually—you will have great energy as a matter of course.

Many of the chapters in this book have direct implications for overall health—eating and drinking, for example. Or supplementation. Or exercise. But that said, there are still a couple of entries on the list of 150 ways to boost energy that don't fit neatly into those categories.

Hence this chapter.

THE PLAYBOOK FOR ENERGY: STRATEGIES THAT WORK

In this section you'll find health-related strategies that can significantly bolster your overall energy and well-being. Making sure your hormone levels are where they should be, for example, certainly can (you'll find sections on some of the big guns in the hormone energy interplay, including the thyroid and the sex hormones estrogen and testosterone). You'll also find a couple of treatment modalities that aren't commonly thought of as having a direct relationship to energy—chiropractic, acupuncture, and reflexology—but which in fact can make an enormous difference to your state of mind and overall sense of energy and well-being. And finally, because how you hold yourself actually affects the amount of energy you spend during the day trying to keep your body "aligned," I have a section on posture to round out the group.

You'll probably discover energy secrets in this section you didn't know about before now. Maybe you'll find a few connections you hadn't considered relevant to your energy, too.

And if you hadn't thought about any of these connections to your energy before now, this is a great time to do so!

#102

Revive Your Qi with Acupuncture

My dear friend Randy Graff is a Tony-award winning actress and a popular fixture on the Broadway stage. She's also frequently enthusiastic about nontraditional, alternative health practices, from acupuncture to Bach flower remedies. So when she first told me twenty years ago about this amazing acupuncturist she was seeing, I kind of silently rolled my eyes.

"Every time I leave his office, I feel completely relaxed and energized at the same time," she'd tell me.

Fast-forward a couple of decades and I now see that Randy was ahead of the curve.

Acupuncture is now accepted as an effective healing modality for a host of conditions. (I wrote about it as an effective aid for fertility in *The Most Effective Natural Cures on Earth*, but that's just the tip of the acupuncture iceberg.)

Now I'll be honest with you—I'm not an expert in traditional Chinese medicine (TCM), but I do have an incredible respect for the wealth of wisdom in this ancient body of knowledge, which is believed to have begun as far back as the Neolithic Stone Age, around 6000 B.C. And I've always been impressed with the ability of trained TCM doctors to diagnose conditions using tongue analysis, pulse analysis, and other tools so foreign to our Western, high-tech way of thinking.

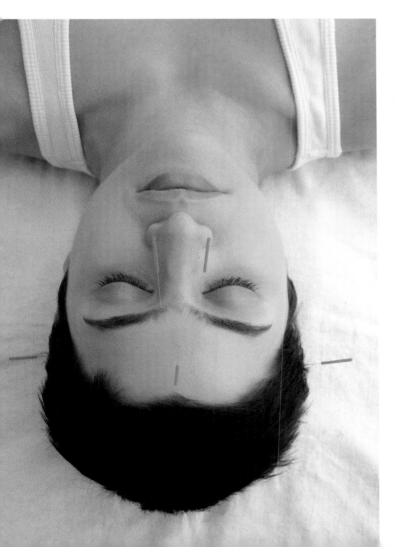

One thing I know for sure—at the very center of TCM (and many of the other Eastern traditions, for that matter) is the concept of energy. In China it's called qi (or chi); in Japan, ki; and in India, prana. They all translate to a single term that's really the subject of this whole book: *life force*.

Energy pulses through us (and everything else in the universe), and when that energy force is depleted or disrupted, then our health (and our energy, as in vitality) suffers. Conversely, when our qi is at optimal levels and flowing smoothly, we're ready to take on the world. Spiritually, emotionally, mentally, and physically, we're strong, healthy, and energized.

One way to balance that qi—or, if you prefer the more Westernized version, to increase your energy—is through acupuncture. I can tell you that the dozen or so times I've tried it I've left the sessions feeling both relaxed and energized, a combination that sounds strange on paper but feels quite terrific and not at all paradoxical.

I'm not alone. Acupuncture has helped people for centuries. Acupuncture needles were probably first manufactured during the Shang Dynasty (1766–1122 B.C.), when bronze-casting technology was first developed. So this stuff has been around for a long time.

THE CONCEPT OF QI

Acupuncture is based on the precepts of TCM: that the body and mind are inextricably linked; that vital energy—or qi—regulates a person's spiritual, mental, and physical health; and that each of us is a delicate balance of opposing and inseparable forces—yin and yang—and when that balance is disrupted, vital energy becomes blocked or weakened.

According to TCM, qi flows through the body along an interconnected network of pathways, called *meridians*. There are twelve main meridians that correspond to the twelve major organs or functions of the body (as well as eight extra meridians where qi can be stored) that can be accessed through more than 400 (some sources say 2,000) acupoints—where qi is believed to flow close to the surface of the skin.

The goal of acupuncture is to maintain health by ensuring that energy circulates effortlessly throughout the body. When qi is blocked or weakened, an acupuncturist stimulates meridians at carefully selected acupoints—generally by inserting and manipulating thin metal needles—to balance energy and allow the body to heal itself. Because the effects of acupuncture correspond to the meridian that is stimulated and not necessarily the location of the needle, an acupoint used in treatment may be in a different part of the body than the symptom. For instance, a point in the foot may be used to treat the eye.

Recent neuroimaging studies have shown that certain acupoints stimulate areas in the brain that correspond to their intended target. For instance, acupoints associated with hearing and vision light up the auditory and visual centers of the brain.

GETTING ON YOUR NERVES

Although Western medicine hasn't been able to figure out the exact biological mechanism of acupuncture, some researchers theorize that it influences the body's electromagnetic fields, thereby causing responses in nerves cells, the pituitary gland, and parts of the brain, which release proteins, hormones, and brain chemicals that control a number of body functions. That may explain how acupuncture affects blood pressure and body temperature, and boosts immune system activity.

Many studies provide evidence that opioid peptides—the body's natural painkiller—are released during acupuncture, which may account for why people receiving acupuncture feel so terrific (and so energized). Scientists here and abroad are currently studying the efficacy of acupuncture for a wide range of conditions.

Today, acupuncture is used for a wide variety of conditions, including pain management, relief from postoperative nausea and vomiting, and treatment for addiction. For all those energy-draining conditions, people undergoing acupuncture report feeling a lot of relief. Research has demonstrated acupuncture's effect on various biological systems, including the digestive tract, cardiovascular system, immune system, and endocrine system. All I know is that after a session, I'm walking on air.

If calm, focused energy is what you're after, acupuncture is definitely worth a try.

———— **WORTH KNOWING** ————

There is no one who's more of a coward when it comes to pain than I am. I get nitrous oxide (laughing gas) when I get my teeth cleaned. So when I tell you that the needles used in acupuncture are absolutely, completely painless, you can take that to the bank. The only thing weird is knowing they're in there. Half the time if you didn't see them sticking out (which you won't when they're in your back) you wouldn't even know they're there. Seriously.

103

Go to a Chiropractor and Adjust to New Energy

I've always had a special place in my heart for chiropractors for three reasons.

First, I don't like bullies. And, much like naturopaths, nutritionists, and even psychologists in the early twentieth century, chiropractors have always been bullied by mainstream medical organizations that consistently mounted mean-spirited public relations efforts to marginalize them. (I myself grew up in the 1950s, when every respectable household considered chiropractors "quacks," thanks to the excellent lobbying efforts of the American Medical Association.)

Second, because during the ten years I spent as a personal trainer in the 1990s, chiropractors were our greatest ally. They helped our clients, they gave workshops to the trainers, and they seemed to have a profound understanding of the

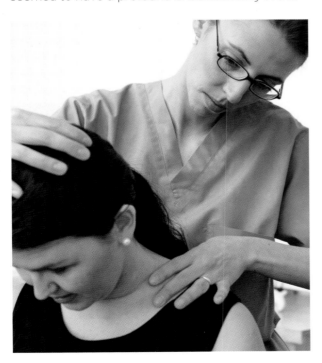

way the body worked as a whole. (I guess when you're not allowed to prescribe medicine, you have to look a little deeper into the body's natural healing abilities.)

And third, because over the years I've come to know more than a few chiropractors who are on the cutting edge of nutritional therapies. Perhaps because their training is more holistic than that of conventional medical doctors, they are, as a profession, far more open to the role of nutrition, diet, and lifestyle, and they seem to intuitively connect the dots when it comes to energy, vitality, and physical health.

So believe me when I say that if you want your energy to go through the roof, you might want to check in to having a chiropractic adjustment.

"Energy loss is first and foremost a sign of a malfunction of some system in the body," my friend, holistic chiropractor Matthew Mannino, D.C., told me. Mannino is president of Source Trainings in Phoenix, Arizona (www.sourcetrainings.com), a company whose tagline is "Where science and spirit unite!"

"If there's a malfunction, energy now has to be used to sustain and maintain health and fight off disease," Mannino continues. Even minor misalignments or distortions in the curvature of the neck or spine can create bigger demands on the muscles and physiology, resulting in lost energy, he says.

"You want the body to have to put out the least amount of effort to keep the musculoskeletal structure in its place," he told me. "When you move away from that effortless, natural balance, it can absolutely lead to people feeling tired all the time."

Think about it. The nervous system is the master control system in the body, and it functions on electrical impulses. "The core of all health and healing is the transmission of electrical energy through

Out of Line and Out of Energy

Chiropractic deals with imbalances in the body that can lead to low energy, imbalances that are the result of structural misalignments. They call these basic structural misalignments *subluxations*. A subluxation is when one or more of the bones of the spine are out of place and create pressure or irritation on spinal nerves, the nerves that come out from between each of the bones in your spine. If there's pressure or irritation on those nerves, they malfunction and interrupt signals traveling over the nerves to the rest of the body. If you interrupt those signals—or somehow interfere with their optimal transmission—it's like driving your car on a road filled with huge potholes. You'll get there, but the journey won't be smooth and you won't be traveling very fast.

A chiropractor can help using a tool called an adjustment, a hands-on technique that restores the body's natural alignment and corrects subluxation. "An alignment ensures that you have the ideal nerve flow into the tissues and that you have optimal energy and well-being," explains Mannino.

Another chiropractor, Lauren Nappen of Mechanicsville, Pennsylvania, puts it this way: "A chiropractic alignment is about connecting the brain to the body and the body to the brain, and letting the magic of life unfold around you. Life force pumps and flows ever more freely—ready, willing, and able to move you toward well-being."

the nervous system," Mannino told me. "The nervous system is the link between spiritual man and physical man because it contains that force—electricity—that allows the cells, tissues, and organs to function properly." If those nerve transmissions aren't firing properly, bye-bye energy.

YOUR THOUGHTS AFFECT YOUR ENERGY

There's also another component to all this that's worth really thinking about. We know that what you think about affects your physiology. (Your heart speeds up when you watch a scary movie, even though you haven't left your seat. The examples are endless.) But according to Mannino—and I agree completely—this feedback loop can work both ways.

So if your physiology isn't working right, if you have a subtle misalignment, your nerve impulses aren't firing on all cylinders, you experience a slight irritation on a nerve or even some minor pain that you're "putting up with," it can profoundly affect your emotions, thoughts, and—most of all—your energy.

When I was a little kid, my mother used to take me to get my ears cleaned. I always thought my ears were fine, but after the doc did his little wax removal thing, I'd always be astonished at the difference in how clear and loud everything sounded. It was like opening up the musical bandwidth from deepest bass to highest treble.

A chiropractic adjustment is like that. You may think you're operating at a sufficient energy level (just like I thought my hearing was fine), but get yourself an adjustment, get your body in alignment, and you'll know what real energy can feel like. It's pretty cool.

104

Do a Posture Check

My grandmother used to love to tell me the story of how my father (her son) once came to her in his twenties and said, "Mom, it's really amazing. As I've gotten older, you've gotten so much smarter."

I wish she were around today so she could see that the acknowledgment of her wisdom was passed on to a second generation. It's just amazing how many things your grandmother (and mine) were right about.

Here's one of them to add to the list: Stop slouching. It has a lot more to do with your energy than you might think.

SLOUCHING TOWARD FATIGUE

When you're hunched over a computer all day, your rounded shoulders and compressed trunk promote shallow breathing. That, in turn, can reduce oxygen intake significantly.

"It's simple mechanics," says Christopher Kauffman, UCSD orthopedic surgeon. "Being bent over decreases the space in the (lung) cavity." Shallower breathing means less oxygen is available to both nourish your body and fuel your energy. Less oxygen means less energy. Poor posture can also lead to muscle fatigue, strain, and lower back pain, all well-known drainers of every kind of energy and vitality on the planet.

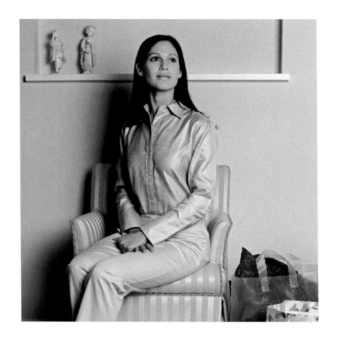

If you want a little extra motivation for taking a posture inventory, consider this: When your back is hunched, your head is thrust forward and your abs protrude. Let's just put it this way: Attractive it's not. When your body is aligned properly, you look thinner, younger, and more confident.

Bad posture can also be the first sign that something in your body is badly misaligned, which can lead to a whole host of energy drains. (See Go to a Chiropractor and Adjust to New Energy on page 189 for a more thorough discussion of this energy connection.)

Meanwhile, let's start with the basics.

"Energy loss is first and foremost a sign of a malfunction of some system in the body."
—Matthew Mannino, D.C., holistic chiropractor

THREE STEPS TO GOOD POSTURE

Step 1. Awareness. Each time you hear the ding of an email, or your phone rings, do a posture check.

Step 2. Move. Don't stay in any one position for very long. Stand up while waiting for a Web page to load, and take frequent breaks to walk or stretch.

Step 3. Exercise for posture improvement. Here are five seated or standing posture-strengthening moves to work into your workday.

Polish the Air

- Sit up straight with your elbows at your sides and bent to 90 degrees, with your palms facing the floor.
- Squeeze your shoulders together without raising them.
- While keeping your elbows at your side, move your hands as though polishing furniture.
- Do this for twenty seconds. Repeat four times.

Tighten Up

- Sit with your back supported against the back of a chair.
- Tighten your abdominal muscles as though you expect to be punched.
- Press your fingers into your abdomen and tighten your abs even more to resist the pressure of your fingers.
- Keep breathing throughout the exercise.
- Hold for fifteen seconds. Repeat five times.

Make Wall Angels

- Stand against the wall with your feet shoulder-width apart, and your weight evenly distributed.
- Gently press your lower back against the wall.
- Place the back of your elbows, forearms, and wrists against the wall.
- While keeping your elbows in contact with the wall, slowly move your arms up and down in a small arc as though making snow angels against the wall.
- Do this ten times.

Slide Down the Wall

- Stand with your buttocks and back against a wall, with your weight evenly distributed and your arms by your sides,
- Keeping your back against the wall, bring your feet out about 12 inches from the wall.
- Keeping your abs tight, lower your body until your knees are bent to about 60 degrees.
- Raise yourself back up to where your knees are slightly bent.
- Do three sets of ten reps.

Sit and Stand

- Sit at the edge of a chair with your feet slightly behind your knees.
- Stand up while keeping your neck and spine erect. Your back should not bend forward.
- Immediately return to a sitting position, but don't put your full weight on the chair.
- Do three sets of ten reps slowly.

#105

Check Your Thyroid–Seriously!

Imagine this: You type the URL of a website (say, just for example, www.jonnybowden.com) into the address bar of your browser. And you wait. And wait. If you're on a PC, the little blue hourglass starts to pour. And pour. If you're on a Mac, the little rainbow wheel of doom starts to rotate. And rotate. (You fellow Mac users know what I'm talking about!)

So what do you do to make your computer go faster?

You learn to type faster!

Sound ridiculous? Well, when it comes to energy, that's what a lot of us do. We take potions, drugs, stimulants, and anything we can find to overcome lethargy, depression, and lack of energy, which is the energy equivalent of learning to type faster on a slow-as-molasses computer. Typing faster is a great idea, but if you're frozen in cyberspace, it ain't gonna get you where you want to go any quicker. For that you need to go to the source of the problem—the computer itself.

In your body, your hormones are like the computer.

If they're not functioning optimally, you can "type" as fast as you like, but it's not going to make any difference. The email isn't going to arrive any quicker, the website won't load any faster, and every so often the screen will freeze. Hormones are the master control center for your body's energy factory. If they're not in tip-top shape, you won't be either.

The sad part of all this is that not all doctors know how to help their patients achieve optimal hormonal functioning and many, even sadder, have no idea what optimal hormonal functioning actually looks like. Physicians can read the chart that tells you whether hormone levels are normal, but falling within a constantly shifting range of lab values for normal hardly tells you whether your levels are optimal. It's like telling you that you make an average income or are of average intelligence. We'd never accept that "diagnosis" in the areas of money or smartness, but we blindly accept it when it comes to our health.

But don't get me started.

HORMONES AND ENERGY: A MARRIAGE MADE IN HEAVEN

A full discussion of the way that various hormones can and do affect your energy levels (not to mention the rest of your health) would fill not one, but many books. It's way beyond the scope of this one.

So I'm going to briefly mention just a few hormones in this chapter that can have really profound effects on your energy, with the caveat that there's a lot more to this than I can possibly cover here. (If I left out your personal favorite hormone, please forgive me. They all work together in a giant, interconnected system, and I couldn't go over all of them. Apologies to the ones such as DHEA, the adrenal hormones, human growth hormone, and all the other fan faves that I omitted to keep this book shorter than *War and Peace*.)

Hormones are the master control center for your body's energy factory. If they're not in tip-top shape, you won't be either.

What I'm hoping is that this information gets you thinking enough so that you dig into hormonal health a little deeper and think twice before blindly accepting a diagnosis of "everything's normal" from your physician, especially when you think it's not.

The Body's Energy Engine

The thyroid is the motor that keeps your energy system running. It's what Richard Shames, M.D., and Karilee Shames, Ph.D., R.N., call "your energy throttle."

"How much energy people have, how well they get up in the morning, how well they sleep, and how much stamina they have for the day is directly related to their levels of thyroid hormone," they say. The Shames ought to know. As the authors of *Thyroid Power*, they're two of the leading experts on thyroid, and they have been sounding the bell as consumer advocates for better thyroid testing for many years.

"As of 2006, experts estimate that as many as 59 million Americans have a thyroid condition, and the vast majority are hypothyroid—and have an underfunctioning, slow, or sluggish thyroid," writes the highly respected Mary Shomon, thyroid expert for about.com. Add the Shames, "This runaway thyroid epidemic seems to be striking menopausal women harder than any other group of patients. By age 50, one in every twelve women has a significant degree of hypothyroidism. By age 60, it is one woman out of every six."

The main hormones released by the thyroid are triiodothyronine, abbreviated as T3, and thyroxine, abbreviated as T4 (the 3 and the 4 refer to the number of iodine molecules in each thyroid hormone molecule, so don't go wondering about where T1 and T2 are; they don't exist). The main job of these hormones is to deliver energy to all the cells of the body. When your thyroid isn't doing its job properly—or when the hormones aren't getting to where they're supposed to get—you wind up with the energy equivalent of that slow-as-molasses computer.

An underperforming thyroid is your worst energy nightmare. According to the Shames and other leading lights in the holistic hormone replacement business, this underperforming thyroid is massively underdiagnosed.

QUESTIONS TO ASK YOUR PHYSICIAN

So why the epidemic of this underdiagnosed energy drainer? Partly it's because the standard tests that everyone uses present, at the very least, a somewhat incomplete picture of what's really happening.

The standard test for thyroid is a blood test for something called TSH (thyroid stimulating hormone). TSH is like the rider on a horse; when you want to go faster, you kick in your heels and give a little slap to the rump of the animal. TSH is the "rump slapper" of the thyroid gland. When levels are low, it cranks up the "giddyaps."

So when TSH levels are high, it's assumed that's because the thyroid is underproducing. Problem is, no one totally agrees on what "good" TSH levels are. Up to 2003, the "normal" range for TSH was 0.5 to 5.5. In 2003, however, the American Association of Clinical Endocrinologists finally recommended narrowing the range to 0.3 to 3, but many labs and physicians have not gotten the message that a TSH of 4 or 5 might indicate a real problem.

Most labs in the United States still use the old range, and in many cases, doctors have deliberately chosen not to follow the new guidelines and will not diagnose low thyroid until they see something in excess of 5, says Shomon. So people with an extremely high TSH of 5 could be told "everything's normal" by their doc, as they drag themselves home wondering why they have no energy.

Shomon and other experts recommend that if your energy levels are low and your doctor says "your TSH is normal," you should ask three critical questions:

1. What was my exact TSH test result number?

2. What is the normal range at the lab where my test results were processed?

3. What normal range do you follow in diagnosing and managing thyroid disease?

RATING THE TEST

The second area of contention is whether the TSH test is sufficient to identify a problem. Many integrative physicians don't think it is.

"We cannot simply rely on TSH or Free T4 blood tests, even though this is the industry standard," Richard Shames says. "Instead, we need to do a more complete panel of blood tests, which would include Total T3, Free T3, and thyroid antibodies."

Antibodies aren't normally requested on a thyroid panel, but if antibodies are high, it may mean your immune system is attacking your thyroid and you may have the autoimmune form of the disorder called Hashimoto's thyroiditis, an energy drainer if there ever was one.

Also, you should know, T4 is actually not an active hormone, but T3 is. About 80 percent or more of the body's output is T4, but for it to actually accomplish anything it needs to convert to the active T3. Problem is, we're finding out that not

everyone does that very well. So you could have perfectly normal levels of T4, but your conversion stinks. Result: Your energy is still in the toilet because your body's not converting enough of the inactive T4 into the energy-enhancing T3.

If your eyes aren't glazed over by now, listen to this: When you're under a lot of stress, the body conserves energy by putting the brakes on conversion of T4 to T3, and instead makes a kind of "dummy" inactive product called *reverse T3*. Now, the testing for reverse T3 is controversial, and specialists debate its value, but there are some practitioners who firmly believe that it is important, and there is even a name for the thyroid malfunction in which your body continues to produce too much reverse T3 and not enough of the "real" thing—Wilson's syndrome.*

The point is, if your energy is chronically low, and you've ruled out all the usual suspects (such as sleeping only three hours a night), get your thyroid tested. But get it tested by someone who knows what he or she is doing—a hormonal specialist who takes a holistic approach. (Quick example: The inactive T4 hormone won't convert to T3 without the important mineral selenium, which is another reason you're better off with a doc who actually knows something about nutrition!)

DO-IT-YOURSELF HORMONE TESTING

Meanwhile, there's a nice, easy, at-home screening test you can do yourself just to see whether there might be a thyroid component to your low energy. Legendary American physician Broda Barnes, M.D., Ph.D., (1904-1988), who spent his life researching and treating endocrine diseases and specialized in

*It's worth pointing out that Wilson's syndrome remains highly controversial and not all medical experts believe in it as a visable diagnosis.

the thyroid, first developed it. It's called the basal temperature test, and here's how to do it:

1. Get yourself a basal thermometer (underarm thermometer), shake it down the night before you use it, and leave it on your bedside table.

2. First thing in the morning, before getting out of bed, tuck the thermometer under your armpit and lay still for about 10 minutes.

3. Record your temperature for at least three days. If you're a woman and menstruating, don't do this during your menstrual cycle.

The normal underarm temperature is between 97.8°F (36.5°C) and 98.2°F (36.7°C). According to Barnes, if your temperature is consistently below this level, get an evaluation. "Be aware," he wrote, "that (thyroid) tests are often normal even though the thyroid gland is malfunctioning. That's because the tests show only how much (hormone) is circulating in the body and tell nothing of how well the hormones are functioning on a cellular level." Barnes also cautioned that you could lose up to 70 percent of thyroid function before the standard tests start showing anything of interest to the average doctor.

So if your energy is in the toilet and you've ruled out everything else—or even if you haven't—find a good hormone doc and get yourself checked.

"The thyroid is the gas pedal for your body's energy flow," says Shames, "but you need fuel and spark for the gas pedal to accomplish anything. Fuel would be optimal nutrients, and supplements add the spark." Supporting the thyroid is not just a way to increase energy, but also a strategy for healthier living.

#106
Harness the Energy Power of Testosterone

When it comes to antiaging clinics touting their high-end programs for reversing aging, increasing energy, upping libido, and generally turning back the clock to a time when your "get up and go" hadn't "gone up and went," human growth hormone (or HGH) gets the lion's share of attention. But as far as I'm concerned, when it comes to hormone replacement for increased energy and overall well-being, testosterone is the king of the hill.

We all know testosterone as the hormonal engine that provides men with the sexual drive needed to guarantee the continuation of the human race. (It's also critical to *female* libido, which is why so many integrative docs who work with hormone replacement now give small amounts to postmenopausal women—it not only increases their libido but also does wonders for their energy. I'm just saying.)

If sexual desire were the only thing that testosterone was responsible for, that would be plenty reason enough to care about it. But testosterone is responsible for far more than just giving your mojo a kick-start. Testosterone is the spark plug that gives men vitality, all the while helping to maintain muscle, skin, bones, sperm production, and immune function. Let's face it: Testosterone gives you energy.

Big time.

THE TESTOSTERONE-ENERGY CONNECTION

Testosterone normally remains high until a man reaches his early thirties. At this point (or somewhat later, if you're lucky), this libidinal lightbulb begins to gradually fade, and, over the next few decades, it will, sadly, continue to decrease.

By the age of seventy, a man typically has half the testosterone he did when he was thirty. Individual differences being what they are, many men lose it more quickly (and some retain pretty high levels well into their sixth decade and beyond—think Hugh Hefner or Sylvester Stallone). Invariably, energy will decline in lockstep with testosterone.

Loss of testosterone used to be accepted as inevitable, as a consequence of aging. But with advances in the science of aging, many thousands of men now enjoy youthful vitality and energy due in part to the increasingly popular (and increasingly sophisticated) therapy of hormone replacement.

"In my ten-year experience doing hormone replacement for both men and women, I've found that the two hormones that significantly increase perceived energy are human growth hormone and testosterone," says my friend David Leonardi, M.D., director of the popular Leonardi Executive Health Institute in Denver, a well-regarded antiaging clinic that routinely provides responsible hormone replacement therapy.

An obvious sign of low testosterone is a decrease in sex drive and other types of sexual difficulties, such as loss of morning erections, but there other signs, loss of energy being prime among them. Others include decreased muscle and bone mass, increased body fat, a decline in cognitive skills such as concentration and memory, and higher cholesterol levels. There is also a notable decline in overall well-being and vigor. Men with reduced testosterone levels are like the Old Gray Mare—they just "ain't what they used to be" in terms of stamina, exercise performance, libido, well-being, or energy.

But it's not just men in Porsche 911s with "midlife crisis" written all over them who experience deficiencies and low energy. Because testosterone is made in the ovaries, women—especially after menopause—suffer from low testosterone levels and have a similar reduction in sex drive and energy. Women might notice symptoms such as droopy eyelids, sagging cheeks, thinning and dry hair, and mild depression. Many of these symptoms are often significantly improved when small amounts of testosterone are added to their hormone replacement regimen.

By the age of seventy, a man typically has half the testosterone he did when he was thirty. Invariably, energy will decline in lockstep with testosterone.

TESTOSTERONE ROBBERS

Because some symptoms are common to other conditions that drain energy, researchers think that low testosterone is a possible contributing factor in chronic fatigue syndrome and fibromyalgia, two other conditions whose defining signature symptom is the loss of energy. In both males and females, chronic fatigue and fibromyalgia are associated with low levels of sex hormones.

The endocrine system is like a giant email chain letter, with one message setting off another in a closely woven matrix of interconnections and chain reactions. Chronic fatigue sufferers, for example, have a disrupted chain of hormonal reactions that begins with cortisol, which in turn can reduce levels of estrogen and testosterone.

Other conditions, from HIV to diabetes to excess body fat, can also provoke a testosterone deficiency. Even medications come into play in this intricate hormonal dance. Cholesterol-lowering medications—specifically Lipitor, Mevacor, Zocor, and Pravachol—are considered "antiandrogenic" and will lower testosterone levels (not to mention conenzyme Q10, a well-known energy spark plug that is invariably diminished with this class of medication).

The moral of the story is that *everything is connected*. (Studies show that when "high-identifying sports fans"—people whose personal identity is intertwined with a sports team—watch their team win, their levels of testosterone rise significantly.) Your body is engaged in a giant game of "Six Degrees of Kevin Bacon." Almost anything you do or don't do, from taking medication to not getting enough nutrients to watching the Lakers lose (if you live in Los Angeles, that is), can have an effect on your hormones, which in turn have an effect on your health.

"These hormones are far reaching in the body," says Leonardi. "There are receptors for testosterone in every organ, from the skeletal muscles to the brain." The end result of low levels—often the symptom you notice first—is a profound loss of energy and vitality.

TEST YOUR TESTOSTERONE LEVELS

Really low levels of testosterone can have serious implications. Deficiencies can increase the risk of heart disease, prostate cancer, and Alzheimer's. When in doubt, take a hormone test. (On a blood test, a testosterone level greater than 70 nanograms per deciliter [ng/dl] is desirable.)

You may also want to consider salivary hormone testing. According to Pamela Wartian Smith, M.D., M.P.H., this type of testing is the best method because it will measure the *bioavailable*—or most active—form of testosterone in the body, not just the free circulating testosterone in the blood.

Salivary testing also provides a perspective of what testosterone levels are doing on a daily basis, whereas a blood test will only measure testosterone levels at one point in time—the time of the test. There are individual variances with any of these options, however, so even if you're asymptomatic, checking testosterone now will help gauge how you're doing down the road.

Smoking, excess alcohol consumption, and drug abuse can reduce testosterone levels, as can stress. Household chemicals and environmental toxins such as pesticides have all demonstrated antitestosterone effects, another reason to do a detox from time to time.

Because zinc is needed for the metabolism of testosterone, make sure that you have at least the recommended daily amount of 18 mg in your diet. (But don't exceed more than 50 mg per day as a supplement on a regular basis). Foods such as seafood (especially oysters), meat, eggs, and black-eyed peas all contain zinc.

One obvious way to increase low levels of testosterone is through responsible* hormone replacement therapy. (Don't confuse responsible, physician-monitored, physiological doses of hormones you may be low in with the kind of thing you read about when sports figures are caught using testosterone and human growth hormone along with the more garden variety steroids. These guys are getting stuff illegally and using massive amounts—a very different situation from what I'm talking about here.)

Testosterone replacement therapy is not terribly expensive, and it gives you an enormous bang for your buck in terms of improved energy (not to mention mojo). "Since it increases lean muscle mass and accelerates fat loss, that would increase energy as well," adds Leonardi. "By increasing lean muscle mass, you raise your metabolic rate."

Leonardi adds that it would be criminal not to point out that low-glycemic nutrition and exercise are both key factors in getting the full benefit from hormone replacement therapy.

HOW TO NATURALLY BOOST TESTOSTERONE

There are also some natural ways to impact testosterone, though admittedly the effect is not nearly as profound as with replacement therapy. One way to get a quick boost of testosterone is simply by exercising. A study in the *Journal of Strength and Conditioning Research* reported that 30 minutes of treadmill running increased testosterone by

27 percent, with levels returning to normal 30 minutes after the run.

Weight lifting is also beneficial. I remember back in the 80s a popular bodybuilding method was the Bulgarian system, which was based on doing two fairly short (under 45 minutes) heavy workouts a day. It was predicated on the belief (probably accurate) that this was the way to get the largest increase in testosterone in the shortest amount of time. Protein shakes are a nice idea as well. They include key amino acids for testosterone production: arginine, leucine, and glutamine.

If, after all, you decide to try testosterone therapy, do it in partnership with a responsible, experienced physician who knows about hormone replacement therapy. Remember that replacing diminished sex hormones is a form of steroid treatment and can have unwanted side effects.

Using natural, as opposed to synthetic, hormones can greatly decrease the risks involved. Natural testosterone can be prescribed as a pill, a cream, injections, or a patch. According to the *Journal of Urology*, dermal patches best approximate the natural cycles of testosterone release, though this opinion is not unanimously held. (Many experienced physicians, including Leonardi, prefer the shots, which aren't as scary as they sound.)

Note: To get an idea of whether you're deficient in testosterone, try this quiz from St. Louis University: www.slu.edu/adam/maletquiz.pdf.

*Responsible as in "administered by a conscientious physician" as opposed to "bought in a pharmacy in Tijuana and given to me by my trainer at the gym."

#107

Balance Your Estrogen Levels

I'll never forget attending a seminar by the great Jeffrey Bland, Ph.D., on the topic of balancing female hormones with nutrition. Bland started the eight-hour workshop with this comment: "We're here to talk about female hormones today, and we only have eight hours so we'll only scratch the surface." He then paused for effect. "If the subject were male hormones, we'd be outta here in 45 minutes."

If you think women are the more complicated sex, welcome to the club.

It would be difficult to explain the effects that estrogen has on energy without a little background, so please indulge me a bit. Just for openers, there are three different kinds of estrogen (more on that later). Estrogen has about 400 different functions in the human body. (Did you get that? *Four hundred.*)

Among other important jobs, it increases metabolism, works as a sleep aid, enhances energy, and decreases depression and anxiety. It regulates the menstrual cycle and promotes cell division. It lifts mood and promotes a feeling of well-being. Estrogen is produced primarily in the ovaries and the adrenal glands, but the body has receptor sites for it everywhere—in the brain, muscles, bone, bladder, gut, uterus, ovaries, vagina, breast, heart, lungs, and blood vessels. Estrogen is ubiquitous in the human body. (And yes, men have it, too.)

UNBALANCED ESTROGEN IS AN ENERGY DRAIN

In hormones, as in Goldilock's porridge, it's all about balance: not too high, and not too low, but just right. An imbalance in either direction (too high or too low) can set off a number of reactions and subsequent conditions ranging from the semi-mild to the very serious (the bumper sticker "I'm out of estrogen and I have a gun" says it all).

Too much estrogen, particularly the wrong kind of metabolites, can increase the risk for hormone-dependent cancers. Too little estrogen may increase the risk for osteoporosis. Hormone balance is the key to reducing breast and other cancers, halting menopausal symptoms, reducing body fat, and maintaining libido.

One of the hallmark signs of a low estrogen state is hot flashes, but there are other symptoms, including a fatigued feeling that gets worse as the day goes on. Because fatigue is such a frequent accompaniment to our busy lives, many women might ignore this symptom altogether, or attribute it to another cause, with the result that a suboptimal estrogen level goes unchecked and untreated.

Low estrogen can be and frequently is linked to all sorts of conditions. A short sample list: poor sleep, depression and anxiety (probably due to low serotonin levels), interstitial cystitis, and PMS. Low estrogen levels can raise LDL cholesterol (the horribly named "bad" cholesterol) and lower HDL ("good" cholesterol). Women with a low estrogen level also tend to have low blood pressure, thin hair, and poor memory.

The Good, the Bad, and the Weak

Most of us recognize estrogen as one female hormone, but the word *estrogen* is actually the name of the *family* of hormones that make up estrogen. There are three members of that natural family: estrone, estradiol, and estriol. To make matters more complicated, these subcategories of estrogen have various metabolites with names you probably don't even want to think about. (Samples: 2-hydroxyl estradiol and 17 beta-estradiol. I warned you.)

Estrone is the main estrogen that the body makes after menopause. Many researchers believe that this estrogen may be the hormone related to an increased risk of breast and uterine cancer. The more body fat you have, the more estrone you make. Frequent alcohol consumption can also keep estrone levels higher than desired.

Estradiol is the strongest of the three estrogens. It is the main estrogen that gets produced *before* menopause. Estradiol, among a load of other responsibilities, helps increase serotonin levels (serotonin keeps you calm and happy), improves sleep quality, decreases fatigue, and helps maintain a healthy cholesterol profile.

The third estrogen, *estriol*, is a weaker estrogen, but it has been shown to be protective against breast cancer. Estriol's benefits are in the digestive tract and in controlling all those annoying symptoms of menopause, including hot flashes, insomnia, and vaginal dryness.

But the term *estrogen* can also include other estrogenic *compounds*, such as animal estrogens, synthetic estrogens, phytoestrogens (plant estrogens), and xenoestrogens (environmental estrogens). All of these estrogens play a role in the management of energy to varying degrees, and this role becomes even more important as we get older.

Your job is to ensure you have the right combination of the three natural estrogens, and eat the kinds of foods that act as "traffic cops," sending estrogen metabolism down the good pathways and away from the potentially carcinogenic ones (think: broccoli).

You also want to manage your exposure to environmental estrogens by making good lifestyle (and dietary) choices, which is your best prescription for decreasing menopausal symptoms, not to mention protecting against disease and decreasing fatigue.

BONE TIRED FROM LOW ESTROGEN

Once a women hits menopause around the age of fifty and estrogen levels are not checked, some symptoms may get even worse. When estrogen levels drop, they have a negative effect on another hormone—the stress hormone cortisol. (Paradoxically, too *much* cortisol can *lower* your estrogen levels.)

The combination of low estrogen and constantly elevated cortisol may lead to a condtion called crashing fatigue. Crashing fatigue is a common and disturbing symptom of menopause. It makes women feel deeply exhausted even though they haven't made any physical effort. Similar to chronic fatigue, crashing fatigue can be debilitating as overall stamina declines and is worsened by physical or mental activity. It's an endless feeling of tiredness, all because natural levels of estrogens have declined. Bye-bye energy.

Because the symptoms can be so varied, it may be beneficial to keep a symptom log to determine whether low estrogen levels are the contributor to a lack of energy. Some signs to look for include panic attacks, migraines, and palpitations that occur for one to two days around ovulation or around menstruation. For those with chronic fatigue or fibromyalgia, be on the alert: If symptoms are worse the week before a period—or if there is decreased vaginal lubrication—low estrogen is most likely the culprit.

ESTROGEN DOMINANCE

On the other side of the coin are the problems with *elevated* estrogen. When estrogen levels are too high, you're looking at anxiety, weight gain, water retention, headaches, poor quality sleep, and fatigue. Certainly nothing likely to boost your energy.

How can you wind up with too much estrogen? It's not hard. We're accustomed to thinking of declining levels of estrogen as an accompaniment of aging. It seems counterintuitive that estrogen levels might rise as we age. But in fact, this somewhat weird paradox probably happens more often than you might think.

How can this be? It's certainly not because women are producing more estrogen internally. Rather, it's because our environment is now chock-full of weird chemicals and compounds that actually act like estrogen. There's even a term for them—estrogenic mimics. These estrogenic compounds, sometimes also called *hormone disrupters*, are all over the place (one recently discovered source is plastics). And they can be fiendishly difficult to get rid of. Many women (and men!) have a difficult time eliminating these exogenous (outside the body) estrogens because of damaged metabolisms and sluggish livers. Nutritionists and researchers call this condition *estrogen dominance*.

THE YIN AND YANG OF ESTROGEN

One of the results of estrogen dominance is fatigue. Here's how it works: Estrogen is what's known as a pro-growth hormone because it stimulates activity. But like everything in the body, it has a counterbalancing force, which in this case is another hormone, *progesterone*.

Progesterone works antagonistically with estrogen to maintain homeostasis, or balance. (Remember the Goldilocks mantra: not too hot, not too cold.) When estrogen increases during the menstrual cycle, progesterone decreases. When estrogen decreases, progesterone increases, in a lovely hormonal version of a seesaw. They work in perfect harmony throughout each month, or at least they do *theoretically.* (I have some friends with severe PMS who might argue differently, as would their husbands and boyfriends.)

Everything moves along pretty swimmingly until around age thirty-five or so. Somewhere around this point or later, at the start of what's called perimenopause, estrogen and progesterone both begin to decline. In an ideal world, they would decline at the same levels, to maintain that optimal ratio, but like most situations that start out with the preface "in an ideal world," this rarely happens. In fact, while estrogen levels will decline about 35 percent through menopause, progesterone levels will take a virtual nosedive, declining a whopping 75 percent. That peaceful seesaw starts to look like one side has a two-year-old on it and the other side has an elephant.

Perimenopause can last anywhere from two to ten years, and although most women may notice some symptoms, they are often told by their oh-so-helpful doctors that there is really nothing that can be done about them. "It's just the way it is" is a common refrain. The less sensitive have been known to mumble under their breaths, "Oh, just live with it!"

To make matters worse, many doctors only check blood levels of estrogen (if they check blood levels at all, something they unfortunately don't always do). Assuming symptoms are simply caused by declining estrogen, many will recommend birth control pills as a way of raising estrogen levels. This may provide some temporary and much-needed relief from symptoms but can further upset a rapidly devolving delicate balance. Over time, synthetic drugs such as birth control pills may further deplete women of necessary nutrients and can ultimately create even more hormonal imbalances.

By menopause, the total amount of progesterone made is extremely low, while estrogen is still present in the body at about half its premenopausal level. Estrogen dominance is the result, and the effects are rarely pretty.

HEAVE THE HORMONE DISRUPTERS

It gets worse. Remember those estrogen mimics we talked about? Commercially raised cattle and poultry are loaded with them. They're in the very food eaten by the livestock that aren't pasture fed and organic, meaning they make their way into the meat we eat as well (yet another in the hundred or so reasons I keep urging anyone who will listen to try to eat only grass-fed meat. I know it's more expensive—just eat less of it!).

Pesticide residues have chemical structures that are similar to those of estrogen, making them estrogen mimics; we sometimes refer to them as *xenoestrogens* (xeno meaning "foreign"). Produce known to contain the highest levels of pesticides are strawberries, peppers, apples, spinach, and celery. And xenoestrogens are all over the place, not just in our food: they're also found in plastics, nail polish, cosmetics, glues, and adhesives, as well as dioxin-containing foods such as the aforementioned meat, milk, eggs, and fish.

Both caffeine and alcohol can raise estrogen levels. Ovarian cysts or tumors can and do make extra estrogen. Stress will ultimately *reduce* progesterone levels.* (Stress overall can do much damage to *many* hormonal systems that are regulated through the adrenal glands.) Too much stress and a reduction in progesterone will further upset the delicate estrogen/progesterone balance. When this happens, we experience insomnia, anxiety, and an even greater depletion of energy.

*According to Robert Sapolsky, Ph.D., too much stress can also reduce estrogen.

BALANCE YOUR ESTROGEN, BALANCE YOUR LIFE

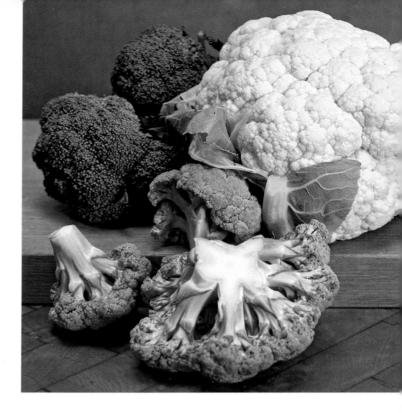

Even a cursory reading of the above material makes it clear that balancing hormones in a healthy way can be a real challenge. But it's absolutely essential to having a ton of energy. No kidding. And there are lots of lifestyle guidelines that women can follow to minimize the onslaught of some of the unhealthy estrogens.

Fill up on fiber. A plant-based, unprocessed, whole-food diet is the best diet for a healthy metabolism and healthy hormonal balance. Try to include *at least* 20 grams of fiber each day, through flaxseeds, fresh fruits and vegetables, and even fiber supplements. The fiber will help you metabolize excess estrogens. If you eat animal products, including dairy, make sure they are organic and free of hormones as well as pesticides.

Drink plenty of filtered water to help your body eliminate excess toxins and environmental estrogens. Avoid high-glycemic foods such as refined sugar, and alcohol or drugs that can damage the liver, which will lead to an increase in estrogen due to the lack of estrogen breakdown.

Choose lots of cruciferous veggies such as Brussels sprouts, broccoli, cauliflower, cabbage, kale, and soy. These foods, all of which (except for soy) are in the brassica family, are vegetable royalty. They contain phytoestrogens, compounds that are similar in structure to estrogen but much, much weaker in potency. Which is a good thing. Phytoestrogens occupy the "parking spots" reserved for estrogen (called estrogen receptors), but with much less bioactivity. By occupying the estrogen receptor sites on cell membranes, they

essentially block the stronger, natural estrogen from occupying the space. Those who have estrogen dominance may therefore experience relief of symptoms and a renewed sense of energy.

These foods pack a double whammy. All members of the cabbage family contain plant chemicals called *indoles*, which actually act as estrogen traffic cops, helping to direct estrogen metabolism down the pathways to the less harmful metabolites—such as the innocuous 2-hydroxy-estrone—rather than the much more potent 16-hydroxy-estrone, an estrogen metabolite that can be a real problem, especially in hormone-dependent cancers.

Helpful Supplements

The best way to increase energy depletion that has been the result of an estrogen imbalance is to support the liver in detoxifying some of the environmental estrogens. Below is a list of some supplements that are helpful:

DIM: Diindolylmethane, or DIM, is an isolated substance found in cruciferous vegetables that balances estrogen levels. (It's actually a refined, improved version of one of the indoles, or estrogen traffic cops, mentioned above.) DIM increases the good, protective form of estrone (2-hydroxy-estrone) while also raising progesterone levels when necessary. DIM also induces certain liver enzymes to block the production of the toxic estrogens and enhance the production of the beneficial forms. A recommended amount is 70 to 400 mg per day.

Calcium D-glucarate: Calcium D-glucarate is found in all fruits and vegetables, with the highest concentrations in apples, grapefruit, and broccoli. This is one of the most important nutrients to help enhance liver function, so it will help rid the body of toxins and remove excess estrogens and xenoestrogens. The suggested dose is 250 to 1,000 mg per day.

Liver support nutrients: Antioxidants, such as alpha-lipoic acid, N-acetyl-cysteine, and silymarin (the active ingredient in milk thistle), help clear estrogen from the liver and support the detoxification process.

Grapeseed extract: Grapeseed extract contains proanthycyanidins (PCOs), which are powerful antioxidant nutrients from the bioflavonoid family of plant compounds. By scavenging free radicals, PCOs can help fortify an important part of the liver detoxification process, increasing estrogen clearance.

Green tea extract: Green tea extract (known as EGCG, for epigallo-catechingallate) is a powerful antioxidant. It increases the detoxification of carcinogens and even increases the activity of other antioxidants. (See page 129 for more information.)

Curcumin (turmeric): Curcumin is the yellow pigment of turmeric—one of the chief ingredients in curry. It is a powerful anti-inflammatory and antioxidant agent that works to inhibit all steps of cancer formation—initiation, promotion, and progression. Curcumin also helps eliminate cancer-causing estrogens and environmental toxins. The recommended dosage is 50 to 100 mg per day.

I know people, both regular folks and doctors, whose practices center around responsible hormone replacement therapy, who swear that correctly balancing hormones is the absolutely most important thing you can do for yourself to increase your energy (and sense of overall well-being). Don't underestimate the roles of these hormones. Figuring out what you need to do regarding the restoration of hormonal balance, and then doing it, may be the biggest energy booster of them all.

Get rid of the xenoestrogens. Reducing reliance on plastics and pesticide-laden foods, and eating plenty of organic vegetables, will ensure that you are also reducing the xenoestrogen load. Water in plastic bottles can contain residues of polycarbonate plastics called phthalates, which are clear endocrine disrupters. Pure water is a must if you're trying to decrease your exposure to xenoestrogens. Unfortunately, grabbing any old bottled water doesn't guarantee that you're getting anything good; the rules governing the regulation of all water sources are more complicated than a 750-page government manual. Just do some due diligence and get the best water you can afford, or install a reverse-osmosis filter (RO) system in your home.

Maintain an ideal body weight. Fat cells increase estrogen production. We used to think that fat was just this inert, passive substance whose only purpose was to sit on your hips and thighs and annoy you. But it's way more complicated than that. We now know that fat is an endocrine organ, and fat cells release all kinds of compounds, including hormones, and especially including estrogen. They're little estrogen factories (which may be part of the reason we're seeing puberty so early these days, especially in overweight kids). So do as much as you can to lose the fat.

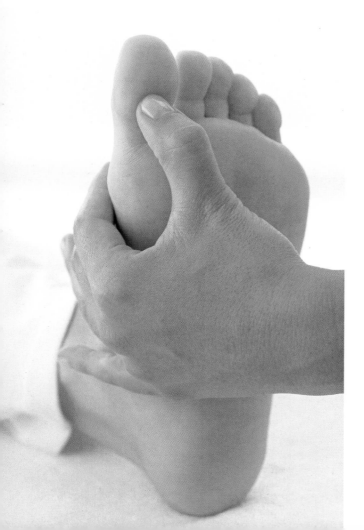

#108

Have Your Map Read

Reflexology is a hands-on healing art based on ancient Chinese therapy. Like acupressure, it works with the body's energy flow to promote self-healing and maintain balance. The practice involves the manipulation of certain areas of the foot (and sometimes the hands and ears) that are believed to correspond to specific parts of the body. By alleviating muscle tension and stress, reflexology can leave you feeling energized.

"The theory of reflexology is based on a kind of map of the human body," explains Bill Flocco, one of the leading practitioners of reflexology in the United States. "Imagine dividing the body into ten wide vertical strips—one for the thumb and big toe, all the way over to one for the small toe and small fingers. Then imagine a similar division into horizontal zones. The reflexologist determines where the stress in the body is and then goes to work on the corresponding zones for the hands, ears, and feet."

For instance, the ball and pad of the foot relate to the chest, and the soft sole of the foot corresponds to the upper abdomen. When the reflexologist applies a particular kind of nurturing touch and pressure to these areas, says Flocco, "the nerve pathways go directly to the brain and then outward to a specific part of the body that corresponds to that area of the hands, feet, or ears." The result, he explains, is a cascade of chemical events that alleviate stress and pain and frequently increase energy.

"The nerves become soothed, and as nerves become soothed, muscles relax. As muscles relax, circulation improves, capillaries open up, and more blood is carried to the cells of the body," says Flocco.

All of this is good news if you want to see your energy boosted. "More oxygen and nutrition are taken to the cells, and as the cells get more oxygen and nutrition they're better able to produce the thousands of chemicals, including endorphins, that are carried around the body and that support the healing process."

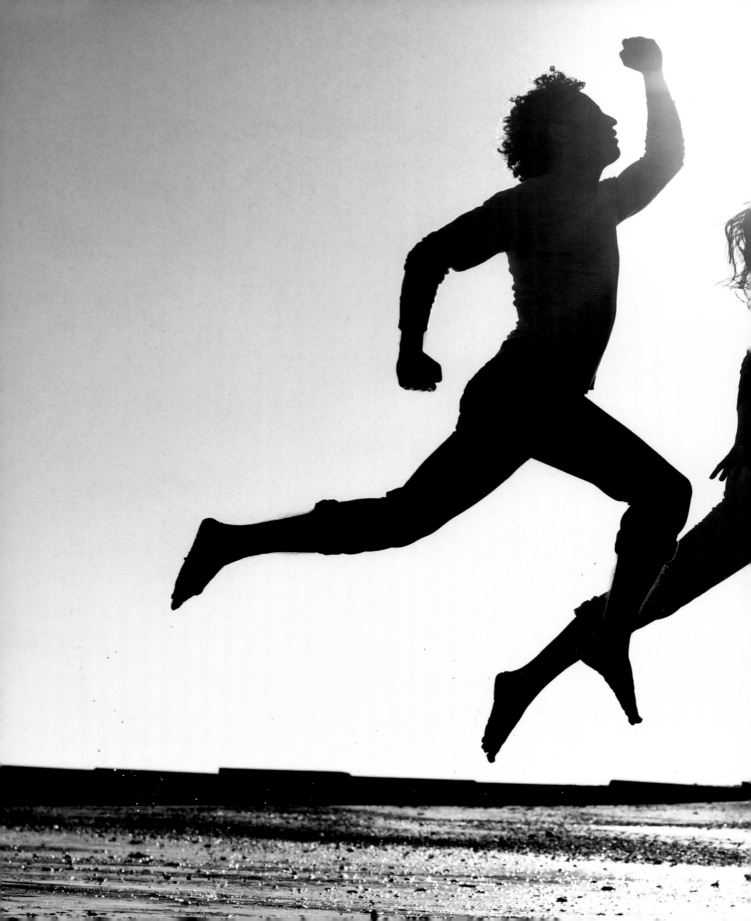

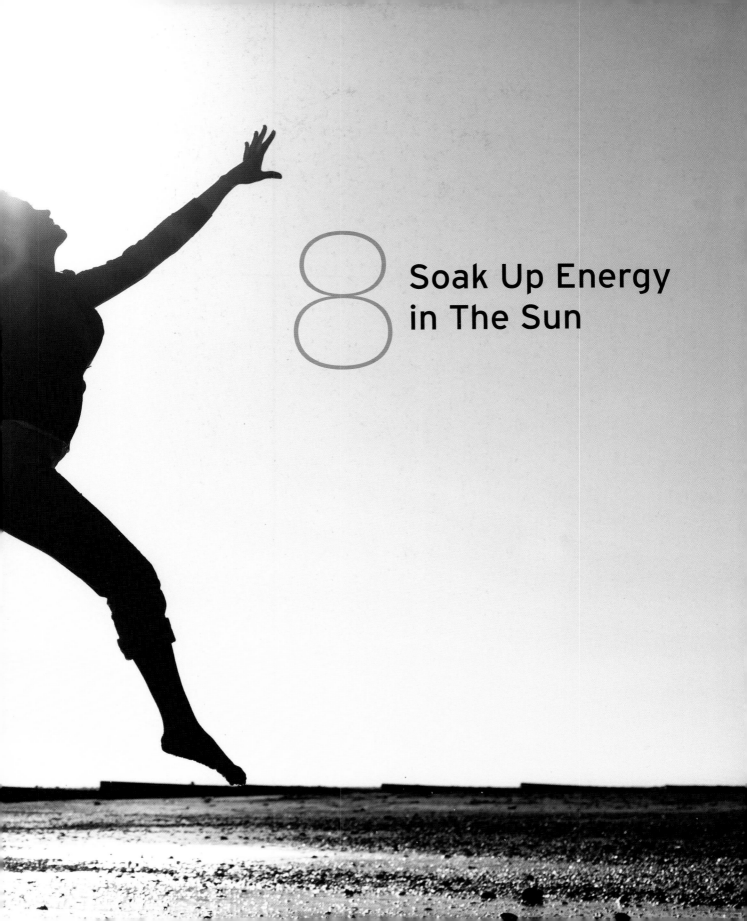

8 Soak Up Energy in The Sun

I call sunshine the underappreciated energy vitamin.

In fact, it's more than underappreciated. In some circles, it's downright underdiscovered. We avoid it at every potential encounter, slathering 45 SPF all over our bodies if we even have to venture out for a bottle of milk. We act as if 5 minutes of exposure is going to condemn us to a lifetime of wrinkles and skin cancer. We treat the sun as our mortal enemy. And we're paying the price—in energy and in health.

It's time to rethink our relationship with this brightly burning star.

YOUR OWN SOLAR ENERGY TRANSFUSION

The sun has been providing energy for about five billion years (and scientists figure it's got at least another five billion to go, just in case you were worried). The sun's energy drives the water cycle—rain and snow—and it drives the winds. The sun is the source of our weather.

Remember photosynthesis? In case you forgot, it means that plants get their energy from the sun.

Maybe you should, too.

"The sun gives you strength, lifts your spirits, and is a source of energy," says my friend, Al Sears, M.D., C.N.S., author of *Your Best Health Under the Sun.* Like a growing body of health experts, Sears thinks we've become so sun phobic that we're missing out on the myriad mood-boosting and energy-enhancing benefits that the sunshine vitamin has to offer. Part of the key to these benefits is vitamin D (see page 213), but part of the benefits also come from the naturally energizing light and its ability to help counter the depression and mood changes that are so common when daylight is shorter or sun exposure is minimal (see page 215).

In this section, you'll learn about some of the energy-enhancing properties of the sun and how to harness the powers of this undiscovered (okay, underappreciated) vitamin for your own personal energy transfusion in a perfectly safe way. Nope, you won't get skin cancer (if you follow the recommendations carefully), and no, you won't turn into a wrinkled mess.

But you just might feel a lot more energetic than you have in years.

#109

Get 10 Minutes of Sun Every Day

So now that we've established (I hope) that some sunlight will boost your energy, the question on everybody's lips is: How much?

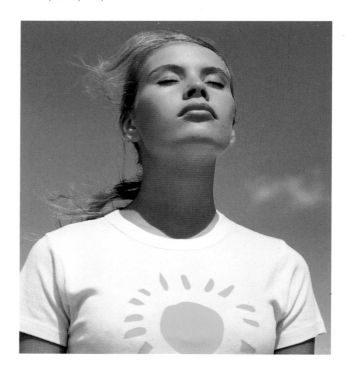

First of all, let me be perfectly clear: I am not advocating a return to the days of basking in the sun drenched in baby oil. There's no doubt that chronic, excessive exposure to sunlight can increase the risk of basal or squamous cell cancer (non-melanoma skin cancers that are rarely fatal). We all know that long periods of exposure to the harsh sun, particularly during the noonday hours and especially without sun protection, is not a smart thing to do. We don't want our skin to age. We don't want all those wrinkles. And we certainly don't want to get skin cancer, not even the nonfatal kind!

So I'm not saying that sun protection isn't important; what I *am* saying is that we've gone so far overboard that we've become sun phobic, and that's starting to increase some of the health risks that come when your body doesn't get enough sun and therefore doesn't make enough vitamin D.

First things first: it's virtually impossible to get enough vitamin D from your diet alone. Very few foods contain vitamin D; it's mostly in oily fish such as salmon (wild, not farm-raised) and mackerel, which you'd have to eat three to five times a week to get your vitamin D requirement. Cod liver oil is another good source, but let's face it, most people aren't going to run out and buy cod liver oil, let alone start taking it every day!

EMBRACE THE SUN SENSIBLY

So what do we do about it? Simple. We get *sensible sunlight*.

Think about it: We evolved in sunlight, points out Michael Holick, M.D., Ph.D., a recognized expert on vitamin D and the author of *The UV Advantage*. We were bathed in sunlight; we feel better in sunlight. And sunlight provides us with a gift, which is vitamin D. We can use the sun's power to generate activated vitamin D in our bodies, which can help protect against various kinds of cancer and other diseases. We're also finding it may also help regulate insulin, which is a huge factor in diabetes and obesity. And it can definitely help with mood and energy.

Here's another thing to think about: Ever notice how you have a lot of energy-draining muscle aches and pains during the winter? And how a lot of people attribute that to the cold weather? Well, vitamin D is very important to muscle function. People who are vitamin D deficient are prone to muscle weakness, more likely to fall, and more likely to experience bone fractures.

So how much sun are we talking about? What could you do right now to harness the power of the sun to improve your life, your health, and your well-being? Well, it depends a lot on the pigment of your skin and where you live. Holick says that for most Caucasians who live where there is sunlight, exposing about 10 percent of your body for 5 to 10 minutes two or three times a week is enough to get your vitamin D requirement. Dark-skinned people and people who live in the northern latitudes need more. (After that, put on the sunscreen and relax!)

The sun offers life. It offers the ability to make a life-enhancing vitamin that most people are deficient in, and it offers the ability to regulate "feel-good" chemicals in the brain so that your sense of well-being and happiness is improved, along with your energy! The bottom line: Don't be sun phobic.

#110

Try Light Therapy

Light affects the receptors in the brain that produce serotonin, the "feel-good" chemical. When you have low levels of that "happy" neurochemical serotonin, you're usually not very energetic. Instead, quite the opposite. You're cranky, subject to cravings, feeling down, and generally not a lot of fun to be around.

Easily fixable with some light therapy.

Here's how it works. When you don't get exposed to light—I'm not talking fake florescent light here, I'm talking what's called *full-spectrum light*, like you get from the sun (or from the machines mentioned below)—you're probably not making enough serotonin. And if you're not making enough serotonin, your energy suffers. It only takes about 30 minutes a day of exposure to full-spectrum light to get a nice energy-boosting dose, and you can certainly get that at a time when the sun doesn't do any real damage to your skin.

We've already established that the sun is good for you for a whole host of reasons (see page 210). But maybe you're in a place or a season where there really isn't much access to the sun, or maybe it's too cold out, or maybe I still haven't persuaded you that getting some daily sun is a good idea. That's fine; there are other alternatives.

CAN'T GET OUT? BRING THE LIGHT TO YOU!

The Circadian Lighting Association, formed in 1993, is an international association of reputable manufacturers that supply lights for circadian applications, including improving winter mood. "I've recommended these kinds of light machines to my clients for years," says nutritionist to the stars and antiaging guru Oz Garcia, Ph.D.

Light boxes have been well tested and have been shown to help people with depression (and, by extension, with energy). These are rectangular fixtures that house several fluorescent tubes. They have been around for about ten years and have proven very effective. Light boxes come in different sizes and styles. Most experts feel that a 10,000-lux* light box is best, but smaller 5,000-lux light boxes can work, too, although they require more time to be beneficial.

If you travel a lot, a **light visor** may be more practical. It's a head-mounted light source that looks something like a tennis visor. The visor is designed to give people mobility during light sessions and portability for travel situations. It's been on the market for a number of years and has proven very effective for many people. Because of its efficient design—it puts the light source nearer to your eyes, explains Kirk Renaud, CEO of BioBrite—it requires only 3,000 lux to produce benefits comparable to a 10,000-lux light box.

Then there's the **desk light**. No ordinary desk lamp, this one. Rather, it's a special extra-bright version that functions much like a light box. The desk lamp model can produce 10,000 lux if it is oriented properly to the eyes, and its design can be less obtrusive for office use.

For more information on the different types of light machines, log on to the website of the Circadian Lighting Association (www.claorg.org). One company I've found that consistently produces great products in all these categories is BioBrite, located in Bethesda, Maryland, which you can find at www.BioBrite.com.

The metric unit of measure for illuminance of a surface is called lux.

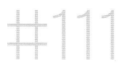

Take Vitamin D for Peak Performance

Recently, a nutritional newsletter I subscribe to had the following headline:

"Vitamin D Improves Physical Performance."

That got my attention.

I've long felt that vitamin D is one of the most underrated vitamins on the planet, for reasons I'll discuss in a bit. I've also long felt that most of us are far too sun phobic for our own good, as the sun is our best source of vitamin D.

But as great as I think both sunlight and vitamin D are for health and for the prevention of disease, I wouldn't have spent all this time on them in this book if they didn't also have an important connection to energy. Three recent studies indicate that they do.

A STUDY IN EFFECTIVENESS

One 2005 study by Netherlands researchers, reported at the American Society of Mineral and Bone Research's 27th annual meeting in Nashville, showed that low levels of vitamin D were associated with low physical performance.

"This study shows that neuromuscular performance in (people) with lower levels of vitamin D was significantly lower than those with adequate levels," said Ilse Wicherts, a doctoral candidate at the Vu University Medical Center in Amsterdam, and one of the researchers on the study. "The change in performance scores with increasing serum (vitamin D) was significant," she said.

Granted, this study was done on older people, where physical performance is a matter of some urgency; the folks whose physical performance is impaired literally can't get up out of a chair without help. But there's no reason to think that the effect of vitamin D that they demonstrated in this older population doesn't happen with young 'uns as well. Why would it not?

Even more recently, researchers writing in the *Journals of Gerontology Series A: Biological Sciences and Medical Sciences* analyzed data from a study known as the InChianti study (Invecchiare in Chianti, Italy). The InChianti study is a large, population-based study of older people aimed at identifying risk factors for late life disability, something every one of us wants to avoid like the plague.

The study looked at more than 1,000 participants aged sixty-five and older in the Chianti area of Italy. It found that vitamin D status was inversely associated with poor physical performance. Those with the lowest levels of vitamin D performed the worst on a battery of physical performance tests, including handgrip strength, balance, and the like. Those with the highest levels performed the best. Interestingly, nearly 30 percent of the sample had vitamin D levels that would be considered deficient. We can only guess at how many had vitamin D levels that were less than optimal.

SPRING TO LIFE WITH VITAMIN D

Although the effect of vitamin D on physical performance is documented, you might think we'd have to play connect-the-dots to make any assumptions or reach any conclusions about energy and well-being. But we don't. Researchers writing in the prestigious *Nutrition Journal* specifically investigated the effect of vitamin D supplements on well-being.

First, they gathered outpatients in an endocrinology clinic who, by any measure, had levels of vitamin D in their blood lower than what is considered desirable by even the most conservative estimates. Current opinion is that desirable vitamin D concentrations should *exceed* 70 nmol/L, and these folks had levels of less than 61 in spring and summer, and those levels were expected to drop to concentrations of less than 40 by the winter. They gave the participants one of two doses of vitamin D supplements—either 600 IUs per day or 4,000 IUs per day.

The subjects were asked to fill out the Seasonal Health Questionnaire, a standard instrument to screen for seasonal affective disorder, as well as an additional ten questions that functioned as a well-being questionnaire, which could easily have been labeled an "energy" questionnaire, since well-being is pretty much a synonym for energy and vitality. They answered the following questions both before the start of the supplementation program and after the completion of the three-month research project.

1. Has your general health been less than average lately?
2. Have you felt less rested upon waking from sleep lately?
3. Have you experienced a down feeling or inappropriate guilt?
4. Have you felt less socially active lately?
5. Have you been indecisive lately?
6. Have you felt less productive or less creative lately?
7. Has your appetite increased or decreased?
8. Have you experienced any cravings for carbohydrates (bread, pasta, rice, sugary foods) more than normal?
9. Has it been more difficult to deal with daily stress?
10. Have you felt irritable or anxious lately?

The well-being score for this part of the study was simply the total number of "yes" responses. The lower the score, the better the well-being.

Both vitamin D groups exhibited highly statistically significant (meaning dramatic, and almost definitely *not* coincidental) improvement in well-being. The response was greater with the *higher* dose of vitamin D than with the lower dose, but there was improvement with both doses. The only group that did *not* improve was a subgroup of participants who had been consuming the higher dosage (4,000 IUs) since the previous year, and that's because they were already so high on the well-being scale to begin with.

In case you're wondering, the authors clearly state that, based on a ton of research, "vitamin D consumption in the amount of 4,000 IUs per day is safe and physiologic for adults." Did I mention that the current Recommended Daily Allowance is 400 IUs? (Actually, I didn't. I just wanted to make sure you were paying attention.)

SUN OR SUPPLEMENT

So the connection between vitamin D, energy, and well-being is pretty clear. Patients in the northern United States who show up at doctors' offices with diffuse musculoskeletal symptoms have low levels of the vitamin in their blood. Women in Saudi Arabia who have low back pain do, too (and they respond well to supplementation of what we would consider a very high level of vitamin D—5,000 to 10,000 IUs per day). Depression scores in the northern latitudes are worst between December and February, when vitamin D levels are at their lowest. And one study of healthy students concluded that as little as 400 to 800 IUs of vitamin D supplementation per day for only five days during the winter improved mood.

Given that many of us don't actually go in the sun at all or don't have a lot of access to it, I think it makes sense to take a vitamin D supplement. In fact, I think it's a no-brainer. Not only can it improve your energy and performance, but it clearly has anticancer activity as well. And most of us are massively deficient.

Here's something else to think about, particularly if you're overweight. Vitamin D is stored in your body fat, so if you have enough of it in your cellular bank account, you can always release it when you need it, such as in the winter. But in obese people, vitamin D gets sucked into the fat cells and it can't get out. Research by Michael Holick, M.D., Ph.D., of Boston University Medical Center, suggests that because of this, overweight people are much more prone to vitamin D deficiency; their vitamin D bank account system just doesn't work as well. So if you are overweight, that's all the more reason why you should supplement with an even higher dose of vitamin D if you want to get all the great-anticancer fighting benefits of this vitamin.

You can give your energy and your health a boost with a daily does of vitamin D. I conservatively recommend 1,000 IUs a day (but truth be told, I take 2,000 IUs). Best of all, they're tiny supplements and easy to swallow, and even the best brands, including the ones I carry on www.jonnybowden.com, are dirt cheap.

Beat SAD with These Six Tips

When I lived in New York City, come January, I noticed a significant drop in my energy. This wasn't exactly helped by having to take my three beloved dogs down twenty-five flights in an elevator to walk them three times a day in absolutely dismal, freezing, windy, February weather when it got dark around noon. (Okay, I exaggerate, but that's what it felt like.)

Turns out I was far from alone in feeling that significant winter drop in energy.

Come the gloomy months of winter, lots of people walk around like the living dead, not really knowing why. For an estimated 10 million Americans, the short, dark days of winter bring a cloud of depression. Turns out there's a reason, and it's named Seasonal Affective Disorder, or SAD. SAD typically begins in fall and ends in spring with the return of longer, sunnier days. People who live in northern climates are at higher risk for SAD. And let me tell you—SAD can and does drain your energy like nobody's business.

Symptoms of SAD include:

- Depression
- Fatigue
- Lack of interest in normal activities
- Loss of energy
- Increased sleep
- Feelings of hopelessness
- Social withdrawal
- Lethargy
- Carbohydrate cravings
- Weight gain
- Difficulty concentrating

Okay, granted, some of those symptoms can come from other causes, but don't discount the possibility that the drop in energy you're feeling in the winter months is directly correlated to the lack of sunlight. As seasons change and days become shorter, lack of sunlight disrupts the circadian rhythms, and it hits some people a lot worse than others. The disruption of the body's internal clock can lead to depression.

Melatonin, a hormone that helps regulate our sleep-wake cycle (see page 82), is usually released at night when darkness falls. It's turned off by sunlight. That balance is very important. If there's no sunlight—or greatly reduced sunlight—melatonin doesn't get the memo to turn off production, and higher melatonin levels make it harder to get out of bed. Also, reduced sunlight can lead to a drop in serotonin levels, which, in turn, can lead to depression.

HELP IS ON THE WAY

What to do, what to do? Try these tips to combat SAD:

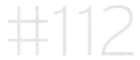

Take vitamin D

Some studies indicate that high levels of vitamin D help alleviate the depression and fatigue that accompany SAD.

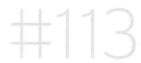

Get outside

Take a walk in the park, or bundle up and sit outdoors, and soak up what little sun there is. Trust me, it makes a difference.

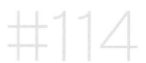

Let the light shine in

Brighten up your house. Open the blinds, and keep rooms well lit.

#115

Get moving

Exercise can also help alleviate stress and anxiety, two by-products of SAD. No kidding.

#116

Head for the sun

If you have the time and resources, a mid-winter vacation to sunnier climates will do wonders for alleviating symptoms of SAD. I can attest to this one from personal experience. Bonus benefit: reduction in stress, increase in energy.

#117

Make connections

When you're feeling down, reach out to your support network. Push yourself to socialize with friends. Really. I mean it.

———— WORTH KNOWING ————

A sun lamp may really come in handy when it comes to combating SAD. See page 212 for more information.

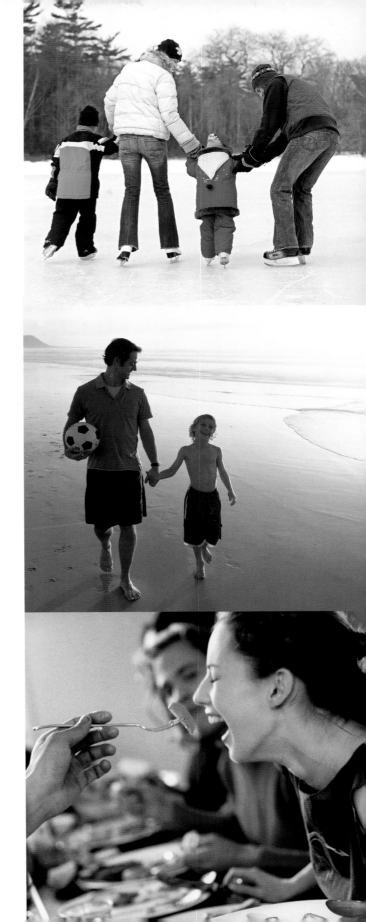

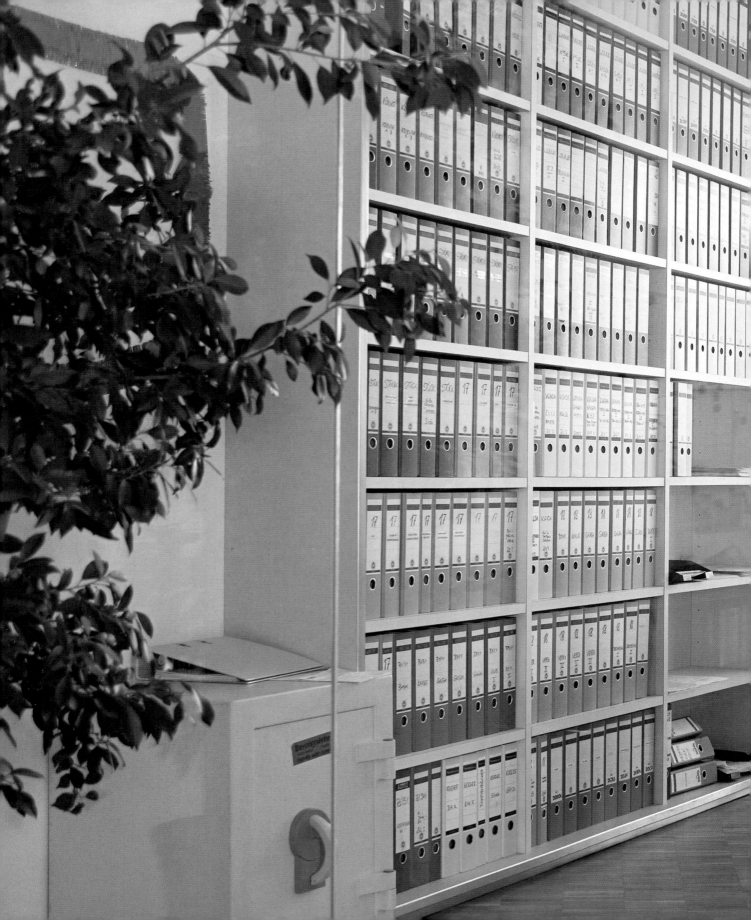

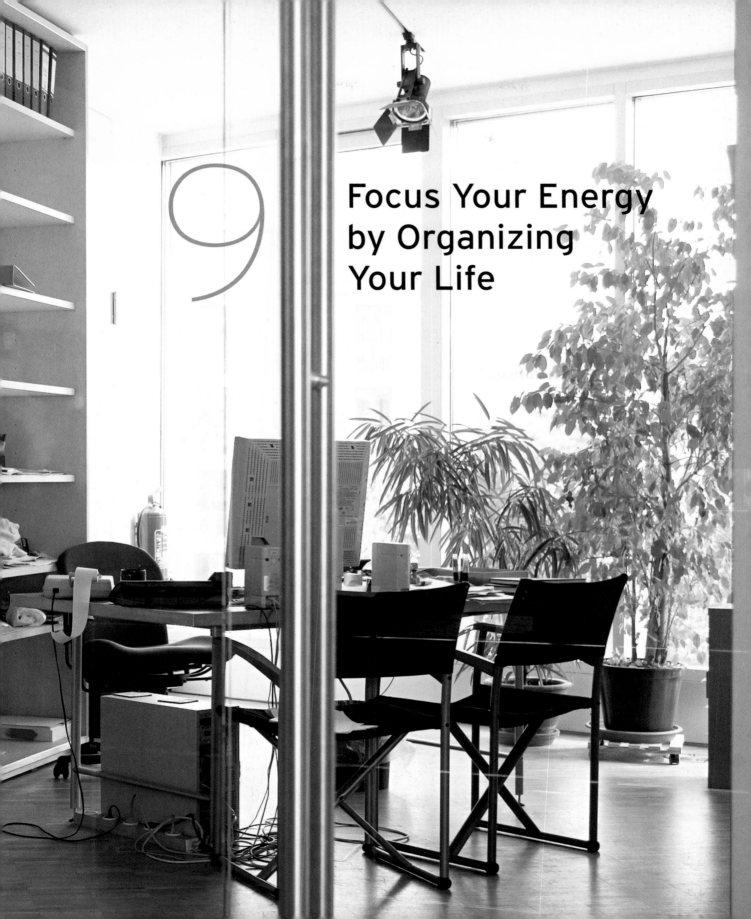

9 Focus Your Energy by Organizing Your Life

put this chapter in the book because of a personal discovery: When my life is organized, I have more energy.

And I'm talking *all the time*. No kidding. I usually have several projects going on at once and, unfortunately, I find it all too easy to sit by and watch them kind of morph into one huge overlapping mess of to-do lists. I wind up spending valuable energy (not to mention time) just trying to put out fires and sort out what needs to be done and when.

On the other hand, when I'm organized, my day just flies. Including my energy. I literally feel an energy boost just from having my desk, email, and various projects "decluttered." Which is no wonder, because if energy were a budget, I would've just freed up about a million bucks.

Personally, I believe the key to the connection between organization and energy can be explained in one word: focus. When you're scattered all over the place, so is your energy. Despite all the emphasis these days on multitasking, I believe that people can only do so many things at once, and the number of things we can attend to at once is probably smaller than most of us believe. When there are a zillion tasks on your desk that need attention in one big unorganized mess, your energy is subtly scattered all over the place. It's like having twenty programs open at once on your computer desktop—everything runs slower. When that desktop is your brain, your energy suffers. A lot.

When I speak around the country on weight loss, one of the take-home messages in my presentation is this: *The way you do your weight loss program is the way you do your life*. My pal T. Harv Eker, visionary author of *Secrets of the Millionaire Mind*, likes to say, "The way you do one thing is the way you do everything." And progressive thinker and educator Werner Erhard used to say, "The way you do anything is the way you do your life." Translated to the currency of energy, I think the message is this: If your life is a mess and your desk looks like your life, you can be pretty sure your energy level is in the same state.

So let's start by getting your projects on track. You'll be amazed at how much energy you'll free up just by getting organized, whether it's your email, your desk, your home, or other areas of your life.

And there's a bonus benefit in the mix: Use some of the "tricks of the trade" I'm about to tell you about how to get better organized, and you may just discover a new clarity when it comes to identifying your life's purpose.

That's a pretty big side benefit.

And probably the biggest energy booster on the planet.

#118

Eat That Frog!

Brian Tracy is an internationally known motivational speaker and best-selling author who is also a pretty high-energy dude. He has a concept that's been a huge help to me in organizing my days for maximum energy.

It's called "Eat That Frog," which is actually the title of one of his best-selling books, *Eat That Frog! 21 Great Ways to Stop Procrastinating and Get More Done in Less Time*.

I know it doesn't sound terribly appetizing as a culinary choice, but read on.

FINISH THE "INCOMPLETES"

For most people I know, procrastination is a huge energy drainer. Many of us spend a ton of energy putting off the things we don't want to do—tasks we find unpleasant, uncomfortable, too challenging, not challenging enough, beneath us, over our heads, fill in the blank. The result is that we have little energy to do the things we actually enjoy.

Tracy's concept is elegantly simple: Do the biggest, ugliest, most distasteful task first. Get it out of the way. (Hence, *eat the frog*. What metaphor could be more disgusting?) The idea is that once you've done the thing that you're spending the most energy avoiding, what's left is psychic space (and relief) and the ability to really focus your energy.

I've found that when I do this, the world literally opens up. Not only do I feel freer and more liberated, but I also feel like I could take on the world. (Of course, I don't always do it, but when I do, look out!)

I've spent a lot of time in this book talking about how "incompletes," whether they are tasks or communications, can take up psychic space, preventing you from being your energetic best. Those incompletes, especially when they're uncomfortable or difficult, tend to be high on the procrastination list. (Why wouldn't they be?) Now, you basically have two choices about how to liberate all that energy bound up in these events. You can spend your time analyzing why it is that you procrastinate—interesting but not very action-oriented—or you can focus on exactly what needs to get done, and then do it.

Tracy suggests starting each day tackling the item, task, project, or conversation that is the most onerous (but necessary). In other words, eat the symbolic frog. Get it over with first thing in the morning, and by comparison, the rest of the day is a breeze. It's as simple—and difficult—as that.

An aside: People often ask me whether it's better to exercise in the morning or at night. The answer is that from a physiological point of view it doesn't matter, but from a psychological point of view it may. I find that people who exercise first thing in the morning set the tone for the day by "getting it out of the way," creating space and energy and setting themselves up with a positive feeling of accomplishment that tends to linger and spread throughout the rest of the day's events. It's actually one of many ways you can eat the frog.

CHOOSE ACTION

Remember, a basic principle of this book is that our thoughts influence our emotions and our emotions influence our actions. Procrastination involves a process that includes magnifying the negative aspects of the task you are avoiding, and giving those thoughts the power to throw emotional roadblocks in the road to success. But remember, procrastination is, after all, a *choice* (see Make Peace with Your Gremlins on page 258).

Guess who does the choosing? You.

Once you hear that familiar voice chanting all the reasons to avoid the task at hand, just jump in and push the override button. How? With action. Decide what you *need* to accomplish, and what you *want* to accomplish.* Some tasks will have pressing deadlines, others will be open-ended. If you have a tendency to put off those one-step tasks (such as making that unpleasant phone call

*Many organizational experts recommend making a list and giving each task a priority rating (1, 2, or 3), with number 1s being those that have to get done today. You can usually find your frogs among the number 1s, even though they often wind up being put off until tomorrow, a surefire energy drainer if there ever was one.

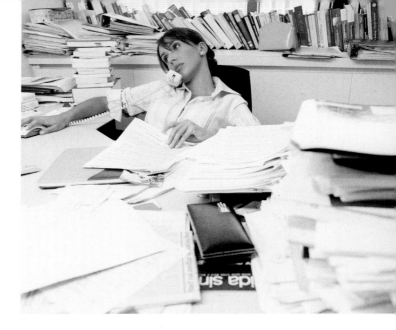

or writing a memo), then prioritize your day so you *start* with the task you least want to do and work your way to the more pleasant assignments.

If it's the long-range projects that tend to overwhelm you, then break them down into concrete, manageable, and achievable steps, and schedule those steps into your calendar. Look, if you decided to run a marathon, and you waited until a week before the race to train, obviously you'd set yourself up for failure. But if you planned well, and started your training early enough, you would gradually build your endurance to a point where running 26.4 miles, and crossing the finish line, is actually achievable.

The same goes for those long-range fear-provoking tasks, such as preparing a presentation for next month's conference. Divide it into small steps, and start your day by accomplishing the tasks you are most likely to delay. You'll conquer your fears and avoid the energy-draining guilt that is a by-product of avoidance.

Approaching your day with an "eat the frog mentality" will not only increase your productivity but will also increase your energy.

#119

Clear Your Desktop

When I was in graduate school, I used to always hear about how high-energy, highly productive people were so well organized. They'd have their desks neat and clean (unlike mine!). They'd know where everything was. They'd have a place for everything.

Can you imagine how productive and energetic you'd be if your desk reflected that level of organization? It'd be like the workaday equivalent of Marine boot camp, where everything was spit-shined and in its place, you could bounce a quarter off the bed, and everyone was raring to go.

Then someone showed me a picture of Jean Piaget's office. Piaget was the noted Swiss scientist and philosopher whose work in the mid-twentieth century was absolutely seminal in understanding child development.

His office looked like Hurricane Katrina had just passed through it.

So much for that theory.

Okay, so there are exceptional people who manage to be both energetic and highly productive in an office of stunning chaos and disorganization (the great conservative writer and founder of the *National Review,* William F. Buckley, was one such person). Thing of it is, you probably aren't one of them. Neither am I.

For us mortals, a clean and uncluttered desk is a great help to focusing our energy. And the rubble of disorganization usually reflects the mind of the owner of said desk, and the scattering of his or her energy. I know it does for me. When my workspace is clean and efficient, I'm able to marshal my energy and focus on the task at hand. I feel more like a laser and less like a low-watt lightbulb, which casts a little bit of light over a large area, but truly lights up none of it.

So, at the risk of sounding like your mother, clean your desk.

REAP THE BENEFITS OF MINIMALISM

Is your desk crowded with knickknacks; trays of paper clips, rubber bands, and other office supplies; and filled with files, books, magazines, and so many papers that the inbox is invisible? All these things demand attention, making it that much harder to focus, which leads to energy-sapping stress that can't be fixed with a double espresso.

It's time to take action. For a less stressful workspace, become a *minimalist*.

Start by piling everything on your desk in your inbox. (You do have an inbox, don't you? It's there somewhere. I know it is.) If you need more space, use the floor. Begin with items that can easily be put away; scissors, the staple remover, tape, and all other office supplies should have a designated drawer. They don't? No problem. Give them one. Or find some easily accessible but out of sight place to store them.

Books go on the bookshelf, and magazines get thrown out, passed along, or neatly filed. Sort through all the papers—every *single* one of them—and dispose, delegate, file, or take action (or add that to your to-do list and file the paper). Resist the temptation to put aside any papers—that just leads to an overflowing inbox (or to relocated junk).

On to knickknacks. You may think you're inspired by your collection of Pez dispensers, but really it's just another concentration spoiler. Get rid of it, or at least get it out of sight. For minimum distraction, try to keep your desk clear of everything except your computer, phone, and maybe a photo or two.

When my workspace is clean and efficient, I'm able to marshal my energy and focus on the task at hand. I feel more like a laser and less like a low-watt lightbulb, which casts a little bit of light over a large area, but truly lights up none of it.

ORGANIZE THE DESKTOP DISTRACTIONS

Now once you've cleared up your desktop, it's time to clean *up* your desktop—your computer desktop. Is it crowded with icons and folders? Do you have a system for all incoming files? (I truly felt more energy once I did this. My computer desktop was a constant drain. I think, at its worst, it had 110 icons on it, so that many were starting to double up.)

If you don't have a logical filing system, then take the time to devise one. Arrange work by projects, clients, or time frame (current projects, past, future, etc). As long as it's intuitive to you, it doesn't matter what your system looks like. Try to minimize your desktop folders to one or two. Keep the dock with all your program items hidden. Now maybe you can see your screen saver. Is it something soothing, such as a mountain, a seascape, or some other view of nature? (If it's not, change it, unless it's a treasured family picture that truly soothes you.)

Now downloads. I suggest designating one folder to contain all downloads in your computer's inbox. At least once a day go through and sort items, then file, take action, forward, or discard.

Once you've cleared your desk and desktop, the best way to keep it from getting cluttered again is to get into a routine. When you're dividing your day into blocks of time, reserve time for housekeeping. If you don't stay on top of your inbox—both real and virtual—you'll soon be inundated with files. Managing your paperwork, information streams, and clutter will go a long way toward alleviating workday stress.

And, unless you're Piaget or Buckley or some other one in a million genius, less stress, less clutter, more organization, and more space translates into more energy.

It definitely does for me. It should work for you as well.

If it doesn't, at least you'll get a neat desk out of the deal.

#120
De-Clutter and Deep-Six the Energy Drain

Here's a rule I've found to be a universal truth: Your energy has a perfect inverse relationship to the accumulation of stuff you don't need. The more unwanted, unused, unneeded stuff you have cluttering up your life, the less energy you have.

Let me explain. Although there are no actual scientific studies on this, there's also no shortage of examples that illustrate how uncluttering your

You may think you're inspired by your collection of Pez dispensers, but really it's just another concentration spoiler.

space can refocus, sharpen, and increase your energy. One woman, for instance, spent three grand to hire three women to come and clean out her entire home because she literally could not get from room to room, an energy-drainer if ever there was one.

In the two cities in which I have lived for any length of time—New York and Los Angeles—professional organizers are a huge cottage industry, and those I've spoken to invariably mention increased energy in their lists of client benefits. Bootsie Grakal, owner of Organize by Boo in Beverly Hills (www.organizebyboo.com), says, "I've consistently noticed that when my clients have clutter in their life, their energy is drained. Once we get them organized and clutter-free, we can literally 'see' and 'feel' the increase in their energy."

And on a personal note, I can tell you that when my space is cluttered (which is more often than I'd like), I walk from room to room constantly distracted by things that are lying around demanding attention. After awhile, all that clutter can almost seem like it's mocking you or daring you to do something about it. You wind up doing nothing, surrounded by an increasing mound of unattended-to tasks, projects, or just outright junk, until ultimately you simply collapse in a sigh, turn on the TV, and give up.

Okay, maybe I'm exaggerating just a little. But not by much. Clutter can not only drag down your energy, but it can also divert important psychic resources that could be better used elsewhere. It's like filling up the buffer zone of your computer, or having a thousand programs open on your desktop. Everything winds up moving slower. Your computer has less "energy" when this is the case—and when it's the case in real life, so do you.

WASTED TIME AND ENERGY IN SEARCH OF A STAPLER

When I lived in Manhattan, I would often see a billboard that read "Mini-storage can change your life." The folks who wrote that were on to something. Now maybe that particular saying has more meaning to those who reside in apartments the size of walk-in closets than it does to people who live outside of Manhattan, but I think it holds a universal truth. No matter where we live, most of us have too much stuff. Way too much.

In fact, the amount of stuff we accumulate only grows as we increase the square footage of our living spaces. So this advice holds for all: Clear the clutter. In your closets, your drawers, your desk, your bedroom. Whether it's hidden away or in full view, clutter takes up energetic space.

And time. How many hours a week do you spend looking for a stapler, or a pair of scissors, your keys, that book you were reading, your favorite earrings—because there isn't a place for everything, so everything can never be in its place? And how much money do you waste buying items that you know you already have—somewhere? It's stressful, frustrating, expensive, and exhausting.

REDUCE STRESS, FREE UP ENERGY

It's time to edit out the extraneous, the irreparable, the unused, and the unsightly; it's time to get down to basics. If you have difficulty letting go of things, you might want to enlist a friend to lend support during the de-cluttering process. ("No, I don't think you'll ever wear that muumuu again; toss it, Will.") And although I usually advocate tackling the job you most want to avoid first, this may be a case where you need to condition yourself into de-cluttering shape by starting with the area that has the fewest emotional strings attached.

As you weed through clothing, accessories, books, paperwork, products, utensils, tools, and knickknacks, be brutal—when was the last time you wore, used, or needed the item in question? Do you have another? Is it out of date or in need of repair? Does it make you happy or your life simpler? Do you have room for it? If in doubt, throw it out (or give it away). What's left gets categorized, then organized. Put like items with like items, then determine whether it belongs in a closet, drawer, or file cabinet—each item has to have a home.

If your closets are a jumble of different types and colors of hangers, invest in new ones—all the same shape and color. Arrange your closet by items (pants, shirts, skirts), then colors. It will make the morning rush to get dressed so much easier.

Also, determine where incoming mail, keys, umbrellas, important papers, and the kids' artwork will go. Once you develop a system, stick to it. The goal is to keep the place clutter-free in a way that will save you time and energy.

By investing some time and energy in creating and maintaining a clutter-free home, you'll be taking steps toward reducing stress and freeing up energy for the important things in life.

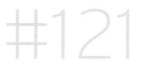

Go Ergo

Just as being physically out of alignment can sap your energy and vitality (see Go to a Chiropractor and Adjust to New Energy on page 189), having a workspace that's "out of alignment" can do the same.

Enter ergonomics.

Ergonomics is the applied science of equipment design, usually referring to the workplace. Its purpose is to maximize energy and productivity by reducing the fatigue and discomfort that comes from poorly designed equipment and workspaces.

If you're a desk jockey, then you're probably familiar with the eyestrain, muscle aches, and fatigue that come from spending too much time in front of a computer. Not much high energy there. So, even if you never consciously thought about it before, you probably know intuitively that badly designed or arranged workstations are a huge energy drain. Fortunately, there's a relatively easy solution to plug this particular drain and to promote energy in the bargain: Go ergo.

"When my clients have clutter in their life, their energy is drained. Once we get them organized and clutter-free, we can literally 'see' and 'feel' the increase in their energy."

—Bootsie Grakal, owner of Organize by Boo in Beverly Hills, California

HOW TO GO ERGO

Here are ways to achieve an ergonomically correct workspace.

- First principle of ergonomics: Arrange your desk so that frequently used objects are close at hand.
- Create space and get rid of clutter. Overcrowding your computer work area is a big, fat energy drain. (You knew that, didn't you?)
- If possible, choose a work surface with a matte finish to minimize glare and reflections.
- Keep the area underneath your desk clear so you can stretch your legs.
- Allow 2 to 3 inches (5 to 7.5 cm) of clearance between your thighs and the underside of your desk.
- Place the phone on the side of your nondominant hand (i.e., left side if right-handed, right side if left-handed). This makes a big difference. No kidding.
- If you spend a lot of time on the phone, get a headset. You have no idea how much energy you lose just by keeping that phone propped up between your neck and your chin. Neck strain means no energy.
- Practice dynamic sitting, which is just a fancy way of saying don't stay in one position very long. Take frequent breaks to stand and stretch. Bonus energy points: It'll increase the oxygen to your brain and muscles!
- Adjust the height of the backrest to support the natural inward curve of the lower back. For a little postural assistance, use a lumbar cushion or rolled towel to support your lower back.

- If your feet don't rest flat on the floor, use a footrest.
- Set the backrest at an angle that allows your hips to be at a 90- to 115-degree angle to your torso.
- Sit upright so your shoulders and lower back touch the backrest. Your thighs should be parallel to the floor and knees at about the same level as the hips, with 2 to 3 inches (5 to 7.5 cm) of space between the edge of the seat and the back of your knees.
- Position the computer monitor directly in front of you about arm's length away (20 to 26 inches, or 51 to 66 cm) and adjust it or your chair so the top of the screen is at or just above eye level.
- To reduce glare, position your monitor so it's perpendicular to the window. If that's not possible, use a glare filter.
- Keep your screen clean, and adjust the monitor for optimal brightness and contrast. Increase font size, if necessary, to avoid eyestrain.
- Position the keyboard directly in front of and close to you. Adjust the keyboard height so your shoulders can relax and allow your arms to rest at your sides.
- Place your mouse adjacent to the keyboard and at the same height. Don't bend your wrist upward to use it, and don't rest your hand on the mouse when you're not using it.
- A trackball uses different muscle and tendon groups than a mouse, so if possible, mix it up.
- Keep you forearms parallel to the floor (approximately a 90-degree angle at the elbow).

- Adjust the slope of the keyboard so your wrists are straight, and not bent back, while you're typing.
- Use a light touch on the keyboard. Keep your shoulders, arms, hands, and fingers relaxed.

Speaking of creating an energy-friendly work environment, consider this: If you're willing to be a little daring, try what my friends at Joe Polish's Piranha Marketing (www.joepolish.com) in Tempe, Arizona, do (and trust me, those are some of the highest energy folks I've ever dealt with!). They sit on exercise balls while they're at their desks. No kidding. It engages your muscles, keeps oxygen flowing, and supports mental alertness.

Joe told me that some of the folks at his office actually work while walking on treadmills. I know it sounds radical, but it works.

When I was a radio host on www.eyada.com in New York City, I used to do my two-hour daily show standing up. I learned from some top radio professionals early on that the "energy" you project (and the energy you *feel*) is very different when you're standing than when you're sitting.

You may not want to stand up at work, or walk on a treadmill while you're reading office reports, but at least create a workspace that's fun, creative, energizing, and ergonomically correct.

Your energy will soar.

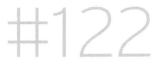

#122
Mono-Task to Accomplish More

Forget multitasking. It's so yesterday. And it's also a secret robber of energy.

Unfortunately, we're in the age of maniacal multitasking. Fuggedaboutit. Multitasking is the enemy of mindfulness, and mindfulness is your greatest ally in reclaiming your energy and focus.

It's time to mono-task.

Mindfulness is one of my favorite subjects (and one of my biggest challenges, as it is for most people I know who practice it). Yet the rewards are immense, not only in terms of your energy but also in terms of your relationships and your health. Mindful eating is both the enemy of mindless snacking and a powerful tool in weight loss. Mindful conversation keeps you engaged with the person you're talking to, instead of scanning the room to see whether someone more interesting is about to walk through the door.

When you're mindful, you're *present in the moment*. You can bring all your energy to bear on the task at hand, whether it's eating, watching television, having a conversation, or even meditating.

Mindfulness equals energy. It's that simple.

And that difficult. In an era when you don't feel productive if you're not doing three things at once, eliminating extraneous distractions and concentrating all your energy on one thing at a time can be difficult. But man, is it worth it. You'll actually get in touch with your own power and energy in a way you may not have done in a long time.

So how to practice? Simple. When you're on the phone, don't read your emails, don't rifle through files, don't instant-message your spouse, don't surf the 'net and . . . *please don't drive.*

Instead, talk, listen, and participate in conversation. Become *engaged* in whatever it is you are doing, something that's nearly impossible when you're dealing in multiples.

DO LESS TO DO BETTER

Mono-tasking *saves* energy (not to mention your sanity). In fact, studies show that multitasking is less productive and more stressful than concentrating on the task at hand. A 2005 study funded by Hewlett-Packard and conducted by the Institute of Psychiatry at the University of London found that checking your email while performing another creative task decreases your IQ in the moment by ten points. That's more than twice the amount when smoking marijuana, and the equivalent of not sleeping for 36 hours.

In a terrific essay aptly titled *The Myth of Multitasking*, *New Atlantis* magazine senior editor Christine Rosen argued that when you're doing a bunch of things at once, there's a good chance you're doing all of them poorly. She was hardly the first to notice this essential truth.

Back in the 1740s, Lord Chesterfield wrote these prescient words: "There is time enough for everything in the course of the day, if you do but one thing at once; but there is not time enough in the year, if you will do two things at a time."

Former eight-time National Chess Champion Josh Waitzkin, author of *The Art of Learning: An Inner Journey to Optimal Performance*, calls multitasking "a virus." One of the most inspiringly energetic people I've ever interviewed is best-selling author Timothy Ferriss, who wrote *The 4-Hour Workweek*, a book in which he extols the virtues of "single-tasking." Coincidence?

"Multitasking forces the brain to share processing resources," says Mark Bauerlein, Ph.D., author of *The Dumbest Generation: How the Digital Age Stupefies Young Americans and Jeopardizes Our Future*. He explains that even if the tasks you're doing don't use the same brain regions, there is still some "shared infrastructure" that gets overloaded.

Edward Hallowell, M.D., author of the self-explanatory title *CrazyBusy*, calls multitasking "a mythical activity in which people believe they can perform two or more tasks simultaneously."

Bottom line: By doing less, or at least by doing fewer things at any one given time, you can actually increase your energy for the task at hand and, in the end, get more done.

#123

Tame The Email Beast

I'm hoping by now I've convinced you that every step you take toward organizing your life frees up more energy for you and helps close some of the energy sinks that can drain even the highest energy person.

One such organizing tip that virtually every professional organizer I've ever known has stressed is doing something about your email. Reading every email as it arrives can derail your concentration faster than you can say "What were we talking about?" Instead of attending to each one as it pops into your inbox, batch your mail. Set aside blocks of time twice a day (if you just have to do it more often, try once every other hour) to read and write emails.

Another key to managing email is keeping your inbox empty. (This may take some time to accomplish initially, but it will save you lots of time in the long run.) It also does wonders for your frame of mind. I'm telling you, whenever I see a number such as 416 in my inbox I can literally feel my energy drop when I think (even subconsciously) about all the unattended little tasks that number represents.

So here's what to do about it.

DON'T LEAVE EMAIL UNATTENDED

When you open emails, process them immediately. Either delete, forward, respond, or if you don't have an answer, move the email into a follow-up folder. Before you move on to another task, be sure you've deleted or archived every incoming email.

Now evaluate all the newsletters you subscribe to. Are they all worth your time? Or do they clutter your inbox? The easy solution: There's a little button at the end of every newsletter that says "unsubscribe." Learn to use it.

Next, tackle the jokesters. Do you have friends who forward you *every* stupid joke or link to every silly YouTube video they watch? Ask them—politely and respectfully—to please take you off their forwarding list.

While you're at it, talk to the well-meaning people who really feel you need them to stay well informed. I had a friend once who went on the Atkins diet for three days and for the next three years her mother forwarded every article ever written about anorexia. I'm sure you can relate.

There, you've just saved yourself from opening ten emails a day.

When you open emails, process them immediately. Either delete, forward, respond, or if you don't have an answer, move the email into a follow-up folder. Before you move on to another task, be sure you've deleted or archived every incoming email.

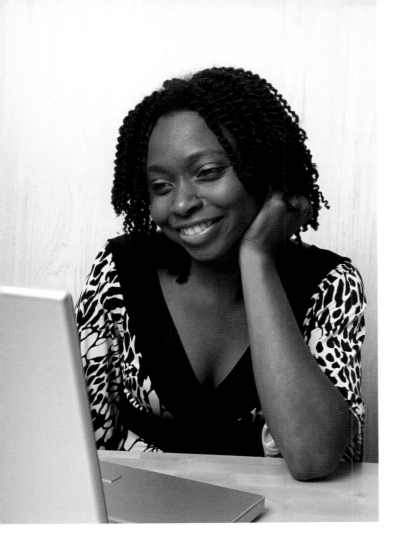

DITCH THE DELIBERATION

When it's time to answer your email, don't waste time trying to be clever or profound; make your point and move on. Deliberating over email can eat up big chunks of your day. If putting what you want to say in an email is difficult, then pick up the phone and have a conversation.

It may seem like small potatoes, but this email organization thing has profound implications for the rest of your energy balance sheet. Not to put too metaphysical a point on it, but the more things we leave "undone" in our mental inbox, the more we drain our psychic (and emotional and ultimately physical) energy. You can start plugging those energy holes by facing up to the challenge of email.

Before long you'll be treating the distractions of your bigger life in the same way: Deal with now, delegate, or delete. What an energizing concept!

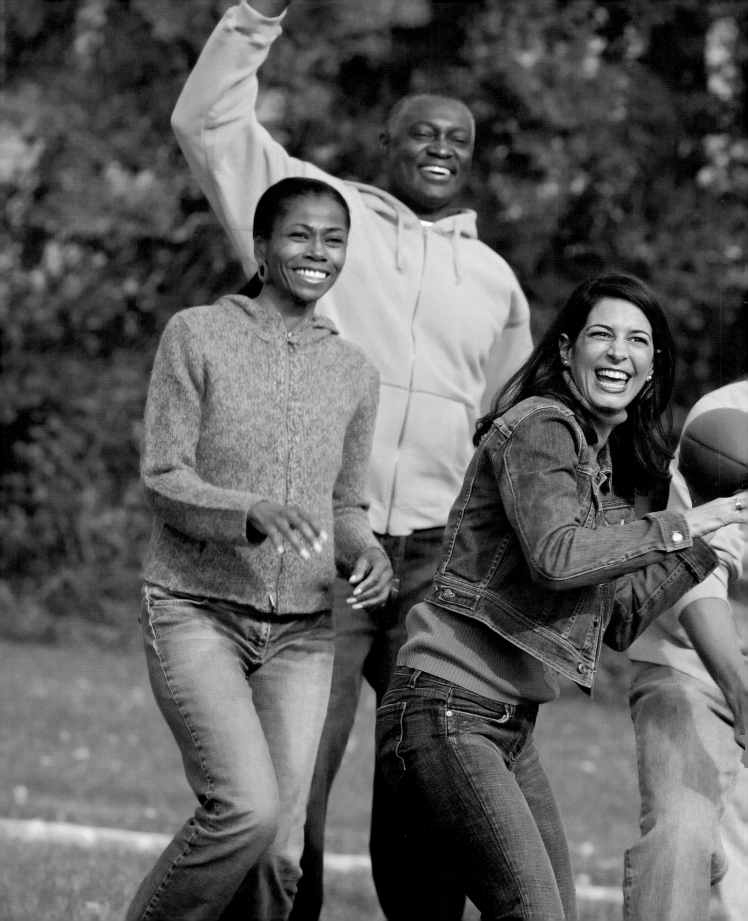

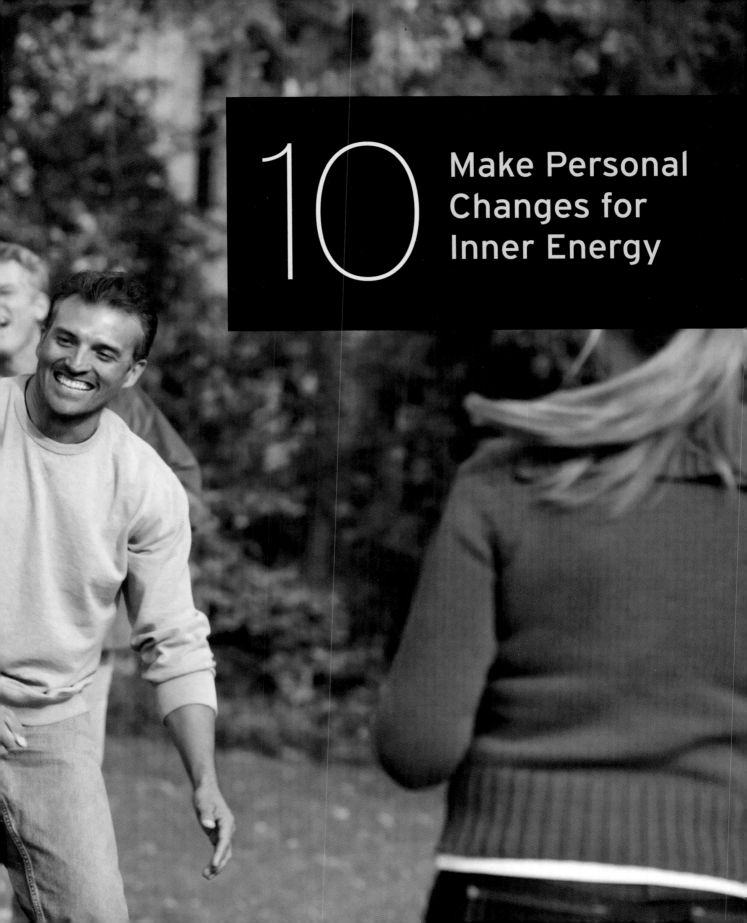

10 Make Personal Changes for Inner Energy

Back in the 1990s, there was a famous saying bandied about in American politics. Democratic political consultant James Carville coined it, using it to keep his candidate (Bill Clinton) on message about the single most important issue in the campaign. The slogan was this: "It's the economy, stupid!"

Well, to paraphrase that classic slogan, when it comes to energy, "It's the whole person, stupid!"

Of course it goes without saying that I'm not calling you stupid. What I *am* saying, however, and have said numerous times throughout these pages, is that energy doesn't just happen. It comes out of everything that makes you unique as a person. It's a by-product of your physical, mental, and emotional life. Energy is what shows up naturally when you remove all the obstacles to well-being, whether these obstacles come in the form of bad food, bad nutrition, or bad choices.

So a big theme of this book has been the removal of those energy blocks from your life. In this chapter, we're going to concentrate specifically on ways to liberate your energy from the toxins of bad relationships, unmet needs, unexpressed communications, and other obstacles to your full self-expression as a high-energy person, brimming with joy, enthusiasm, and optimism.

Yes, I'm talking about you.

THE HIGH-ENERGY YOU

If you don't recognize yourself in that description (here it is again, in case you forgot: *brimming with joy, enthusiasm, and optimism*), the reason might well be because you have neglected critical aspects of your own personal and spiritual growth. If that's the case, I hope the techniques and suggestions found in this chapter will help get you back on track.

The tips and suggestions in the following pages focus on removing *personal* toxins rather than chemical ones, but make no mistake, the former can be as toxic as the latter, and they can be (and frequently are) even more of a drain on your energy. These tips and suggestions also focus on ways you can apply "Miracle-Gro" to your best instincts by volunteering, looking outward, helping others, practicing forgiveness, and communicating more honestly.

In many ways, this chapter is the most important one in the book.

If "brimming with joy, enthusiasm, and optimism" sounds like a good definition of a high-energy person, that's because it is. And it can be a perfect description of you. In fact, it probably already is. You just may have forgotten how to be that person.

I hope this chapter will help you remember how.

#124

Lose the Energy Vampires

Here's the definition of an energy vampire: Someone who sucks up all the oxygen in the room. Someone who leaves you depleted. Someone who, when you interact with him or her, leaves you feeling less than good.

These people drain your energy. Lose them.

The world-famous Framingham Study demonstrated that we are, in large measure, the average of the three people we spend the most time with. If three of your best friends are obese, you have a 50 percent greater chance of being obese. Many motivational speakers have expanded the maxim to five people, but the point remains. If you want to see how you're doing, look around at the five people you spend the most time with, says Jack Canfield, author of *Chicken Soup for the Soul*.

It's the same thing with your energy. If the people you spend the most time with are sucking you dry, there's no supplement, food, or exercise in the world that's going to give you that lost energy back.

So lose the vampires.

JETTISON THESE FOUR ENERGY DRAINERS

Not sure who your vampires are? Here's a quick definition. They're the friend, relative, or coworker who drags you down with negativity, and leaves you feeling angry, deflated, somehow incomplete, and nearly always drained of energy. They're part of a relationship that's both unsupportive and unrewarding. Sometimes, sadly, but not surprisingly, they're found in your own family.

Toxic friends come in various packages. Here are a few examples of the various subgroups, and how to identify them:

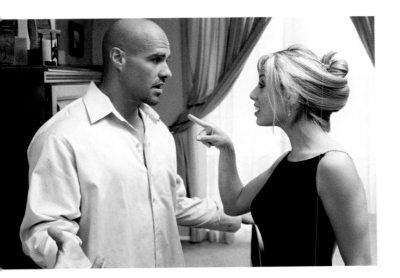

- Crosses every boundary. There's no end to the favors she will ask or the time she'll take up. Don't expect much in return.

- Blames first, asks questions later. Assumes everything wrong in her life is someone else's fault. Refuses to take responsibility for her own actions. Constantly complains and expects you to listen. Endlessly.

- Is known as "the tornado." His life is chaos, every situation is a crisis, and every encounter with you is just another opportunity to replay the drama of the day. Best characterized by the old joke about the actor who talks endlessly about his performance and then says, "But enough about me! What did *you* think of my performance?"

- Is called "the downer." You tell him your child has been having headaches and he tells you about his friend's niece who died of a brain tumor. You stop at your bank's ATM machine on your way out to dinner and he launches into a 30-minute diatribe about credit card companies and the government's stranglehold on the middle class. Even if you agree with him, he's annoying as hell, and you're drained by his negative energy.

Get the picture? I can almost *feel* you nodding emphatically. We all know these folks. (And if you're still unsure of the definition of an "energy vampire," use this one, direct from the cliff notes: Someone who leaves you feeling angry, depressed, or worn out.) Once you've identified her or him or them, ask yourself this: Why is this person in my life? Is this the kind of friendship/relationship I deserve?

REDRAW THE LINE IN THE SAND

One way to boost your daily energy is to lighten your load, and these folks are weighing you down. Fire them. If they're family members and you can't do that, renegotiate the boundaries. My friend Jada did that recently and the results were very positive.

Jada's mother had a habit of not returning phone calls for weeks at a time, and Jada felt like she just wasn't that important in her mother's life. So Jada finally had a "powerful conversation" with her mother in which she explained, as honestly and noncritically as she could, that she felt very badly when she didn't get a return call for weeks, and that it wasn't okay with her to have their relationship continue this way. Her mother explained that her phone manners didn't mean she didn't love her daughter—she was just absentminded and scattered. They agreed to a 48-hour rule except in rare cases of an emergency. Setting a new boundary was quite empowering to Jada, and she felt very good about it.

Every time you communicate to someone what is and isn't okay with you, you are setting a boundary. Most of us don't bother to do it and just steam inside when others cross our invisible and unstated lines. That drains energy. It's empowering—and energizing—when we speak up for ourselves, and even more so when we do it in a way that doesn't diminish or blame the other person.

Setting a boundary with someone doesn't have to be a difficult and uncomfortable conversation. In fact, you may be able to do it alone just by rethinking what you will and won't put up with. That's a powerful and energizing conversation, even when you have it with yourself. At the same time, cultivate healthier relationships. Learn to say no and to enjoy time alone.

If, after assessing the relationship in question, you realize it will never be anything but an energy drain, then it's time to unplug the connection. Believe me, nothing increases your energy like lightening your load.

#125

Have a Powerful Conversation

The 1990s were an exciting time to work in fitness. The fitness boom was just hitting big, and clubs were opening all over the place. Right in the middle of the Upper West Side of Manhattan, a club called Equinox opened its doors for the first time. (It went on to become one of the biggest and most successful high-end fitness club chains in the United States, with fifty locations and counting.)

The owners, Danny, Lavinia, and Vito Errico, were hands-on operators, in their early thirties, and completely driven by a love of all things having to do with fitness. They were also smart

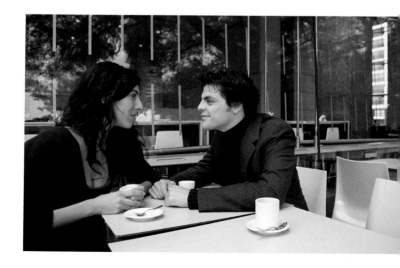

enough to hire the absolute best people in the business, including Bob Esquerre, Chris Imbo, Kacy Duke, Rocco Greco, Patricia Moreno, Annette Lang, Molly Fox, and Rich Baretta, many of whom went on to become household names in New York fitness circles and others of whom remain to this day the elder statespeople and teachers of whole generations of fitness professionals.

They also hired me, in my first professional job as a personal trainer. Through a combination of luck, chemistry, and hard work, I joined the "inner circle" of the people steering the Equinox boat.

Equinox *was* energy. There was a real sense of being on the cusp of something truly big. Equinox was in the news, every single day. We were designing and developing programs that were cutting edge, from trainer certifications (the Equinox Fitness Training Institute), to rock-climbing programs, to the first yoga-based group fitness classes (courtesy of Molly Fox). It was impossible to walk into the gleaming, shining, immaculate structure that was Equinox and not feel your pulse race.

In those days, I used to have weekly meetings with Danny Errico, one of the three owners of the club. Every Tuesday at 9:00 a.m. we'd discuss programs we were developing, kick around ideas, and discuss new equipment, teachers, classes, and ways of making the trainers better and the clients happier. And I noticed something very interesting happen.

No matter how tired or spent I felt when I walked in, no matter how little sleep I had gotten the night before, no matter what fight I may have had with my then-girlfriend (whom we shall affectionately refer to as "The Demon"), no matter what was going on in my life, when I left those meetings I felt turbocharged with energy. I'm talking ten cups of Starbucks Americano energy.

I'd leave those meetings like I could take on the world, like I couldn't wait to get started on the next project, like there weren't enough hours in the day to do all the terrific things I wanted to do.

And I was *never* tired.

So how did this happen?

COMMUNICATION: THE GREAT ENERGIZER

At first I actually thought there might be something in the water we were drinking. The feeling was that profound, pronounced, and palpable. It wasn't until much later that I put it all together and came to discover what I now call the "power of the powerful conversation."

What did we talk about in those meetings? Well, ideas for the club for sure. Programs. New equipment. New ways of getting people healthier. All subjects that have a certain energy on their own, but it was more than that. There was *acknowledgment* in those conversations. There was the sense that you were being heard. The sense that you made a difference. That your ideas were great and people appreciated them. That you were being listened to and that your ideas were going to actually be translated into action and, even better, that those actions were going to change people's lives for the better.

No wonder I left those conversations feeling high.

And right there I discovered something about energy, even though I wasn't able to put it into words until years later. That discovery led me to a principle that I truly try to live by, and try to incorporate into my life as often as I possibly can, and it's this: Powerful conversations energize.

A powerful conversation is one in which you tell the truth (more on that on page 239). When you really listen. When you really feel heard. When you're connected to the emotion and spirit of what you're talking about. The conversation can be something personal, or it can be related to business or your relationship or your plans for the future, or anything you feel passionate about. It can be a conversation with your loved one about something that hasn't been discussed before—anything from "when you come home and go right to the computer, I feel a little abandoned"—or a passionate exchange of ideas with a partner about developing a new business. The key ingredients for maximum energy enhancement are honesty and acceptance in a supportive environment and a true desire to communicate at a deeper level (and yes, your professional dreams for a business can certainly count as that).

I'm not always able to, but I try hard to have one breakthrough, powerful communication a day. Whenever I do, I feel an energetic high. A powerful conversation is the diametric opposite of mindlessness. It's focused, laser-sharp, honest, revealing, visionary, intense, and, well . . . powerful.

Try it. And watch your energy soar.

#126
Make a Promise

Just for fun, I asked one of the top life coaches I know, Laurie Gerber, what she thought was a great energy tip.

She didn't miss a beat. "Make a promise to yourself and keep it," she said.

There are few more energizing things on the planet than to experience your own personal power, according to Gerber. I have to say, I agree completely. "There's no better way to feel powerful than to make a promise and keep it," she says. "Your energy level will soar."

Some of the ways you do that is by keeping your word. By living a life you're proud of. By bringing what you say and what you do into alignment (it's called *integrity*, which, when you think about, is a close relative of integration or wholeness, and an antonym of separateness or breakdown).

"When you make a promise to yourself," Gerber told me, "you're giving your word to yourself about something that's important. Something you care about. Some component of the kind of life you want to create for yourself, the kind of life you can be proud of." She's right. After all, we never promise to watch soap operas and eat bonbons. We promise ourselves to stop smoking, to lose weight, to tell the truth, to clear up a misunderstanding.

And how great—and energized—we feel once we do it. Making a promise might be as simple as saying, "I'll learn something new every day," or, "I'll get out of bed by 7 a.m." Or Gerber's favorite: "Tell someone something that you've been avoiding saying." Bonus points for promises that push you to the edge, or in some cases, well beyond, your comfort zone.

There's no better way to feel your power, and your energy, than to make a promise and keep it. Werner Erhard, a great teacher of mine, once said the following: "If you keep telling it like it is, and you keep saying it like it is, and you keep promising it like it is, and you keep making it happen, your word becomes law in the universe."

I get energized just thinking about it.

#127

Tell the Truth

A lot of energy gets lost when you hold things in.

That goes for suppressed emotions and feelings (see EFT, page 175), unspoken communications, unmet needs and desires, and what we in the self-help movement used to call "withholds." A quick definition: A withhold is a communication that you're not delivering. Something you'd like to say but aren't. And it winds up costing you energy.

So if you want a really quick energy booster—a cup of espresso for the soul—try this: Tell the truth.

"If there's someone you don't want to talk to, if there's something you don't want to do, or if there's something you're just plain uncomfortable about, nine out of ten times there's some truth that hasn't been spoken, and that kills your energy," says life coach Lauren Zander. Most people just don't ever really lay their cards out fully on the table, Zander says, and this has everything to do with the amount of energy a person can feel, experience, and enjoy in a relationship and in life.

"Consider," she asks, "how you feel when you're around someone and suppressing yourself. Or when you want something and you're not getting it. How do you feel?" Her point is well taken. One thing you *don't* feel in those circumstances is full of energy. The equation is a simple one: Relationships dictate our moods, and our moods dictate our energy. "That's the formula here," Zander explains.

THE TRUTH WILL SET YOUR ENERGY FREE

In another section, I talked about how having a "powerful conversation" could be an incredible energizer (see page 236). But the converse is true as well—one bad (incomplete, unsatisfying)

conversation and your mood can shift, and not in a positive way. Stuff is left unspoken and unresolved. Your energy is diminished. Your vitality is drained. "The only thing that will actually get that vitality back and enhance your energy is the liberating act of going back and telling the truth," Zander says.

She's right. If you accept this premise—that we leave our energy on the table when we get hurt, or when we don't get what we want, or when we don't speak up for ourselves—Zander suggests taking the following steps:

1. **Ask permission.** It's as simple as saying, "Would it be okay if I told you how I really felt the other day when [fill in the blank] happened?" Zander suggests some good ice-breaking openers, such as, "I'm nervous that if I tell you this I might feel worse, but if it's okay with you I'd like to share," or "I don't know if you even know this, or meant it when you said it, but can I tell you my reaction to [fill in the blank]?"

   "It's also critical that they say yes," says Zander, "and that they have the time to discuss it. If they don't, you're not going to get taken care of, and the energizing power of telling the truth will be lost. Pick a time when they can actually be present for your communication," she advises.

2. **Start the conversation with "This is how it is for me."** As any marriage and family counselor will attest to, you'll never get anywhere with a conversation that puts the blame on the other person. It's not "you make me feel bad" it's "this is how I feel when [fill in the blank]." This opens the door to being heard and understood— a surefire energy

en-hancer. It also keeps your listener out of the uncomfortable position of being on the defensive, which is almost guaranteed to accomplish exactly nothing.

3. **Spill the beans.** Tell the other person your truth, the way it really is for you. No blame, no saying that person was wrong, just an honest, self-revealing picture of what you didn't communicate that you'd like him or her to know.

"Whatever they say, the most important point is being proud of your own bravery," says Zander. The energizing power of telling the truth actually has less to do with whether your listener "gets it" than it does with not suppressing your feelings and expressing what you feel in your own voice. "We lose vitality because we cower," Zander says.

We can reclaim our vitality by speaking in our voice. From the heart. With the truth. There are few things I know of that are as certain to increase your energy instantly.

#128
Ask Yourself These Four Questions

A lot of us wait for a change in energy like we're waiting for a bus—we expect it to drive right up, stop, and wait for us to hop on board. When it doesn't appear, we get frustrated, bored, or depressed. And our energy wanes.

I saw this kind of thing a lot early in my career when I worked with actors, first as a personal trainer and then as a nutritionist. After all, acting is a profession where your big break can come when

you least expect it—and usually does. You could be on the unemployment line, when all of a sudden your agent calls and you've got the audition of your life, and voilà, you've landed a major role in the next Spielberg movie. If that happened, your whole life could change.

So I understand that feeling of waiting for something to happen. But I also understand that change rarely happens like that, and even if it does, all the luck in the world won't mean anything if you're not prepared for the opportunity.

Now what does this have to do with energy? A lot, actually. If I gave you the proverbial bottle with a genie in it, and the genie jumped out and offered you three wishes, and you got your three wishes fulfilled immediately—what do you think that would do to your energy level?

Don't think too hard. I'll answer it for you: Your energy would go through the roof. So having what you want—in life, in relationships, in fitness, and in health—is a huge part of having a lot of energy. It's easy to get weighed down and drained when you're laboring in a life you feel you didn't choose, don't really want, and aren't particularly happy with. That's not exactly a prescription for high energy, at least not where I live.

MOVING YOUR LIFE FORWARD

This entry is about getting what you want so you can have all the energy that comes with feeling fulfilled and satisfied. One tool I've found to be particularly useful for getting that life (and the energy that goes with it) is to use what I call "The Four Questions."* Start by writing them down, preferably in a journal, where you can make entries on a regu-

*These questions have been in the toolbox of motivational speakers and life coaches in one form or another for many years. I'm indebted to my friend Jack Canfield for this version of them.

lar basis. This isn't an exercise that you do once; it has maximum impact on your energy and well-being when you do it on a regular basis.

Here are the four questions:

1. What did I accomplish today?

2. Why is that important to me?

3. What further progress can I make in that area of my life?

4. What specific action can I take to further my progress?

You can do this in every area of your life. What you accomplish in one day won't be limited to just work, play, or health.

Let me give you an example. Maybe you helped your child with his homework today, which is definitely accomplishing something. Now ask yourself: Why is that important to me? (Here's a sample answer: Because it furthers my relationship with my child and supports him at the same time. It makes me feel connected to an important member of my family.) Then ask: What further progress could I make? (How about doing it again tomorrow?) What specific action could I take to ensure that will happen? (How about checking your calendar and writing in a time to work with junior on his homework?)

AN ACCOMPLISHMENT ENERGY PILL

It's not all that complicated, but it allows you to take inventory of what you've actually accomplished in a given day. Believe me, being reminded of that, acknowledging it, feeling good about it, can be like taking an energy pill.

You finish a report at work, pay some bills, take your daughter to soccer practice, walk your dog, go to the gym, read a book, give a presentation at work, and attend a staff meeting. All these things are accomplishments. But this isn't just about listing them so you can feel good, though that's a part of it. It's about connecting what you did with your larger purpose, consciously examining the actions in your life in a context.

We can call that context *direction*. What have you done? Why are you doing it? Why is it valuable? What's the goal, what's the purpose, and if that's a value and a purpose that you love and embrace, what more can you do to further your movement in that direction?

What we're talking about here is very different from waiting at the bus stop for the "energy" bus to arrive (or an actor just waiting for his big break to come out of nowhere). Now we're talking instead about an actor who's *prepared* for the big audition, whenever it comes. We're talking about taking charge of your life and making your actions *meaningful* and *purposeful* and *conscious*. There's nothing more energizing that knowing you're moving in the right direction.

So remember—four questions. Answer them every day, in every way. Four columns on your page: What did I accomplish today? Why is that important to me? What further progress can I make in that area of my life? And what specific action can I now take to further my progress? Answer those questions every day for thirty days and you'll be amazed at what you get done, what you accomplish, and how you've moved toward your ultimate goals: Creating the life you want and the life you love. And that's a life that will keep you excited and energized.

#129

Acknowledge Someone Daily

Now I'm going to give you a tip that's easy to do and that will not only make you feel better and more energized, but will also make the people around you feel better. You'll be giving a gift that doesn't cost anything, and it's something that every single person on the planet wants. You're intrigued? Great. Here it is:

Acknowledge someone. Every single day.

After years of working with thousands of people, I really believe that underneath it all—the defense mechanisms, the rudeness, the unproductive or self-destructive behavior—the vast majority of people just want to make a difference in life. And they want to be recognized, appreciated, and acknowledged.

When you tell people that you appreciate them—whether it's because of their kindness, sense of humor, or problem-solving ability—I'd be willing to bet that every cell in their body experiences a different energy, and you can clearly read the effect of your words on their faces.

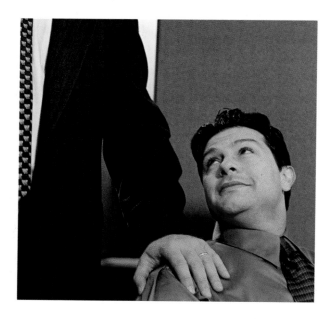

POSITIVE ENERGY SWELLS FROM ACKNOWLEDGMENT

An acknowledgement is a simple statement of someone's value. It's a way of telling someone how he or she has made a difference to you. It doesn't have to be anything major, such as, "Thanks for pulling me out of that burning building. I really appreciate that you saved my life."

It might be as simple as "Thanks for being so patient with me. I know you were under a lot of stress, and I really appreciate that you took the time to help me out," or, "I really admire how kind you are, even to strangers, including that new waitress we had last night."

Now you might think that the only beneficiary of your words is the person you acknowledge, but you'd be wrong. That person's definitely going to get something out of it, no doubt about it, but the other person who benefits is you. Believe me, every time you put out a kind, generous, or gracious word or deed, it reverberates throughout your body, sending positive energy into every cell.

So every single day acknowledge someone for something. The positive energy you give will be energizing, both to the person who receives it and—guaranteed—to you.

#130

Practice Forgiveness

If you've ever had chronic, low-level pain, you've probably held your body in a certain posture to avoid the discomfort of bending, or favored one leg or arm, because putting weight on the other one is just a little more uncomfortable.

Emotionally, we do this *every day* when we carry around the unexpressed and unresolved pains of past heartaches and experiences that cause us resentment and anger. Unexpressed and bottled-up feelings of anger and resentment take up psychic space, just like the dozens of incomplete projects on your desk, but unlike the projects, feelings of anger and resentment can poison and pollute your soul—your outlook on the world is smaller, more suspicious, less trusting, less open and giving.

It's hard to be energized when you are holding on to toxic emotions.

So you want more energy? Practice the art of forgiveness.

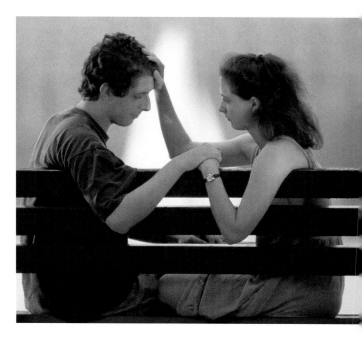

ONE OF THE MOST IMPORTANT LISTS YOU'LL EVER MAKE

Start by making a forgiveness list. When you start thinking about all the people and situations you resent, you may find that you have a really long list. It may go back to grade school to the kid who bullied you in the schoolyard or the girl who rejected you at the dance. Maybe your list includes someone who never returns your calls, or a back-stabbing coworker, or the woman who pushed ahead of you in line at Starbucks, or the guy who cut you off on the freeway. And of course your list probably includes family members, because some of those hurts and disappointments and wounds go very deep indeed.

It's important to start with what you feel you can handle. For example, it might be difficult to start practicing forgiveness for the first time with the partner who swindled you out of your business and left you bankrupt, or with the person who divorced you and broke your heart. But maybe you could handle forgiving that supermarket clerk who was smarmy to you on the checkout line when you brought thirteen items into the twelve-item express lane. Forgiveness is, after all, an emotional muscle, and you have to work up to the heavy lifting.

Pick three people on your list and then, one person at a time, allow yourself to feel whatever anger and resentment that comes up related to that person. In fact, I want you to try to *increase* that feeling of anger and resentment. (It shouldn't be hard.) Think of the *injustice* of what he did to you, of how *small* it made you feel, of the *unfairness* of the way he treated you.

Let that sit and simmer for a minute.

Now take a deep breath, close your eyes, and release that anger, annoyance, or irritation, or in some cases, your rage and your hurt. Just let it go.

Do it again—take a deep breath and release it. Try to imagine what it's like to *be* that person whom you resent. What might she have been feeling at the time she hurt you? What might his point of view been (remember, you don't have to agree with it or even like it—just understand what it might have been). What is his day like? What is it like to be her? Just put yourself inside the other person's skin for a minute.

And then wish the person peace.

Some healers suggest imagining the person or the situation that caused you pain in a pink bubble, surrounded by white light. Then imagine the whole scene floating away in a cloud of serenity and forgiveness.

IT'S ABOUT YOU

Now if you're new at this, you might be skeptical. I know I was, the first (and second, and third) time I tried it. The first impulse for many of us is to think, "I don't want to forgive them. What they did was wrong!" Which may (or may not) be true, but it is irrelevant to this practice. The practice is about *you* letting go of an energy-draining emotion; it's not about letting other people off the hook.

Remember, if you carry around a little hot ball of anger, the only person it sears is you. This technique is not for the object of your anger—it's for you. And don't get discouraged if you have to try it several times. In fact, I'd be surprised if you didn't.

If you keep practicing this technique, you'll be amazed at what you're able to accomplish. By letting go of some of the toxic feelings that have been holding you back and weighing you down, you are letting go of negative energy.

And guess what's left underneath when you release the toxic fumes?

Energy. Fabulous, light, "I can do anything," weight-off-my-shoulders energy.

Give it a try. You have nothing to lose but some of the biggest energy drainers on the planet.

#131
Volunteer Your Services

There's a classic series of studies done back in the 1970s in which the residents of a nursing home were each given a plant to keep in their room. Half of them were told they were responsible for the care and feeding of the plant, and the other half were told that the staff would take care of it. By the way, we're talking about one of those plants your grandmother used to have, a snake plant, the kind you can't kill even if you leave it unattended in the back of the garage for a year. So it didn't require a lot of care.

The practice is about you letting go of an energy-draining emotion; it's not about letting other people off the hook.

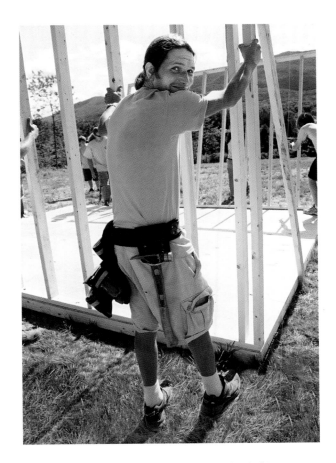

The half who were responsible for taking care of the plant had better medical reports, lower blood pressure, fewer visits to the doctor, and actually died at a significantly lower rate during the study's duration. (You can't have a lot of energy if you're dead, at least the last time I looked.)

This study is often used to illustrate the incredible medical, physical, psychological, and energetic benefits of taking care of something. (It's not by accident that married people live significantly longer than singles do.)

The lesson in this is pretty simple: One way to increase your own energy is by expending energy for someone—or something—else. (Even if it's a plant, although you can probably do better.) My suggestion? Volunteer.

EXPECT A BOUNTY OF BENEFITS

Although being benevolent can do wonders for your self-worth, which, by the way, is *always* energizing, volunteering offers many other rewards. It can be the chance to learn something new, meet like-minded people, have fun, develop leadership skills, build up your resume, or explore a new career direction. And that's just for openers.

Then there are the health benefits. "There is now a convergence of research leading to the conclusion that helping others makes people happier and healthier," said Stephen Post, M.D., a professor at Case Western Reserve University School of Medicine in Cleveland, Ohio.

In fact, studies have shown that volunteers are happier, have higher self-esteem, have a greater sense of control, get more satisfaction out of life, experience better health, and have less depression than non-volunteers. Volunteering can even help alleviate chronic pain. So you can get healthier and happier and create more energy for yourself while doing your part as a citizen of the world.

FIND YOUR CALLING

Whether you are interested in promoting social change, fighting sickness and disease, or cleaning up the environment, there is an agency or association that could use your help. If you decide to explore volunteer opportunities, start by asking yourself what you hope to gain from the experience. This is kind of a cool step, actually.

Back in the day when humanitarian and educator Werner Erhard started the group that ultimately became the Landmark Forum, the group had a rule about "assisting" (which was Forum-speak for volunteering). The rule was this: You have to create at least as much or more value for yourself as you create for the organization by donating your time.

You can make that same rule for yourself when you volunteer, though you may find you don't have to. It kind of happens by itself. The gift to the person volunteering—in health, energy, well-being, and satisfaction—almost always dwarfs the gift to the organization or cause to which the volunteer donates.

Act locally or think globally. Many cities and counties have an office of volunteer service to help you sort through the opportunities available in your own community. Then there are volunteer vacations where you can build a school, teach English, work in a health care clinic, or participate in an archaeological dig overseas.

Volunteering can be exciting, inspiring, and rewarding. It can also help you gain perspective on your own challenges in life. Now, since this is a book on energy, a word of caution is in order: Don't make volunteering just one more obligation in an overcrowded schedule. Be realistic about what you can and want to do. Find the right volunteer opportunity, one that leaves you fulfilled and appreciated, and you'll come away energized. I'll give you my personal, absolute, money-back guarantee on that one.

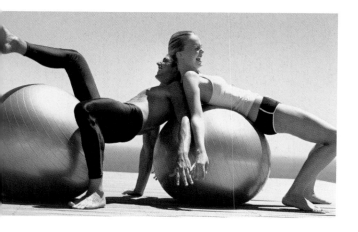

#132

Exercise with Your Mate

Here's a twofer, from an energy standpoint. Exercise with your mate.

Not only will you reap all the mind and body rewards of physical activity (in case you need reminding of the myriad health and energy benefits of exercise, see page 96), but you'll also foster a stronger relationship with the person you love. And if you make a habit of exercising together, studies show, you each stand a better chance of sticking to a routine.

You also stand a better chance of upping your sexual and romantic energy, which is not exactly a bad side benefit. When I interviewed the great sociologist and writer Pepper Schwartz, Ph.D., author of *Prime: Adventures and Advice on Sex, Love, and the Sensual Years*, she quickly drew the connection between energy and relationships: "One major source of depression is when your relationship or marriage is not doing well," she told me. "And that takes away from the ability to mobilize energy." The remedy? "Exercise together!"

"Many people don't get those energizing endorphins going if they aren't physical with each other," Schwartz told me. "Endorphins are a class of brain chemicals that make you feel joy. And once you get them going, it's enormously helpful for getting the whole romance thing going."

AROUSE YOUR PASSION WITH ADRENALINE

Of course, she's right. Early in the 1970s an important article by researchers Elaine Walster and Ellen Berscheid appeared in Psychology Today titled "Adrenaline Makes the Heart Grow Fonder." In it they tell of a study in which one of three groups of men were led to believe they would soon receive a series of three "pretty stiff" electrical shocks.

The experimenters introduced each of the men to a young woman and later casually asked how much each liked her. Those who were expecting the electric shock exhibited more liking for the girl than did a control group with whom the experimenters never discussed the possibility of shocks.

In another study, two groups of young college men were introduced to the same woman under two very different circumstances. In one circumstance, they simply met her as a research assistant. In the other, she greeted them as they finished completing a scary (but safe) task of crossing a rope bridge. In both conditions the young woman gave the men her business card. Far more of the "scared" men rated her attractive and actually called her for a date. Moral of the story: If you want to get your passion and energy aroused (or that of a potential date), get those adrenaline levels up!

Energy is passion, and to love passionately, a person must be physically aroused. One way to produce that arousal is with exercise, and when you exercise with your mate, both of you are often the subconscious recipients of that aroused passion.

CHOOSE YOUR ACTIVITY

The exercise you pick should depend on your goals, fitness abilities, and preferences. If the two of you have different athletic abilities, find a middle-ground activity (this is especially important when one spouse is overly competitive). Playing doubles in tennis, going tandem—kayaking or cycling—and hiking at a pace that works for both of you are all great ways to pair mismatched strengths. (Even walking together could do it— plus it's a great way to start a powerful conversation; see page 236.)

My girlfriend Anja and I like to hike in the nearby mountains (with our highly competitive dogs). Getting away from our hectic lives, even for just an hour, is time for us to catch up, discuss life's mundane details, plan great things for our future, or silently share the sounds of nature. All that, plus breathtaking views and a heart-pumping workout.

Winter activities such as ice skating, snow-shoeing, and skiing can be great ways to bond. (But be forewarned—relationships can hit an icy patch when a downhill newbie is taught to ski by a significant other. Take lessons, and whatever you do, do not follow your significant other down an expert slope unless you know you're ready. Diamonds may be a girl's best friend, but Black Diamonds—or worse, Double Black Diamonds— offer nothing but pain to a beginner.)

You can also practice togetherness at the gym while exercising at your own pace on side-by-side cardio machines. Take a yoga class, pair up for salsa lessons, or get into swimming. Doesn't matter. Get your heart rate up and your (mutual) energy will soar. Your romantic life won't be too shabby either.

Every relationship needs a little variety, so share an athletic challenge—try rock climbing, rafting, or mountain biking. Challenging activities excite our brains, help build new neural pathways, and slow the aging process.

Exercising together promotes good health, reduces stress, increases energy, makes you look and feel better, strengthens your relationship, and may improve your sex life.

What's not to like?

It Doesn't Always Work Out the Way You Hope!

A male graduate student I know was working on a research project in Japan, where he found himself developing a crush on one of his fellow grad students. She, however, didn't seem to be the slightest bit interested in him.

So he hatched a good-natured plot. He was familiar with the research that showed how raising adrenaline levels together often has a positive romantic effect, so he decided to ask her to go with him on an adventure—a rickshaw ride through the streets of Tokyo. She eagerly agreed.

Afterward, excited from the new experience, she turned to him and told him how great the ride had been.

And then added breathlessly, "And that rickshaw driver was so handsome!"

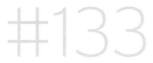

Show Your Creative Colors

One Christmas,* my brother Jeffrey gave everyone in our family an unusual trio of presents—a large artist's drawing pad, a box of sixty-four Crayola crayons, and a Slinky.

There was a method to his madness. He was trying to get us to engage the right side of our brain, the side that doesn't think logically or in a linear fashion, but is instead responsible for creativity and play.

I call the right side of the brain "the great energy liberator."

And evidentially, I'm not alone.

Right around the time of this writing, there was mounting buzz in the blogosphere about a video that was capturing the attention of millions of viewers. Within a relatively short time, the star of the video (about whom more in a moment) had a book deal, appeared on *Oprah*, and became a sensation.

I can tell you this: The video—called "My Stroke of Insight"—is one of the most profoundly moving things I've seen in years. You can view it on the "Technology, Entertainment, and Design" website (www.ted.com). What it has to teach us about energy and the right brain is amazing.

Here's the back story.

A STROKE OF INSPIRATION

One bleak, typically New England winter day in 1996, Jill Bolte Taylor, Ph.D., a thirty-seven-year-old Harvard brain scientist and the star of the aforementioned video, woke up with a throbbing head-

*Sharp-eyed readers may be puzzled by the fact that I've made a number of references to being raised in a Jewish home; however, we were very secular and inclusionary Jews and we had both a Hanukkah menorah and a Christmas tree!

ache. Thinking that exercise would help alleviate the pain, she hopped onto her cardio glider. When that offered no relief she got into the shower. Stepping under what seemed to be a torrent of water, her sensory perception changed. She was struck by a sense of awe as the physical border of her body seemed to melt into her surroundings. "What a bizarre living being I am. Life! I am life! I am a sea of water bound inside this membranous pouch."

She was having a stroke.

Strangely, she didn't panic.

"How often does a brain scientist get to study her own brain from the inside out?" she asks in her now-famous lecture taped at the 2008 TED conference in California.

As she was "enfolded by a blanket of tranquil euphoria," the left side of her brain, the control center of logic, order, language, and "that constant chatter that had attached me to the details of my life," began shutting down. Until that December day in 1996, she had been a work-focused, type-A scientist who spent a lifetime living in thoughts. But now, with the left side of her brain temporarily disabled, she awoke to the peace and grace and energy that reside in the right side of her brain. And her life was profoundly changed.

When you listen to Bolte Taylor speak, which I really hope you will do, you will be struck immediately by her sense of boundless energy. (You may also be struck by her almost spiritual sense of grace and wisdom and joy, but for now, let's just focus on the energy part.) Her message is clear: If you want that energy, and all the other wondrous feelings that go with it, you simply have to do more to exercise that often quiet right brain of yours.

HOW TO AWAKEN CREATIVE ENERGY

The good news is that you don't have to actually go out and have a stroke to tap into the right side of your brain. You just have to work at quieting the left half, where past experiences and future worries can create the negative, judgmental voices that weigh us down, tire our spirit, and limit our potential. Once you learn to access the right hemisphere of your brain—crayons, anyone?—you can awaken creative energy and experience a deep sense of inner peace.

The right side of the brain is the part that lives only in the now. It's not tired. It's not fatigued. It's not exhausted. It's just in the now.* And one way to tap into the power of now is to reach back to your grade school days. Which brings me back to the crayons.

Pick up a pack of crayons and color your world periwinkle blue, pine green, or scarlet red. Don't judge. Don't analyze. Suspend logic. Let go. Vary the strokes and shades; let your imagination get

*It's probably no accident that one of the best-selling self-help books of all time is Eckhart Tolle's The Power of Now.

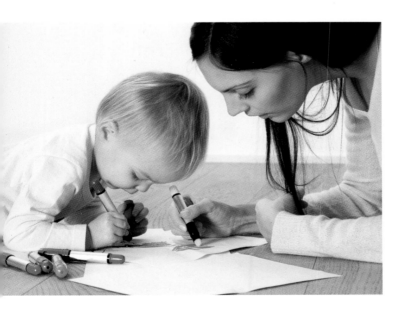

carried away in Crayola. Once you let your left brain nap, you can awaken the artist within. You may want to shift from crayons to charcoal or paint, or maybe your artistic medium is clay or straw. It doesn't matter. By merely making an effort to quiet those limiting, negative inner voices and listening to your creative instinct, you can shift into a really positive energy zone.

The more you practice, the easier it will be to overcome stress, unlock your creative power, and live in the here and now.

Do that, and I guarantee you'll feel energized.

#134

Shift Your Attention

Yesterday I Googled the term *information overload*. There were more than two million listings. So now we're safely in an era of information overload *about* information overload. No wonder America, among other nations, has a serious attention deficit problem.

All that information, and the multitude of ways it comes at us, adds to the clutter in our offices and homes and brains. It makes it more difficult to concentrate on the task at hand when you're worried about all the other things that need your attention.

You try to focus on the budget figures you have to digest for the afternoon meeting, but what with your email dinging and your cell phone vibrating, and all that downloaded research you have to sort through, your mind keeps interrupting you . . . *did you ever return your mother's phone call? . . . hey, you've got to call George and go over these figures before the meeting . . .*

You tell yourself to concentrate on the Excel spreadsheet on the screen in front of you . . . *oh, wait, did you RSVP for that party on Saturday? . . . there's something you're forgetting . . . your feet hurt . . . maybe you shouldn't have walked from the train in spiked heels, and . . . running shoes, did you forget your gym clothes, and was that what you forgot to remember? . . .* You concentrate on concentrating on this budget, you go over the figures for the advertising department . . . and . . . *not another IM, haven't you told your son not to instant-message you at work . . .* You really, really try to focus, but you can't because your brain's spam filter has gone on strike.

Sound familiar?

WHEN YOUR FOCUS FAILS

You, my friend, are suffering from directed attention fatigue (DAF). (Yup, they've even got a name for it.) That catchy term was coined by a husband and wife team of environmental psychologists from the University of Michigan, Stephen and Rachel Kaplan.

"When people talk about mental fatigue, what is actually fatigued is not their mind as a whole, but their capacity to direct attention," says Stephen Kaplan, Ph.D. "Sustained directed attention is difficult and fatiguing." That constant demand for concentration in the face of distractions—internal and external—fatigues our *inhibitory attention system* (translated: the part of the brain that directs our attention so we're able to concentrate and ignore distractions).

Besides an inability to focus, other symptoms of DAF include forgetfulness, impatience, and general crankiness.

FOCUS ON THE FLORA AND FAUNA

But there is something you can do about it—reboot your brain. When you can no longer concentrate, when your stream of consciousness floods your mind with distractions, there's an easy fix: Shift your attention to the outdoors.

See, most of what we experience as mental fatigue isn't really our brain saying, "I need to veg out in front of the TV." Rather, it's our brain saying, "I need to stop concentrating on this task that's been taking up all my mental energy and focus. I need relief!" It's the mental energy equivalent of being full after dinner, but perking up when the waiter brings the Death by Chocolate brownie. Something new? Bring it on! All of a sudden our energy comes back. (How else do you think Oprah has the energy for a TV show, a radio network, a magazine, and Harpo Productions?)

For us mortals, the solution is easy. If you're in a room with a view, pay attention to nature and focus on the greenery outside. Work in a windowless cubicle? Then hang a picture that depicts a beautiful setting. Studies by the Kaplans as well as other researchers in this burgeoning field of environmental psychology have shown that merely having a view—or even a *picture* of nature—can get that inhibitory attention system of ours back on track in a New York minute. In fact, a number of studies have found a correlation between a view of nature and relief from stress, boredom, and anxiety, as well as increased productivity at work and even a speedier recovery for hospital patients.

In other words, nature nurtures us in a multitude of ways.

THE ENERGY OF GOING GREEN

In his book *Biophilia*, sociobiologist Edward O. Wilson proposed that we are genetically hardwired to seek out natural settings. If that's so, and it seems to be, it would account for the restorative effect of living, green environments (think: a walk in the woods).

"For human survival and mental health and fulfillment," Wilson says, "we need the natural setting in which the human mind almost certainly evolved and in which culture has developed over these millions of years of evolution."

For more than thirty years, sociologists, biologists, psychologists, and architects have studied the effect nature has on us and looked for ways to bring nature—or facsimiles of nature—into public spaces, hospitals, and offices. But as great as nature is, there are other ways to take advantage of the energy-boosting properties of attention shift.

EAT THAT ATTENTIONAL DESSERT

While exploring these other ways, remember that your goal is to take advantage of the energy-restoring power of an attention shift. If you've spent hours poring over stock reports, go read a book of Peanuts cartoons. If you've run errands frantically all afternoon, take a hot bath. If you've talked all day, try a half hour of uninterrupted silence. If you've been writing at the computer, borrow your kid's coloring book and go to town (see page 248 on using crayons).

The point is, you can recharge your energy batteries by simply "closing down shop" on whatever task you've been totally focused on, and engaging a new set of skills, changing your focus, moving into a new environment, or taking on a different project. A long, focused bout of attention on one task or project is like doing biceps curls with the left arm only. That arm is going to fatigue after a while, but when you pick up the weight with your right arm, you find it feels pretty light. That's because there's plenty of energy available in the right hand; it's been resting while you've been lifting with its opposite.

In much the same way, there's plenty of mental energy available—the trick is to know how to spread it around.

Bonus benefit: Once your mental energy is restored, you can always get back to your spreadsheets and really focus on those budget numbers. (Or not.) If you choose to go back to the original task, you'll be able to do it with even more energy than before.

Manhattan, I read about a local "guru" who was reported to be able to organize and rearrange your living space so that you could have maximum energy. She practiced some obscure Asian art form whose name I couldn't pronounce at the time, and it was said that when you organized your space according to the principles of this practice, you could not only maximize your own energy, but also attract precisely the things you wanted into your life—love, prosperity, you name it. Donald Trump was said to have had the lobbies of his building designed according to this practice.

The guru in question was a charming woman named Carole Meltzer (www.carolemeltzer.com). I hired her. I found her to be quite a character—a combination of Long Island designer and spiritual guru, and, as I later learned, the first American woman to be trained in China as a Master in this interesting energetic art form, which, of course, was known as feng shui (pronounced fung shway).

Well, it worked. From the moment she applied her magic touch—telling me where the "energy

#135

Flow with Feng Shui

Ever walk into a room and feel like the energy just isn't right? You might not be able to put your finger on it, but something about the space leaves you feeling a little unsettled. Maybe it's too dark or too stuffy or the colors don't work, or maybe it's the placement of the furniture.

It could be you've stepped into a room with bad feng shui.

Here's my personal experience with feng shui and energy. Years ago, when I was living in

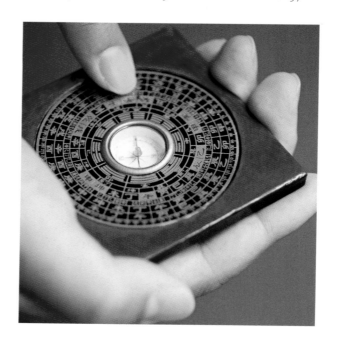

was blocked" in my apartment, creating "flows," changing colors, putting symbolic materials in key places in order to attract love, romance, and prosperity—things noticeably changed. I'm not kidding. It was during this time that I began a new relationship, my income went way up, and the general "feel" of my Manhattan apartment became more airy and open. I swear, I could literally feel my energy rise, and the energy of the apartment was noticeably different, something commented on by virtually everyone who came to visit.

So what the heck is feng shui anyway? And how can it help you with your energy?

Glad you asked.

WELCOME NATURE FOR ENERGY AND HARMONY

Feng shui is the ancient Chinese art of bringing harmony to an environment, based, in part, on tenets found in nature. Through design, the purposeful placement of furnishings and objects, and the use of color, a feng shui Master balances yin and yang, allowing positive energy, or *qi*, to flow freely throughout the space. It's a system built on five elements—fire, water, earth, metal, and wood—and the colors that symbolize each. How those elements interact can impact the energy of the environment in either a positive or a negative way.

Every area of your life is also represented by an area of your home called a *gua* (a feng shui map of a space is called a *bagua*). There are nine *guas*: prosperity, fame and reputation, relationships and love, creativity and children, helpful people and travel, career and life path, skills and knowledge, family, and health and all other life situations not mentioned. Each *gua* also has corresponding symbols, body parts, colors, and shapes.

When a space has bad feng sui, it gives off negative energy. The result could be mental or physical fatigue, stagnation in your career or love life, or a host of other unpleasant consequences. Although I'm hardly a feng shui Master—heck, I could barely pronounce it a few years ago—I do know a few basic principles that can help make your environment more conducive to positive energy, both yours and that of the universe.

TIPS FOR ENERGIZING YOUR SPACE

Start with the room you feel most affects your energy level. The first step is to remove all clutter, which holds stale, negative energy (see page 224). In feng shui, out of sight is *not* out of mind (a principle you've heard me state many times in this book). No matter where clutter accumulates—your attic, a hall closet, or that drawer you'd just as soon never open—it affects the energy of your home. If it affects the energy of your home, believe me, it affects *your* energy as well. In spades. Even if you're not consciously aware of it.

No matter where clutter accumulates—your attic, a hall closet, or that drawer you'd just as soon never open—it affects the energy of your home.

Next, evaluate the lighting. In feng shui, light represents the sun, and a well-lit room promotes vitality and the smooth movement of positive qi. If there's a lot of available natural light, then for goodness sake, let it shine in! If not, use lamps and candles to brighten dark spaces.

Another essential for energy is good air quality. Open windows often to keep air circulating, and use an air purifier or air-purifying plants to help filter out toxins.

If it's the kitchen you're focusing on, you'll be relieved to know that the oven-sink-refrigerator triangle design of most kitchens actually balances water and fire, so it's good feng shui. (By the same token, if you introduce too *much* of the water element, found in the colors blue or black, you might extinguish the symbolic fire of energy, so use those colors sparingly.) As with everything else in feng shui, striking the right balance with color is important. For instance, red represents fire, so introducing it into a room can bring energy, excitement, and passion. But too *much* red may lead to anger or overstimulation. Although you want a calming bedroom, a bit of red—say, a decorative pillow or candle—might spark passion (which, for most of us, is a good thing!).

For the most part, though, your bedroom should be a sanctuary filled with calming yin energy. The best colors for the bedroom are skin tones, anything from white to rich brown—it's no accident that those gorgeous designer bedrooms you see in catalogues are brimming with these warm, inviting colors! Everything in your bedroom should represent love and relaxation.

There should be symmetry in the bedroom, just as there should be in a good relationship. Place your bed in the middle of a solid wall (if possible) with nightstands on either side. Flowers add fresh energy and life to a bedroom. Note to people who use their bedroom as a combination office or exercise room: Anything that takes your mind away from sleep or sex should be banished from the room. Sorry. But trust me, you'll thank me for it later.

Although feng shui is an art that can take a lifetime to master, you can use some of its basic principles now to increase your energy and your overall well-being. By becoming more aware of how furniture placement, colors, and décor affect your mood, you'll be able to make your home more comfortable.

Even if you don't meet your future wife, husband, boyfriend, or girlfriend, I promise that you will have a lot more positive energy in your life.

#136
Change Your Frequency

Every type of energy—electrical, physical, mental, spiritual—has a frequency. And a frequency tune-up can be just the thing you need to get more energy in your life.

Let me explain.

Every living thing—you, me, our pets, even plants, trees, and vegetables—vibrates, if you will, to certain frequencies, and the lower, darker frequencies are perceived as "negative" while the higher frequencies are perceived as "positive." There are color analogies to this—light and dark being the most obvious—and musical analogies (major and minor), but the fact that there is a continuum of "negative" and "positive" energy is not in doubt.

Our feelings and our thoughts are like mixing boards for that energy. They can turn it up; turn it down; add noise, interference, and static; and ultimately crash the system (which is almost always what you perceive as crushing fatigue).

"Emotional stress takes away your energy and drains you," says my friend Aleta St. James, who became a national news item when, in 2005, at the age of fifty-seven, she became the oldest woman in the United States to give birth to twins. Now, at this writing, sixty years old and a single mother of two, she has more energy than most people I know, frequently goes 14-hour days, shows no sign of slowing down, and leaves most people in her wake, feeling like they can't keep up.

St. James knows what she's talking about when she talks about energy. She's a life coach whose stock in trade is something called energy medicine. In her own practice she does what's called energy transformation, helping people make the kind of life shift (also the title of the book she wrote about her experience) that allows them to leave behind most of the energy-sapping negative emotions and generate replacements from the "light" end of the spectrum. Not for nothing do they call the process of giving up anger and stress "lightening up."

"Worry, anger, and stress totally take away your energy and drain you," St. James told me in a recent conversation. "But it's not just about thinking positively and telling yourself everything's going to be fine and that there's nothing to worry about. It's actually learning how to shift yourself out of feeling these negative feelings and to begin to actually reprogram yourself to feel and think positively."

TAKE A DEEP BREATH . . .

I asked St. James for some tips that you might be able to use right now to instantly boost your energy. She suggested practicing deep breathing.

"Most of us breathe very shallowly," she told me. "When we get upset, we hold our breath. Consequently, we get stuck in that feeling of fear or anger, and those two emotions are energy zappers."

Here's how to do it:

- Take long, slow, deep breaths as soon as you start feeling stuck on a negative emotion.
- Breathe in through your nose, filling up your stomach, and then breathe out through your mouth. Do this until you establish a rhythm, like waves of the ocean moving in and out on the shore.
- Connect with what you are feeling so that you can release it.
- Now ask yourself, "What am I feeling that I need to release?"
- Let that feeling surface.
- Is it anger, frustration, insecurity, or something else?
- Allow yourself to really feel it.
- Hold your breath for the count of five.
- As you exhale, imagine that there is an orb of gold light in front of you.
- Release those feelings that are keeping you stuck into the gold light.
- Feel as if the gold light is a powerful vacuum cleaner, pulling all negative emotion from your body, organs, and cells.
- Keep breathing and releasing until the negative feelings dissipate or until the negative emotion feels neutralized. You will feel a shift.

"It is important to release the feelings and then replace them with something else," St. James told me. "This is the step that most of us forget." Here's how to do it:

- Once you have neutralized the negative feelings, begin to visualize how you *want* to feel (joyous? peaceful?). Then begin to bring in those feelings associated with that condition or state.
- For this part of the exercise, imagine an orb of *white* light.

Allow that white light to fill your body and the entire space surrounding you.

"Remember, nature abhors a vacuum, so you need to fill up the space you have just emptied of negativity with gorgeous and beautiful energy and visualizations," St. James explains.

I end almost all my lectures and workshops with a variation on the following words: *"If you can visualize it, you can believe it. If you can believe it, you can do it."* Nowhere is that truer than with energy. If you can visualize the kind of positive, joyous energy you want to fill your life with, you will be on the way to creating it. And that's the kind of energy we all want in our lives.

To learn more about Aleta St. James's "Energy Transformation" system, visit www.aletastjames.com.

Take a Cold Shower

Okay, here's a riddle for you: How can you save energy and gain energy at the same time? Give up? Take a cold shower. It's an invigorating and energy-boosting way to start the day. And since, according to the U.S. Department of Energy, heating water can account for up to 25 percent of your energy bill, taking cold showers will be good for you, your pocketbook, and the environment.

People have used cold water therapeutically to promote health for centuries. It produces a natural analgesic (painkilling) effect that can ease muscle aches and pains. Plus, a cold shower raises your metabolic rate, which can reduce fatigue and increase energy. There's even some evidence that it may help relieve depression, which is pretty high on the list of energy killers!

Exposure to cold water also improves circulation, aids in ridding the body of toxins, reduces inflammation, enhances the immune system, and helps stabilize blood pressure. Not a bad resume

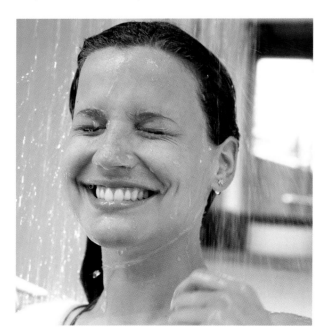

for an energy enhancer that's essentially free! Not only will taking regular cold showers make you feel better, but it will also make you *look* better—it does wonders for your skin and hair.

There is no quicker way to get a blast of energy than by turning the hot water off and spending as little as a few seconds under a cold shower. Scandinavians have long known about the energy-boosting power of a bracing cold shower, and they even build alternating hot and cold showers into their spa treatments. The energizing effect of cold water is as close as your bathroom.

If you're interested in trying this for yourself, here are a couple of things to do to make sure this energizing experience is a pleasant one. First of all, make sure the bathroom is warm. The last thing you want to do is step out of a cold shower and into a freezing cold room. Second, when you get into the shower in the first place, start with the temperature at whatever you consider normal (which is usually warm). Then move out of the water stream and turn the hot water off. Test the water with your feet first, then your hands and face to acclimate. Try to stay in long enough for the shock to wear off. (You may have to build up, starting with as few as 5 seconds. No problem!) Then towel off and start your day exhilarated and energized.

────── **WORTH KNOWING** ──────

If you have any health issues, particularly heart disease or Raynaud's disease, or if you are anemic, you may want to check with your health care professional before getting into the cold shower habit.

Make a Gratitude List

The law of attraction got a lot of attention back in 2006, when an aggressively marketed DVD called *The Secret* took the world by storm and made minor (and sometimes major) stars out of the twenty-five or so cast members. Personally, I think *The Secret*, which suggests that positive thoughts are powerful magnets that attract happiness, good health, and wealth, was terribly misunderstood (and *misused*), and for many people, a very important lesson was lost. That lesson, which I'm going to discuss right now, has a lot to do with your energy levels.

Here is the gist of the law of attraction: What you focus on and what you think about and what you give energy to is what tends to manifest in your life.

You *create* good energy when you *come from* a place of good energy (a more New Agey way of restating Gandhi's maxim, "*Be* the change that you want to see in the world.")

When you come from a place of love, it's easier to generate love. When you *think* and *feel* loving thoughts, it's easier to *attract* loving thoughts. As one of my high-energy friends put it, "It's like listening to a radio. If you're tuned to the rock and roll station, you're not going to 'receive' the smooth jazz station. You have to be tuned to the waves that you want to receive on. If you are tuned to the hate waves, you don't usually attract love."

It's no accident that when an angry drunk walks into a bar looking for trouble, he always finds it. He's tuned to angry, violent frequencies—of course he's going to attract violence.

So if you're thinking about what a crummy day it is and how miserable your boss is and how no one understands you, guess what tends to manifest? More of the same! It's incredible how that happens, isn't it? The point here is that our thoughts have a lot of power. And though we can't completely control our thoughts, we can control our attention and our focus.

So here's the tip: Make a gratitude list. I want you to actually write down ten things in your life that you're grateful for. It can be people, places, things, conditions, or anything you want. On my list I put my relationship with my partner Anja, my new Macintosh computer, my writing opportunities, my amazing health, my friends, my dogs Woodstock and Emily II, my career, my outdoor gazebo surrounded with plants . . . you get the idea. The point is to spend a little time actually focusing on some of the many wonderful things in your life. It can be absolutely anything you want. Just put down the first ten things that come to mind, and put them in a list.

Then read that list every day for thirty days. We're talking about a time investment of fewer than three minutes a day. Just read and reflect on the things you're grateful for. You might even find that as the thirty-day period unfolds you have more things to add to the list. That's fine; write them down. The energy you put into these thoughts of gratitude and appreciation will come back to you many times over. You'll find you have a renewed appreciation for many things you'd been taking for granted.

In fact, in studies on gratitude, subjects who were instructed to keep gratitude journals showed higher levels of positive emotions, life satisfaction, vitality, and optimism, and lower levels of depression and stress than those who didn't. The gratitude group also reported better quality sleep and less pain, and they were more likely to exercise regularly and to have made progress toward achieving important personal goals. That's a formula for high energy.

That's the law of attraction in action. Put it to work for you to increase your energy now.

Make Peace with Your Gremlins

One of the biggest energy drains in the world is the chorus of voices we all have in our heads.

Don't pretend you don't have them. We all do.

The great acting teacher Uta Hagen used to call them "trolls." She'd tell her students the following: "You know every one of you has a little troll who sits on your shoulder and chatters away, saying you can't act." (She understood perfectly the insecurity of actors.) "That little troll tells you, 'You're a fraud, and you're gonna be found out any minute, and you have no business on a stage, who do you think you are anyway, you're no actor!' Every one of you has that little troll on your shoulder," she'd continue. "It's just the nature of being an actor."

Then she'd go on: "Well you know that troll of yours? Here's the bad news: *He's never going to go away.* So the action isn't in trying to get rid of him. That's a hopeless task. But here's what's not hopeless: *making peace with him.*"

Finally she'd pause dramatically and deliver the punch line, slowly:

"You need to be able to say to him, 'Thank you for sharing, little troll. You're welcome to sit there on my shoulder, but if you wouldn't mind, just keep quiet for a few minutes because I'm going out on that stage to act!'"

MAKE PEACE WITH YOUR INNER CRITIC

Uta Hagen called them trolls, some people call them voices, and personally, I call them gremlins. No matter. Make peace with them, however you need to do it. Let them chatter away; they're going to do it anyway. Remember, you can't *will* yourself not to have a thought—it's just *there*. You can't make it go away. You can't *not think* about a thought you're having. It'd be like telling you, "Don't think about a purple elephant."

But here's the good news: You don't have to *empower* that energy-draining thought. You don't have to *act* on that chatter. Listen to it, notice it, accept it as a part of you, which it is, but don't give it any power. That's the power you have in the world. You can't make the gremlin disappear, but you can sure unplug him and take away his ability to hold you back.

We all have doubts and considerations and roadblocks. Even Mother Teresa questioned her faith, but it didn't stop her from doing what she did. Embrace those energy-stealing gremlins just as surely as you embrace every other part of yourself—they're part of your own truth.

Then thank those little guys for sharing, but don't give them the power to bring you down. Quiet the voices of insecurity and self-doubt—realize it's just the mindless chatter of harmless little trolls—and instead, engage your energy.

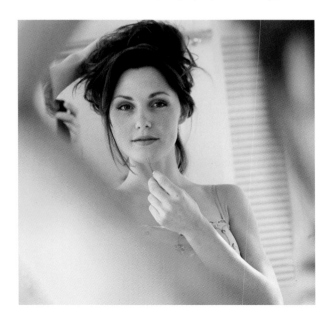

#140

Dress Up!

Do you happen to remember the now quaint compliment, "You look like a million bucks"? Or maybe Vince Vaughn's frenetic exhortations to Jon Favreau in the movie *Swingers*—"Money, baby. You're money!" Either way, what both these expressions have in common is that they implicitly recognize the connection between how you look and how you feel.

One of the constant themes throughout this book is that you can *reverse-engineer* your energy. When you're feeling less than energetic, there are a lot of things you can do to *look and act* like you have energy. Often—if not always—you'll wind up *feeling* exactly the way you look and act, even if you didn't start out that way.

That, by the way, is why top motivational speakers make sure that their audiences get up from time to time and jump around or high-five their neighbors or repeat a phrase out loud with enthusiasm ("I can't *hear* you!"). They know, like any warm-up act in Vegas, that you can *generate* excitement in people simply by getting them to *act* excited.

DRESS FOR SUCCESS

It's the same thing with energy. I remember being a shy teenager who had a horrendous time getting dates. An older mentor made a remarkable and unexpected suggestion to me: Put on your best suit and go shopping for groceries. Sounds ridiculous, right? To me, too—until I tried it. All of a sudden, I felt like a million bucks. People noticed me and smiled unexpectedly, and the cashier winked at me, and right away, I felt sexy. A simple change in my clothing changed my presentation to the world, which in turn changed the world's reaction to me, which in turn . . . Well, you get the picture.

Remember Billy Crystal's perennially tanned character Fernando on the old *Saturday Night Live?* (You don't? Here's a hint: "You look mahvelous.") Holding court in his mock Hideaway, he greeted every guest with the catchphrase, often adding his famous credo, "It is better to look good than to feel good."

Well, you can do both. Start *looking* like energy, and I'm willing to bet you'll have it in short order. No matter how you feel, if you make the effort to look good, then you may just start to feel good. So when you want to rev up your energy, get dolled up. I'm not talking about donning a black-tie outfit (unless, of course, you're heading to a black-tie event), but dig through your closet for those clothes that flatter, the ones that always make you feel attractive, and dress to impress—yourself. Take extra care with your hair and, for women, your makeup. Once you've decked yourself out, stand up straight, gaze into the mirror, and smile. Does your reflection match that of someone whose spirits and energy are low—the way you felt before this mini makeover?

Of course it doesn't. You look good, maybe even great. Pretty soon, your mood and energy level will match.

Bonus benefit: If you happen to be a shy teenager, you may even wind up with a date.

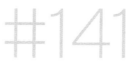

Make a Color Shift

When your energy sags and you need a quick pick-me-up, think red. Deep saturated red, to be precise. Although the color symbolizes different things in different cultures, studies have consistently shown that it has a stimulating effect.

How's that, you ask? Let me explain.

Color *is* energy. It actually has temperature, measured in what's called degrees Kelvin. (Examples: The temperature of direct sunlight is 5,000K, the temperature of a match flame 1,700K.) This all started in the late 1800s, when a British physicist named William Kelvin discovered that if you heated a block of carbon it would glow in the heat, producing a range of different colors at different temperatures.

But I digress.

REV UP WITH RED (OR ORANGE OR YELLOW)

Our experience of color basically happens because light waves of various frequencies are processed through photoreceptors in the retina, then sent as nerve impulses to the cortex, where, voilà, they're translated by the brain into our experience of color. Truth be told, we can only detect three of them: red, blue, and green. Our fabulous in-house computer called the brain then does the color mixing to create the exact hue.

Because it affects our brain, color can be much more than a visual treat. It can be an experience, one that evokes emotion. Color can excite or calm, it can convey a sense of coolness or warmth, it can symbolize strength or purity or romance. The famous psychoanalyst and child psychiatrist

Bruno Bettelheim used to insist on having his clinics painted yellow, precisely because of the effect that color had on the energy of his young subjects.

For thousands of years color has been used as a healing therapy. Today, most color therapists believe it's the different energy frequencies of color that affect us physically and emotionally. Those frequencies stimulate the pituitary and pineal glands, triggering certain hormonal responses. Modern conventional medicine employs some version of color therapy. For instance, infants who are jaundiced are treated with blue light.

Some research indicates that a person's mood and personality are reflected in the colors they choose. Several studies, for instance, found that people who wear dark colors to the exclusion of any other colored clothes tend to be depressed (which, if it's true, would mean there are an awful lot of depressed people living in Manhattan, where black is the new black). You don't have to be a scientist to figure out that spending your days in a drab-colored room will sour your mood.

Generally, colors with longer wavelengths—reds, oranges, and yellows—are thought to be more stimulating than those at the other end of the spectrum, where the greens, blues, and purples reside. (That's why guests on television shows wait in "the green room"—it's calming!)

One commonly held explanation is that we associate warm colors with the energy of the sun and daylight. But there are many variables as to how we perceive and respond to color, including its hue and saturation, the material used, what other colors surround it, and how it's used (a yellow dress may evoke a very different feeling than a room of the same shade). Deeply saturated colors—whether warm or cool—have been shown to be stimulating in some studies. Our reaction to any color may also be its association with memories, and the emotion those memories provoke.

COLOR YOUR WORLD

If you want to give your energy a real boost, experiment with color. If your closet is filled with a sea of black, go wild and try some red. Or maybe a brilliant turquoise will get you going. If you have to ease into color, start with a brightly colored shirt or scarf and see how that makes you feel.

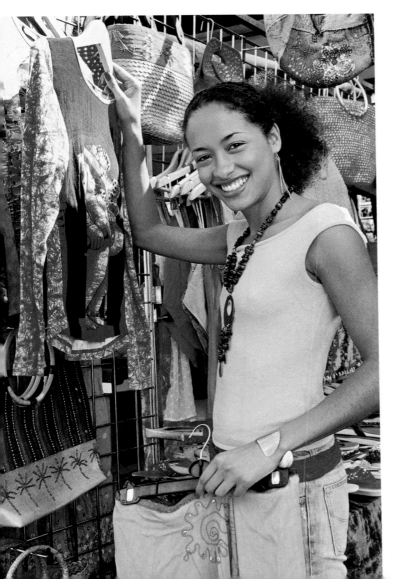

We all have colors that seem to brighten our faces and bring out the color of our eyes (the color your mother always said you looked good in). The mere act of making an effort to brighten your wardrobe is energizing.

Adding some color to your life will boost your energy, but don't overlook the effect a color change can have on others around you. Even if *you're* not feeling it at first (which I'm sure you will), those brighter, warmer, more energetic colors may make *others* respond to *you* in a warmer, more energetic way. If energy is anything, it's contagious!

#142

Free Your Energy by Riding the Horse in the Direction It's Going

Years ago, there was a great teacher named Werner Erhard. Despite withering criticism from a cynical press, Werner—everyone called him Werner—changed the lives of thousands of people. He was one of the pioneers of the whole self-help, personal-growth movement.

Anyway.

Werner was in his heyday back in the 1970s, especially in San Francisco, where his headquarters were. He was a dynamic, mesmerizing speaker, and people came out in droves to hear him. One particular evening, he was scheduled to speak at the Cow Palace, a huge stadium in the heart of the city.

Only problem was, there was an earthquake scare.

Government officials urged people to either evacuate San Francisco or stay home, but at the very least to stay off the roads. Whatever else they did, it was strongly suggested that they *not* head downtown. This didn't seem to stop the thousands of people who got in their cars, headed precisely in that direction, and subsequently packed the sold-out event at the Cow Palace.

The press was astonished. They crowded around Werner, shoving microphones in his face and asking him how he could account for this remarkable behavior on the part of his followers. One reporter said, "Werner, how do you explain the fact that the whole city of San Francisco is on earthquake alert, half the city seems to be evacuating the area, and yet there are thousands of people flocking into downtown here at the Cow Palace to hear you speak? How can you account for this? Is this some kind of cult you're running?"

Werner smiled and replied, "It's very simple. There's not going to be an earthquake. You see, I've *decided* that there will not be an earthquake."

The reporters looked around at each other, convinced they were in the presence of a delusional madman who clearly thought he was God. Then Werner, ever the master of the dramatic pause and the killer delivery, waited a moment, smiled shyly, and added, "But if you happen to hear the earth rumble, you'll know I changed my mind."

I call that "riding the horse in the direction it's going."

RESISTANCE IS FUTILE

Now hold that thought for a moment, and let's talk about lifting weights.

If you've ever tried to lift a really heavy weight, then you know what it's like when your muscles get tired. Whether it's moving furniture from room to room, pushing a piano a few feet for better placement in the living room, or bench-pressing 250 pounds at the gym (I *wish*), your muscles eventually give out and give up from exhaustion. In fact, one classic principle of bodybuilding and fitness training is to do as many repetitions as it takes to hit "failure," i.e., the point at which your muscles are so fatigued that they can't perform another rep. It's not by accident that they call weight training "resistance" training.

Well, the same thing happens to your emotional and spiritual muscles when you *resist* the universe in unproductive ways. The more you resist, the more energy you put out trying to change something that isn't going to change, at least not from the force of you pushing at it. All that happens is that your energy muscles get fatigued. Our language even reflects that. We describe people who "drain" our energy. We refer to people, places, and things that suck the life out of us as "exhausting."

Most of that energy drain comes not from other people, but from our own resistance.

Want proof? Do this exercise. Clasp your hands together as if in prayer, fingers interlocked. Now push with all your might, using the muscles of both arms. Concentrate on trying to move your left arm with your right one, all the while pushing back with equal force. If you're like most people, nothing's going to move (because the left and right arm muscles are of equal force). This kind of exercise is known as "isometrics" (*iso* meaning "same" and *metrics* meaning "movement"). There's a lot of energy expended, but nothing actually *happens*.

Now do the same exercise, but instead of pushing back with the right arm, simply stop pushing back, let go, and lift your right arm out of the way. What happens? Your left arm moves

effortlessly through space and winds up on your lap. No more resistance, no more need to push.

No more energy drain.

LET THE HORSE LEAD

Now back to Werner, the Cow Palace, and the threatened earthquake. Werner had decided to proceed as if there wasn't going to be an earthquake, but not to resist if there turned out to actually *be* an earthquake. The point of his comment was this: It's way easier to ride the horse in the direction it's going.

Contrary to the initial impression he undoubtedly left on many reporters, he wasn't a delusional madman who thought that by a sheer force of will he could act like God and determine that there wouldn't be an earthquake. He was simply illustrating an enlightened principle for dealing with the world—*choose what is*. "If you hear the earth rumble, you know I've changed my mind," is one of the wittiest ways to illustrate this principle, which is at the heart of many Eastern and spiritual philosophies—*choose what is*.

It's about not resisting. It's about moving your right hand so your left hand can travel effortlessly through the air, meeting no resistance. It's about choosing what *is*.

When you choose what is, you are essentially riding the horse in the direction it's going. If you've ever ridden a horse, you know that riding it where it is going anyway takes a lot less energy than trying to force this 1,000-pound headstrong animal to do something it doesn't want to do. Not only is that easier on the horse, but it's also way easier on you. To top it off, if you're willing to take the ride first, rather than fighting the horse at every corner, you have a much greater shot at eventually moving the horse in the direction in which *you* want to go. Fighting takes energy. Hanging on and going along for the ride . . . not so much.

ENERGY CREATED BY DOING NOTHING

Whole systems of martial arts are built on this principle. Aikido, for example, basically teaches you how to get out of the way and use your opponent's own energy to defeat him. You don't resist; you just conserve *your* energy while your opponent uses his to slam into the floor.

You can use this principle to immediately increase your daily emotional and mental energy. Riding the horse in the direction it's going is like plugging one of the biggest energy drains in your life. Think of the amount of energy you expend fighting things that aren't going to change, at least not in the immediate future, and at least not because you're raging against them. (I know what of I speak. Let me remind you that I live in Los Angeles and have to deal with absolutely insane traffic on a daily basis. Guess what I found? Resisting it doesn't make the traffic go faster. Resisting it doesn't make a whit of difference, except, of course, to my own energy levels!)

Think of one thing you spend a lot of energy resisting and, just for today, try this lesson from Werner Erhard: Choose it. Embrace it. Go with it. Go along for the ride. Make up something good about it. (In my case, I bought Sirius satellite radio and learned to look at the traffic as a great excuse to listen to classic jazz for an hour or so a day.

Now, when the freeway is like a parking lot, I simply "choose" traffic and jazz. (Of course, if the traffic moves like the wind, you'll know I changed my mind.)

If it's an evil colleague whom you're resisting, try saying, "Well, that's just Steve being Steve," instead of trying to change him. If it's an airline delay, go read a book. If it's traffic, buy a satellite radio.

There's an old saying from science fiction writer Robert Heinlein: "Never try to teach a pig to sing; it wastes your time and annoys the pig." Couple that with another saying of undetermined origin: *What you resist persists*. The more energy you spend trying to resist what is, the harder the universe will press back. Stop resisting, get out of the way, and what you're resisting will disappear. You'll have freed up more valuable energy for yourself instantly.

Note: For those who are interested, a recent (and mesmerizing) new movie was released in May 2008 called *Transformation: The Life and Legacy of Werner Erhard*. This terrific movie by award-winning director Robyn Simon should go a long way to restoring the reputation and good name of this remarkable human being. Werner Erhard has been thanked in the acknowledgments of every book I have ever written and every book I will ever write for the rest of my life. Every one of us in the "self-help" or "motivational speaking" business owes him an enormous debt. If you want to understand why I say this, I strongly recommend the movie.

#143

Perform a Random Act of Kindness

I feel energized when I do something nice.

And honestly, because I've gotten to know my readers over the years, and they are the nicest people on the planet, I'm going to go out on a very safe limb here and make a prediction—you will, too.

I'm being serious here. For me, maybe it goes back to being a Boy Scout and helping little old ladies cross the street. Who knows? But I've never felt anything but a lift whenever I do something kind, nice, or generous for another person. I'm not kidding when I tell you that kind of giving is a gift to the giver.

I'll give you an example, and believe me I am only telling you this to share the effect that giving has on me, not to tell you what a great guy I am. (Compared to what some people dedicate their lives to, anything I do doesn't even deserve a mention.)

Some days, when my energy is low and I'm not particularly motivated to work, I'll start browsing around the charity sites on the Internet. I'm particularly drawn to International Rescue Committee (which basically does everything good everywhere; check it out at www.theIRC.org); the animal rescue organization Best Friends Animal Society (www.bestfriends.org); and KIVA, an incredible group that makes micro-loans (such as $25 and up) to indigent people around the world to help them start small businesses in their communities and try to work their way out of poverty (www.kiva.org). I have a dozen others, but you get the point.

Then I'll start just hitting the "Donate" buttons. Now listen carefully. The amount is irrelevant. The act is not.

GIVING BEGETS ENERGY

Here's what happens for me: I feel connected. I feel I'm doing something good. I feel like I'm giving something, however small, back. I feel a part of something bigger, an effort to make other people's lives better. It takes attention off myself. It draws my attention to people and situations that have it way, way worse than I ever did. I donate. And it makes me feel good.

Now listen carefully again: Never, never, in all the time I have been doing this do I not finish the experience feeling energized.

You might think, "Well, that's just him," but I don't think so. Bill Clinton wrote a terrific book about the experience and practice of giving (aptly named *Giving*) that kind of supports the feeling I'm describing on a global basis. But you don't need to be Bill or Melinda Gates to make a difference here. Some local, close to home charities and causes would love to have your support, believe me. Find one that touches your heart and give something to it—money, time, or any donation that allows you to connect with something outside yourself. The energy is contagious.

If you don't feel like making a contribution to a charity, put a quarter in someone's meter before the time runs out, and then keep walking. Bring a dog that's waiting outside Starbucks a bowl of water. Visit a senior. Read to a child. Volunteer for something.

I don't really care what it is. The point is, whatever connects you to something bigger, whatever feels like "giving" to you, energizes you on a cellular level. It triggers the release of brain chemicals associated with altruism, community, and alertness. It reduces stress. It makes you feel good.

#144

Have More Sex

Some of us may reflexively laugh at the notion that daily sex will help you live to be 100, but don't be so quick on the draw (no pun intended). There are a lot of serious health benefits to regular sex, not the least of which is increased energy. (In fact, I can hardly think of anything more energizing than a great sex life, but maybe that's just me.)

But what's no laughing matter is that many of us—including couples in committed relationships—go hundreds of days without sex. In fact, erectile dysfunction (ED) affects 30 million men in the United States and half the male population between forty and seventy. According to sexologist Laura Berman, M.D., 43 percent of women reported having some kind of sexual dissatisfaction and one-third of them specifically reported low sexual desire.

Stress, lack of energy, fatigue, depression, anger, and worry are all sexual-appetite killers, and few foods—even the erotic staples such as oysters and chocolate—are going to make much of a dent if your mind is somewhere else. On the other hand, sometimes low libido for men or women has a physical origin. As often or not, it's a mixture of both desire *plus* the ability to do something about it.

What's up with that? And what can we do about it? Read on.

FOOD FOR FOREPLAY

Assuming the "spirit is willing," we still have to make sure the body is able. First order of business: Improve overall circulation. The best way to do that is through exercise. Almost any kind will do, as long as your heart is pumping, blood is flowing through your organs, and oxygen is cleaning out the cobwebs in the brain.

Exercise also raises "feel-good" chemicals in the brain called *catecholamines*, making it far more likely that you'll feel amorous rather than exhausted. Certain yoga postures are said to be fantastic before sex, notably a shoulder stand for men and the butterfly pose for women.

Then there are the sexy foods. Here's my list of the top eight foods that may increase libido naturally:

1. **Almonds (or nuts).** These contain important fatty acids that help the brain work better.

2. **Avocados.** Not only are they a sensual delight, but they also contain important fatty acids that help the brain and the heart.

3. **Celery.** Guys take note—celery actually contains a small amount of *androsterone*, a male hormone released in sweat that's been known to turn women on.

4. **Chile peppers.** Hot peppers contain *capsaicin*, which can stimulate circulation.

5. **Chocolate.** It's no accident that chocolate is the gift of love. It contains *phenylethylamine*, a chemical that's released in the brain when you're in love.

6. **Oysters.** High in zinc, which is essential for male sexual functioning, oysters have been associated with sex since the days of Casanova.

7. **Figs.** Figs are high in amino acids and are believed to increase sexual stamina. Plus, they're sensual, juicy, and sweet—perfect for "food foreplay."

8. **Nutmeg.** According to Daniel Amen, M.D., author of *Sex on the Brain: 12 Lessons to*

Enhance Your Love Life, nutmeg is used in Indian medicine for enhancing desire. In one animal study, an extract of nutmeg had the same effect on mating behavior as Viagra did.

NATURE'S ENERGY APHRODISIAC

High-carbohydrate dishes such as pasta are more likely to lead to snoozing than romancing. Go with energy-producing protein and vegetables, and leave the table just a bit hungry. Some foods, by the sheer nature of their sensuality, can trigger amorous feelings—a juicy peach, for example, or a silky avocado. Foods with luscious textures and tastes are always mood-enhancing. The sheer sensuality of eating them, especially with a partner over a romantic dinner, may lead to even more sensual delights later on.

Finally, to turn on the brain naturally, engage your sense of smell. Almond and coconut are always good bets, and they make great scented candles. Lavender has been shown to be one of the most universal turn-ons, as have—believe it or not—the aroma of pumpkin pie and buttered popcorn for men, and baby powder and licorice candy for women.

There's no aphrodisiac on earth like romantic love—attraction is the ultimate aphrodisiac. It's better than any energy-enhancing drug, better than any supplement, food, or potion. You can't buy it, eat it, or create it out of nothing, but if you have it—and your body is in good shape—you're in for a great time.

Remember: Great sex equals great energy. Trust me on this one.

#145

Get a Coach

What did basketball player Michael Jordan, boxer Muhammad Ali, and legendary opera singer Leontyne Price have in common during the height of their respective careers?

Give up? They all had a coach.

Along with many other top performing athletes and musicians, not to mention business executives, parents, entrepreneurs, and other assorted folks, Jordan, Ali, and Price all recognized the value of a coach. An entire profession—life coaching—has evolved to address the needs of people in all walks of life who can benefit from the astonishing value a coach has to offer.

You can, too. And it will do wonders for your energy.

Here's why. We've talked at length in this book about all the factors in our lives that can drain energy: stress, energy vampires, and toxic relationships (not to mention bad food, and poor exercise and sleep habits). A coach can be a remarkable asset in identifying (and implementing) life strategies that can ultimate free up an enormous amount of energy.

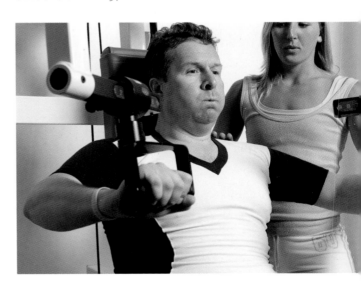

Think about it. If you had someone to bounce ideas off, help you strategize, help you identify areas in which you might be stuck, lend an objective and sympathetic eye to some of your patterns, and to whom you could be accountable for promises (kept and unkept), how helpful would that be to you? A golf coach helps you analyze your swing to see what's working and what's not. A life coach does the same for your life.

At various times in my life I've employed a coach to help strategize, identify patterns that might be sucking up valuable energy that would be better spent elsewhere, hold me accountable, and move me forward to the next level in my life.

Coaching isn't for people who are "broken"—it's not therapy. (Therapy is great; it's just different from coaching.) Therapists tend to ask, *"What happened?"* Coaches help you discover what comes next. There's an old saying in "coach world" that therapists ride in the car looking out the back and helping you figure out where you've come from; coaches ride in the front seat, helping you discover where to go next. This can be invaluable to a person wanting to go, as they say, "to the next level."

Although I can't substantiate this, it's widely believed that a certain president and a well-known international leader both used the services of one of the most famous life coaches of all time: Tony Robbins. Successful people use coaches all the time.

When you hire a financial advisor, he or she looks at your overall financial picture and helps you identify where you might be leaving money on the table; ultimately, they help you make investments that are more likely to pay off. Hiring a coach is like hiring an advisor to help you see where you're leaving *energy* on the table. A good coach can help you identify areas that are more likely to pay off in terms of your stated goals, well-being, and energy.

Coaching is typically done over the phone, usually in half-hour sessions, three or four times a month. I highly recommend it.

#146

Change a Habit

One principle of this book has been that the habits you create for yourself, around food, exercise, and relationships, are the raw material from which you get your energy. Some of these habits will increase your energy, and some will do the opposite. Of course, the trick is knowing which is which.

And that's only part of the trick. Many of us are fully aware of habits that are energy draining, if not outright self-destructive. But changing them is another thing. (I often say in workshops that I've yet to meet a person who smokes because he didn't get the memo that coffin nails cause cancer. He's not smoking because someone forgot to tell him it's a really bad thing!)

The point is, changing an energy-draining habit is about a lot more than just getting intellectual information. It's about *doing*. One thing I've learned from watching dog trainers over the years is that if you want to break a bad habit, you have to substitute another one. (My pit bull puppy, Emily, thinks having a tug-of-war with expensive suede couch pillows is the most fun you can have in the world. It was a lot easier to break her of that habit when I showed her a substitute behavior that accomplished the same goal—tussling with a chew toy.)

Substitution as a technique for changing a habit is actually a principle I first learned in graduate school psychology. Let's say you've got a toddler who tends to have a tantrum in the middle of Wal-Mart when he can't get you to buy his favorite toy. You'll have a much easier time breaking him of that endearing habit if, at the same time, you can offer him a different activity, one that is actually positively rewarded.

Behavioral psychologists call this "extinguishing" and "conditioning"—you *extinguish* the tantrum by removing any positive reinforcement, and *condition in* a replacement behavior that *does* produce a desired reward.

So how do we "extinguish" our own energy-draining habits and "condition in" new, more productive and energizing ones?

Simple. Create a plan B.

REPLACE BAD HABITS WITH GOOD ALTERNATIVES

Pick whatever unhealthy, energy-draining habit you've been trying to wean yourself from as an example. Although you can intellectualize ad nauseam about why you should change your ways, there's a part of your brain that's a screaming two-year-old—it wants what it wants when it wants it, whether that's a cigarette, a pint of Häagen Dazs, a bottle of wine, or carte blanche at Nordstrom. And although we could argue about the wine or the shopping spree, most of the habits we want to break are the same ones that drain our energy and vitality.

I'm sure by now I don't have to tell you that those bad habits can damage your physical, emotional, and financial health; add to your stress levels; and ultimately sap your energy. To effectively change an ingrained habit you need to do three things:

1. Define your reasons to change.

2. Recognize what triggers your behavior.

3. Collect a bag of diversionary tactics to occupy your inner toddler.

Change is hard, but it's doable—with a plan. Start with this advice:

- **Prepare for change.** Before you try to give up the cigarettes, cut out sugar, or control your spending, write down all the reasons you want to change your behavior. Keep the list growing, and reread it often. Plan ways to work around the typical situations, experiences, and feelings that trigger your craving.

- **Take one day at a time.** Give yourself at least a month to focus on changing just one habit. As with any goal, commit to yourself (in writing) and to those around you. Come up with a reward (preferably something healthy, such as a day at a spa) for sticking with it, and build in consequences for giving up (donating your favorite outfit to charity). Plan each step of the process.

- **Out with the old, in with the new.** If you are trying to cut down on the amount of television you watch, for instance, have a prime-time replacement. Make it something pleasurable—reading a novel, playing with the kids, or socializing with friends. If you replace a bad habit with a good one, then you'll have filled the energy drainer with an energy promoter.

- **Spin to win.** You see this all the time in a presidential election cycle. Candidates attempt to lower expectations so that if they lose a primary they can declare victory by moving the goalposts. ("We were expecting to lose by 30 percent, and we only lost by 15 percent—so we actually won!") Believe it or not, there's a valuable lesson in this: *Manage your expectations.*

  This is especially true when you're trying to lose weight. Remember, there are no unrealistic goals, just unrealistic timetables. If you set a goal of losing 20 pounds and after a month you've only lost 4, it's still progress, and don't let your inner voice tell you otherwise. Celebrate small successes in a healthy way.

- **Wait it out.** When the urge to resort to the old behavior strikes—whether it's indulging in a pint of ice cream out of the container or having a cigarette—have a diversionary tactic ready. Those times when you're feeling stressed and suddenly want more than anything in the world to do something you know is going to sap your energy (cigarette, sugar indulgence, fourth slice of pizza), go for a walk, take a bath, practice a few yoga moves, or call a supportive friend. Cravings are remarkably fickle, and if you can wait them out for 15 minutes they usually pass.

A good set of diversionary "plan B" actions can help you make it through. Remember that list you made for the reasons you want to replace an energy-draining habit with a more productive one? Read it. Preferably aloud. Whenever you're feeling "weak," remind yourself that *you* are in charge here. Taking steps toward a healthier life will add up to an improved self-image, a more positive outlook on life, and increased energy.

Some of my fellow teachers in the self-help movement, such as my friends Jack Canfield, Mark Victor Hansen, Christine Comaford-Lynch, and T. Harv Eker, love to say that it takes twenty-one days to form a new habit. I think they're right. But think about it. If you devoted three weeks to cultivating one new, energy-enhancing, life-affirming habit, at the end of the year you'd have seventeen strong new behavioral strategies for successful living.

Imagine how much energy you could create for yourself with that!

#147

Make a List of Goals

Life is full of choices, and some of those choices lead to more energy in your life. Some . . . not so much.

There are, of course, the everyday choices—shorts or pants, sushi or Italian, the 405 Freeway or Sepulvada (okay, that's a Los Angeles inside joke that only people who spend four hours a day stuck in traffic could understand). And then there are the bigger, life-altering decisions—having a child, moving to another city, going to law school.

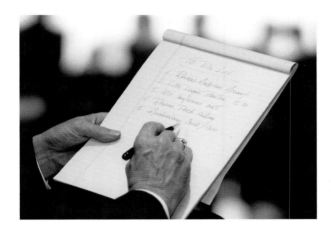

The more mundane choices can be decided by weather, whim, or traffic reports. But to make the really important decisions—those that determine the direction your life will take—you need to know where you are heading by mapping out your future.

There is nothing more frustrating or energy draining than living a life without direction. Fortunately, help is on the way, and it comes in the simple form of a tool called a personal road map.

TAKE THE ROAD TO ENERGY

I first learned this terrific energy-boosting "exercise" from life coach Roz Van Meter, a frequent guest on my old New York radio show (www.coachroz.com). It's a great way to create your own road map, and you start by checking your own internal compass.

Take two sheets of paper and on one write the heading, "What do I want *more* of in my life," and on the second, "What do I want *less* of in my life." If you take the time to really examine these questions, you'll begin to recognize what's meaningful and what's meaning*less*. (Hint: The meaningless stuff drains your energy in direct proportion to how meaningless it is.)

The next step is to use that information and write down three goals in each of the major areas of your life—relationships, career, health, spirituality, financial, and personal. Make them real. Make them specific, measurable, and truly meaningful to you. (Example: Don't just say, "Lose weight"—say, "Lose 10 pounds by May 5 at 5:00 p.m. That's specific, actionable, and measurable, and has a way better chance of being achieved.)

FOOLING THE BRAIN

You know the old saying "I'll believe it when I see it"? Well the first place you have to "see" your goal is in your mind. This is a cornerstone principle of everything I believe about energy, vitality, well-being, transformation, and health. Remember, *everything starts with your thoughts*, everything from weight loss to good health to great relationships to success in business.

It all starts by simply *visualizing* yourself actually *achieving* your goals.

See, the interesting thing about your mind is that at a deep, other-than-conscious level, it really can't distinguish between reality and thoughts. Your subconscious mind is actually kind of dumb. For the subconscious, everything is black or white, on or off, yes or no. It doesn't recognize shades of gray. That's been demonstrated many times by brain scans. If you show someone an actual real-life object, such as an orange, for example, and then you have her close her eyes and *imagine* the same orange, her brain scan will show virtually identical activity in the same places of the brain, whether the object is real or just imagined. At some level, *your brain doesn't know the difference*.

And you can use this fact to your advantage, in myriad ways, not the least of which is to increase your energy.

VISUALIZE SUCCESS

It's really simple. If you set up an *idea* of a goal, *see it* in your mind's eye as though it's happening, and put some *mental energy* and *focus* on it, you've actually sent a message to your subconscious that *helps make the goal more real*. It's the principle of creative visualization in action, and it works. Studies have shown, for example, that basketball players who "practice" shots in their mind without actually touching the ball score more baskets than those who don't visualize.

By committing yourself to living a more meaningful life, and setting goals that move you in the right direction, you'll gain the energy to tackle whatever obstacles you encounter. Many of my clients who've undertaken this exercise look back on the goals they wrote in their journal a few years ago and have been astonished to find that they've achieved a large number of them.

When that happens, it's time to write down some new goals.

So take a tip from the wisest and most successful people on the planet—set goals. Make lists. Imagine. Visualize. Put some mental energy into it.

And then, as you work toward accomplishing those goals, your energy will take off.

148

Practice Mindfulness

I honestly believe that one of the reasons we feel so energy depleted all the time is that we're never fully present for our lives. Let me explain. Multitasking (which we've covered elsewhere; see page 228) is just the tip of the proverbial iceberg. We're so accustomed to having our attention divided that even when we don't think we're multitasking we're still doing it. We do it whenever we pay less than full attention to where we are, what we're doing, and who we're with. In fact, the experience of being fully present—what many spiritual gurus call "mindfulness"—is one of the most energizing skills you can learn.

Remember, attention divided is energy divided, and energy divided is less than optimal energy. You wind up feeling fatigued because you're trying to pay full attention with less than all your senses fully focused. It's like trying to turn up the heat in your house while nine out of the ten vents are closed. You keep turning up the thermostat and wondering why the house doesn't get warm. That's what we do with our energy. Learning (and practicing) mindfulness is the way to open the other vents.

PRACTICE MINDFULNESS EVERY DAY

Mindfulness is a skill that's been mastered by every great spiritual leader and is part of almost every spiritual practice that I know of. It will

Remember, attention divided is energy divided, and energy divided is less than optimal energy.

absolutely boost your energy when you learn how to do it. And good news—you don't have to go to a monastery or a retreat or become a monk to learn it, practice it, and reap its energy-boosting rewards. You can apply it right now, in your own life, in your car, at the gym, at the dinner table, in a conversation with your coworkers or your significant other, or just sitting outside enjoying the summer breeze.

Here's how to do it. For a few minutes every day, give complete and utter attention to being in the moment, to being fully *present* in what's going on around you. If you're talking to someone, listen carefully to every word. Try actually "recreating" that person's experience as he talks to you, as if you're living inside him for a few minutes, understanding what he's saying, both with his words and his body language.

If you're at the gym lifting weights, think of the muscle that's being worked, put your mind into it, imagine it growing, experience the muscle fibers contracting with your effort, the blood circulating through your veins, and your breath filling your lungs with oxygen. If you're eating a meal, notice every taste, every color, and every flavor. If you're walking down the street, start paying attention to what's on the left of you. The right. Notice how loud the street noises are. Hear what people are saying. How many people are in front of you and what color hat is that guy on your left wearing?

MAKE YOURSELF AVAILABLE TO THE MOMENT

Being mindful may feel like a new experience to you. I know it did to me when I first started practicing it. But there's almost nothing I can think of that will so forward your ability to be present for your

life, savor every moment, enrich every interaction, and blow your energy level right out of the water.

The great spiritual masters do this every single moment of every single day. It's called "being high on life." And it all comes from the practice of mindfulness, of focused attention, and of being really *available* for what's true and happening, right now, in this moment.

So practice mindfulness. Even for a few minutes, every single day. It's the energy equivalent of wiping your windows with cleaner. All of a sudden, everything looks clear, clean, uncluttered, and new.

#149

Stay Connected

A recent study finds 65 percent of us spend more time with our computer than our significant other.

That fact does not exactly come as news to my girlfriend Anja, who has oh-so-gently commented on it a few hundred times or so (but who's counting?). In fact, the only surprising thing about that bit of research is that it's *not* surprising. We've become an increasingly tech-tied world, and sometimes it seems like the major way we relate to one another is through the medium of an electronic device. (Not for nothing do they call the BlackBerry a Crackberry.)

Sending text messages is great, but you don't get to look into someone's eyes. And if all our connections live in a virtual world, then, Houston, we have a very big problem.

My LinkedIn and Facebook communities and MySpace "friends" (don't get me started) may number in the thousands, but they can't hold a candle to my relationship with my friend Susan, whom I can actually meet at Starbucks once in a while when she isn't taking care of her three children. Nor can any one of our collective online relationships hold a candle to the relationship we have with the person we call when we get engaged or break up with someone.

No matter how you slice it, spending time with good friends is a surefire stress-buster and a terrific energy enhancer.

It's also a life extender. In his landmark book *The Blue Zone,* National Geographic explorer and writer Dan Buettner reports on four areas in the world where people live the longest and healthiest lives and are frequently active and healthy into their late nineties and often beyond. Absolutely every one of the people he studied listed strong social connections as one of the forces in their lives.

Bottom line: It's hard to have energy if you're not connected.

THE STRENGTH IN NUMBERS ADVANTAGE

Now in this department, women may actually have an advantage. They seem to be hard-wired to connect to others in times of stress. A study from UCLA suggests that the stress response in women isn't limited to just fight-or-flight, which is the typical male response to stress.

The great biologist and writer Robert Sapolsky, Ph.D., of Stanford University, has characterized the female response to stress as "tend and befriend" (a possible explanation for why women go to the bathroom together on a double date!). That's because stress triggers the release of a cascade of chemicals, including oxytocin, a "bonding" hormone that, in women at least, can elicit the urge to connect to others.

The researchers theorize that just as fight-or-flight is a throwback to our hunter-gather days, so, too, is women's tendency to "tend and befriend." In times of danger, the men fled or went for their weapons while women would collect and comfort their children and gather their friends, a strength-in-numbers approach to adversity.

Today, when a woman responds to stress by, say, having dinner with friends, studies suggest that she is further protected from stress by the release of even more oxytocin, producing a calming effect. The researchers even suggest that the seven-year advantage women have over men in longevity may be related to women's tendency to connect to others.

Men create this energy-enhancing effect of connection by bonding over sports, poker, golf, or any of a number of "male" activities, even if they're not aware of the reason. But whether you're a man or a woman, connection increases energy. (Ever see a bunch of guys cheering on the Los Angeles Lakers during playoffs? It's not exactly a low-energy situation!)

AN ENERGY TRIFECTA

So having a circle of family members, friends, and coworkers to swap stories with, lean on, and support is essential for our mental and physical health. Without those connections, stress wears us down more easily, leaving us fatigued, vulnerable to illness, and devoid of energy.

For more than two decades, study after study has documented the protective effect that strong social ties have against disease. Social and family connections lower blood pressure, heart rate, and cholesterol. People with few social connections are far more likely to experience poor mental health and poor physical health, and to die prematurely (the ultimate energy drain).

As we age, strong social ties can also help us maintain an active mind. In a study of more than 2,800 people age sixty-five and older, Harvard researchers found that people with at least five social ties—church groups, social groups, or family and friends—were less likely to suffer cognitive decline than seniors who didn't. People with strong social ties rate themselves as happier, more satisfied, and more fulfilled.

Job stress is a major energy drain. But there's something you can do about it. A study published in the *American Journal of Public Health* found that workers who felt they had colleagues whom they could lean on were better able to handle job stress and far less likely to suffer from major depression than those without supportive coworkers. Cultivating friends at work will not only help you handle stress, but it will also help protect your valuable energy reserves from being drained by the rigors of work.

Good relationships make us healthier, happier, less stressed, and more energized. The prescription is relatively easy: Strengthen the bonds of friendship and take time to spend time with the people you love. If you don't have a circle of close friends nearby, then connect with like-minded people through religious institutions, civic groups, book clubs, volunteer work, political campaigns, or cooking classes, for example.

And don't limit connections to the human variety. Animals offer an energy that can be contagious. (I'm absolutely convinced that having animals around me all the time is a big part of the reason I have as much positive energy as I do.)

Connect with others. It will protect against sickness, lower stress, and extend life. It's truly the energy trifecta.

#150
Compose Your Own Last Lecture

Sometime around January 2008, a video was posted on YouTube that, almost instantly, gained cult status. The subject of the video was an unlikely candidate for the title of "national phenomenon," yet that's exactly what it has become. On the face of it, it was simply a lecture given by a professor of computer science at Carnegie Mellon University. As of this writing, it has generated more than 2.5 million views, an appearance on *Oprah*, a prime-time special with Diane Sawyer on ABC-TV, and a best-selling book.

So what exactly was so special about this video, and why am I writing about it in a book on energy?

Glad you asked.

WORDS OF WISDOM

There's a time-honored academic tradition where professors are asked to pretend that they can give only one more lecture in their career. They're asked what they would want to leave as a legacy, what they would most want people to know about their work, and how they would sum up everything they had to teach. In this case, the professor in question was a wildly popular computer scientist named Randy Pausch, a man of phenomenal energy and contagious good spirit whose courses at Carnegie Mellon were routinely packed to capacity. The video in question was, in fact, titled *The Last Lecture*.

But it was a last lecture with a difference.

Randy Pausch died of pancreatic cancer in July 2008. In September 2007, when the lecture was delivered and recorded, he had been given six months to live. Everyone in the packed crowd that day knew, as did Randy, that this "last lecture" was not a hypothetical exercise. It would, indeed, *be* his last lecture.

Now if you haven't seen it, let me just say one thing: Watch it. As soon as you can. I promise you, you will never forget it, and it may even be a life-changing experience for you.

I want to talk about it in this book because I think Randy had more to teach us about energy and spirit than almost anyone I've ever written about. Although I could never convey the experience of watching the full lecture, I'll try to distill some of the major lessons from watching it.

The first, and perhaps most important, lesson is one I've tried to underscore throughout this book: *Energy is not something you "get," it's a by-product of how you live your life.* How you eat, how you exercise, how you sleep, and how you reduce stress are all the important physical conditions that set you up for a life of energy and spirit, but even more important are the mental, spiritual, and emotional connections and ties that invigorate and empower you to really soar. If you live your "truth," you will have energy.

Randy demonstrated this, even in a body that was racked with an incurable cancer (he started the lecture by doing one-armed pushups). Not for one second do you feel anything but awe for this energetic, evolved, fully realized human being whose message is nothing short of mesmerizing.

Randy summed up the lessons of his life, a life well lived indeed. They're lessons we could all do well to learn and implement in our own lives.

- Never lose the childhood wonder.
- Help others.

- Have fun ("I'm going to keep having fun every day that I have, because there's no other way to do it," he laughed).
- Acknowledge people.
- Ignore everything people say and only pay attention to what they do.
- Tell the truth.
- Apologize when you screw up.
- Focus on others, not yourself.
- Show gratitude.
- Don't complain, just work harder.
- Find the best in everybody, no matter how long you have to wait for him or her to show it.
- Listen.
- Never give up.

What would you say if you could deliver a "last lecture"? What would be your legacy? What would you want your kids, loved ones, and family members to remember about you? What would you teach them?

Prepare your own personal last lecture and you'll discover the true secret of untapped energy that lives within all of us.

Enjoy the journey.

Resources

A word about the resources section. This is a very abbreviated list of resources that were mentioned in the book. I particularly wanted to include some of the lesser-known companies, people, and services that you might not have heard of yet, that you might not have found on your own, or that were not listed in other books. This is like my personal list of "discoveries." Approach this resource list the way you might approach a list of "off the beaten path" vacation spots—terrific places that you would probably not have heard about if a friend hadn't told you what an amazing time he had there.

EXERCISE

Patricia Moreno

For more information about the wonderful Patricia Moreno and her special brand of energy-enhancing exercise, you can visit her website, www.satilife.com. There you'll find a lot of information on what she does, as well as a very cool set of exercise DVDs that are really quite special. She teaches around the NYC area and also conducts workshops and retreats.

X-iser

The X-iser machine I discuss on page 108 can be found through a link on my website, www.jonnybowden.com, in the web store under "exercise."

STRESS REDUCTION AND MEDITATION

Energy Transformation

Aleta St. James, featured on page 254 of this book, has been described as "among the best healers in the world" by no less than Candace Pert, Ph.D., star of *The Secret* and author of the classic text *Molecules of Emotion*. Aleta has wonderful programs for energy as well as some of the best CDs I've ever used for meditation and relaxation. Learn about her LifeShift Experience at www.aletastjames.com.

Qi Gong

There are many great places to take qi gong classes, but if you want a super introduction without leaving home you couldn't do better than to try the two introductory DVDs available from Jeff Primack's Supreme Science Qigong Foundation (www.qigong.com). Jeff also takes his show on the road, holding weekend workshops for the astonishing price of $70. I interviewed Jeff for this book, and it's hard to imagine a more dedicated and committed individual. He's also a natural healer. His DVDs are a great way to get introduced to this remarkable practice.

MEDITATION, RELAXATION, AND YOGA

Rosen Wellness

For individualized wellness programs featuring stress reduction, meditation, yoga, and relaxation for individuals, groups, and corporations, you couldn't do better than to check out Bernard Rosen, Ph.D. (www.brwellness.com). Bernie is also a certified yoga instructor, and he is especially proficient at designing group and corporate programs as well as individual ones.

Yoga Pulse

My friend Anastasia has more than a few things going for her. One, she's a killer tennis player. Two, she's drop-dead gorgeous. Three, she's incredibly humble and modest. And four, and most important, she's developed a really wonderful yoga program for stress that combines nutrition, spirituality, and exercise. Sure, it might be a tad vegetarian for my taste, but overall it's a delicious secret that I'd love you to discover for yourself. Find out about Yoga Pulse at www.yogapulse.net.

Yoga, Stress Reduction, and Ayurvedic Medicine

Suzanne Norman is a gifted healer who is also a registered yoga teacher (RYT) with the National Yoga Alliance, a member of the International Association of Yoga Therapists (Yoga Research and Education Center), a certified Transformation Meditation teacher, a certified Thai yoga massage therapist, and a certified Neuro-Linguistic Programming Master Practitioner. She's also a terrific lady. Learn about her wellness, meditation, and energy programs at www.wellbodymind.com.

DETOXIFICATION: SAUNAS

Infrared Saunas by Life Saunas International

This company makes the best infrared sauna I've ever seen. I have one in my home and I use it constantly. I've met the CEO and the principals of the company, and I can vouch for the fact that they are absolutely first-rate people and that this is a first-rate product. I particularly like the "chromotherapy" feature of their home saunas, which makes use of healing and energizing lights. The saunas have all kinds of cool features (including built-in Sony music players with an MP3 connector), and they deliver amazing value for an affordable price! I have a link to Life Saunas on my website, www.jonnybowden.com, under "shopping."

DETOXIFICATION: NUTRITIONAL PROGRAMS

Elson Haas, M.D.

The king of the hill when it comes to detox diets is my friend Elson Haas, M.D. I've long recommended his book, *The New Detox Diet*, and if you're in the San Rafael area of California you couldn't do better than to check out his clinic, the Preventive Medical Center of Marin, Inc. He's also a natural healer, a superb nutritionist, and a gifted teacher. Visit his website at www.elsonhaas.com.

Food Sensitivity Testing

As I discussed on page 59, identifying food allergies can be a major boon for energy. The two tests that I think are most reliable are the ALCAT and the LEAP tests.

The ALCAT test
www.alcat.com
Cell Science Systems
1239 East Newport Center Drive, Suite 101
Deerfield Beach, FL 33442
Phone: (800) US ALCAT (872-5228)
Phone: (954) 426-2304
Fax: (954) 428-8676
E-mail: info@alcat.com

The LEAP Test (Lifestyle, Eating and Performance)
www.nowleap.com
Signet Diagnostic Corporation
3555 Fiscal Court Suites 8 & 9
Riviera Beach, FL 33404
Ph. 888-669-5327
Ph. (561) 848-7111
Fax. (561) 848-6655

PERSONAL GROWTH AND HEALING

Emotional Freedom Technique (EFT)

I learned about EFT firsthand from my dear friend Glen Depke, who is the prototype of the term *gifted healer*. Depke designed the Nutritional Typing program I discuss on page 175 of this book, and he is one of the country's leading EFT practitioners. I highly recommend him. Check him out at www.depkewellness.com.

Coaching

A great resource for finding coaches is Coach Training Alliance. They are an ICF (International Coaching Federation) certified school with a first-rate curriculum, and you can be very confident of any of their graduates. I know the president of the school, Will Craig, and have great respect for and confidence in him and the school. My instructional programs for Weight Loss Coaches are offered through Coach Training Alliance. They're terrific. Visit them at www.coachtrainingalliance.com.

GENERAL

Balance for life

If the Dali Lama were reincarnated as a woman with a family living in Providence, Rhode Island, she would be Jeanette Bessinger. The author of several successful cookbooks, she's a health counselor who has dedicated her life to helping others, especially families who need to learn to cook and eat well with limited time and money. Jeanette developed the recipes for one of my books, *The Healthiest Meals on Earth*. She's also an ordained nondenominational minister, and one of the most wonderful people I know. Visit her website and get her terrific newsletter at www.balanceforlife.com.

Clayton College for Natural Health

If you're interested in getting a nontraditional education in some of the areas of nutrition and health that aren't routinely covered in conventional programs, this is the place to go. The teachers are wonderful, dedicated people, and Clayton is a leading college in natural health, traditional naturopathy, and holistic nutrition. The focus is on healing without drugs and empowering people with information. Visit them at www.ccnh.edu.

NUTRITION TOWN HALL

Robert Crayhon, M.S., C.N., is one of the people I most respect in the world, not only for his demonstrably encyclopedic knowledge of nutrition and health, but also for his inexhaustible energy, deep humanitarian instincts, huge heart, and desire to make the world a better place. His latest nonprofit project is Nutrition Town Hall, a weekly one-hour meeting where anyone can go to gain support and learn new information to help maintain or achieve health through optimal nutrition and a healthy lifestyle. Robert founded this outreach program to help serve those who couldn't afford to visit a nutritionist. There is no advertising, no marketing, no selling, and no promotion, just first-rate information and support for healthy living. At the time of this writing, Nutrition Town Hall is only in New York City, but knowing Robert, by the time you read this, it will be nationwide. In any case, check out the website at www.nutritiontownhall.com.

WEBSITES AND NEWSLETTERS

www.NaturalNews.com

Natural News is the website and newsletter of one of my favorite people in the field of health, Mike Adams, the original "Health Ranger." Mike has tirelessly worked to bring his readers health news, views, and opinions you won't get everywhere else. I support him so much I occasionally contribute to his site. He's a scrupulously honest, high-integrity guy, and his website is as non-commercial as you can be and still make a living. I have great respect and affection for him. www.naturalnews.com

www.RenegadeHealth.com

Kevin Gianni is another well-kept secret that deserves to be discovered. His site and his radio show—*Renegade Health*—is a fun and entertaining daily health show that covers easy-to-do tips on nutrition, living foods, fitness and, as Kevin puts it, "feeling awesome all the time." His interviews with thought leaders on *Renegade Health* are terrific. There's a bit of a tilt towards raw foods and a vegan lifetyle, but all in all you'll get great information from a variety of experts.

A FINAL NOTE

I've left out far more wonderful people in the field than I've included, largely because I wanted to concentrate on energy, rather than specifically on diet and food. For more specific info on nutrition and diet, be sure to check out four of my favorite blogs:

- Dr. Mike Eades's blog is consistently smart, informed, and informative. I have his RSS feed on my home page and read him all the time. www.proteinpower.com/drmike
- Jimmy Moore is the go-to guy when it comes to interviewing thought leaders and researchers with a low-carb bent. www.livinglavidalowcarb.blogspot.com
- Connie Bennet is terrific for issues relating to energy-draining sugar and sugar addiction. www.sugarshockblog.com
- Regina Wilshire's *The Weight of The Evidence* is always worth checking out for an informative take on dietary issues that can sap energy. www.weightoftheevidence.com.

Image Credits

Cover images from John Ganun and
www.istockphoto.com.

The pictures in this book are used with permission
and through the courtesy of:

Fair Winds Press
from *The Healthiest Meals on Earth*, 2008:
    page 145
from *The Most Effective Natural Cures on Earth*,
    2008: page 291
from *Reflexology Card Deck*, 2008: page 206
from *Tamilee Webb's Defy Gravity Workout*, 2005:
    pages 103, 104

Getty Images: pages 2, 6, 7, 12-13, 20-21, 24, 28, 31,
43, 45, 47, 50, 54, 76-77, 85, 88, 89, 90, 92, 94,
96-97, 111, 114, 119, 120-121, 124, 135, 137, 139, 140,
142-143, 157, 158, 160-161, 168, 170, 174, 177, 179, 181,
187, 189, 191, 208-209, 210, 217, 218-219, 222, 231,
232-233, 235, 242, 243, 245, 246, 249, 252, 256,
259, 261, 267, 271

Jupiter Images: pages 2, 6, 36, 53, 68, 107, 111, 112,
163, 184-185, 236

Life Saunas International: page 151

www.istockphoto.com: pages 82, 204

Glossary

5-HTP (5-hydroxytryptophan)—precursor to serotonin in the brain

Acetylcholine—an important neurotransmitter in the brain; needed for memory and thinking

Acetyl-l-carnitine—the acetylated form of L-carnitine, which may have brain-protecting properties

Adaptagen—any compound that has a normalizing influence on physiology, regardless of the direction of change caused by the stressor

Adenosine—calming neurochemical

Antioxidants—compounds in food that help fight the process of oxidation, or oxidative stress, a factor in virtually every degenerative disease

Asanas—various poses used during yoga

Betaine—also known as trimethylglycine (TMG), a compound that works synergistically with folate to reduce potentially toxic levels of homocysteine

Bioavailable—a measure of the fraction of a compound that actually enters the circulation or reaches its destination in the body

Bioflavonoids—a family of plant chemicals with multiple health and energy benefits

Bisphenol A—toxin used in polycarbonate plastics; studies have show that high doses have an estrogen-like effect on the uterus and prostate glands

Brain-derived neurotrophic factor (BDNF)—a naturally occurring protein found in the brain that acts like "miracle grow" for the brain cells

Catecholamines—brain chemicals that improve mood and help fight depression

Chlorogenic acid—antioxidant particularly effective against a very destructive free radical called the superoxide anion radical; found in sweet potatoes, apples, and coffee

Choline—nutrient found in eggs, needed for healthy brain and liver function and fat breakdown; forms betaine in the body; thought of as a member of the B-vitamin family; needed for the synthesis of acetylcholine

Circadian misalignment—when the body's internal clock is out of sync with the external environment; can cause digestive problems, headaches, and insomnia

Coenzyme Q10 (CoQ10)—ubiquinone found in most tissues in the body; essential for the manufacture of the body's energy molecule, ATP (adenosine triphosphate), and a powerful antioxidant

Cortisol—stress hormone that, in elevated levels, may ultimately age the brain by shrinking the hippocampus

Cucurbitacins—chemicals in pumpkin seeds that may interfere with production of DHT (dihydrotestosterone), an undesirable metabolic by-product of testosterone

Depressant—a chemical agent like a sedative that diminishes the function or activity of a particular part of the body; in medicine, a drug that slows the activity of vital organs

Diindolylmethane (DIM)—isolated substance found in cruciferous vegetables that balances estrogen levels; increases the good, protective form of estrone while also raising progesterone levels when necessary

Dopamine—"feel-good" neurotransmitter in the brain; helps maintain focus and alertness

D-ribose—molecule made in the body's cells and used for cellular function

Electrons—tiny subatomic particles that carry a negative electric charge, which surround the nuclei of atoms

Emotional Freedom Technique (EFT)—simple method for releasing emotions which, in the process, frees the energy suppressed along with your feelings

Energy—general name for life force and vitality

Enzyme—something that speeds the rate at which certain chemical processes can take place

Estradiol—strongest of the three estrogens, which is produced before menopause; helps increase serotonin levels, improves sleep quality, decreases fatigue, and helps maintain a healthy cholesterol profile

Estriol—weaker estrogen shown to be protective against breast cancer; its benefits are in the digestive tract and in controlling symptoms of menopause, including hot flashes, insomnia, and vaginal dryness

Estrogen—family of hormones that perform about 400 functions in the human body; produced primarily in the ovaries and adrenal glands; known as a "female hormone" but is present in both women and men

Estrogen dominance—condition associated with menopause in which both estrogen and progesterone decline, but progesterone declines more dramatically, throwing off the balance of the two hormones

Estrone—main estrogen that the body makes after menopause; believed to be the hormone related to an increased risk of breast and uterine cancer; more body fat causes a higher production of estrone

Fiber—indigestible component of food; associated with lower risks of heart disease, diabetes, obesity, and cancer

Flavonoids—plant compound with antioxidant, anticancer, and antiallergy properties; more than 4,000 have been identified

Free radicals—destructive molecules in the body; can damage cells and DNA

Gliadin—a substrate of gluten

Glutamine–an amino acid that is a natural energy fuel for the brain

Gluten–protein in grains; found in wheat, rye, barley, and to some extent oats

Glycemic index–measure of how much a fixed amount (50 grams) of a given food (like fruit) raises blood sugar

Glycemic load–a more accurate measure of a food's effect on blood sugar than glycemic index, one that takes into account portion size

Glycerophosphocholine (GPC)–phospholipid that has been extensively researched for its effect on mental performance, attention, concentration, and memory formation

Glycogen–the form in which sugar (carbohydrates) are stored in the body, primarily in the liver and muscles

Hippocampus–area of the brain responsible for memory

Homocysteine–naturally-occurring amino acid that can be harmful to blood vessels, thereby contributing to the development of heart disease, stroke, dementia, and peripheral vascular disease

Indoles–phytochemicals found in cruciferous vegetables that are protective against prostate, gastric, skin, and breast cancers; examples include indole-3-carbinole and DIM

Inhibitory attention system–the part of the brain that directs our attention so we're able to concentrate and ignore distractions

Inositol–substance synthesized by the human body that is usually considered a member of the B-vitamin family but is not technically a vitamin

Insoluble fiber–indigestible part of foods that moves bulk through intestines

Insulin–fat-storing hormone that, if raised high enough, long enough, and frequently enough, contributes to diabetes, heart disease, and aging

Insulin resistance–associated with metabolic syndrome and type 2 diabetes

L-carnitine–a vitamin-like compound that escorts fatty acids into the mitochondria of the cells, where they can be "burned" for energy

Leucine–amino acid found in protein

L-glutamine–most abundant amino acid in the human body

Lignans–plant compounds with protective effect against cancers, especially those that are hormone-sensitive, including breast, uterine, and prostate cancers

Low-glycemic food–also known as "slow-burning carbs," they raise blood sugar slowly and not too high

L-tryptophan–amino acid found in protein foods, including eggs, poultry, beef, and tofu

Lysine–essential amino acid that works hand in hand with other essential amino acids to maintain growth, lean body mass, and the body's store of nitrogen, an essential part of all amino and nucleic acids

Macronutrients—protein, fat, and carbohydrates

Massage therapy—covers more than eighty types of practices and techniques; therapists press, rub, knead, and manipulate the muscles and other soft tissues of the body, varying pressure and movement; relaxes the soft tissues, increases delivery of blood and oxygen to the massaged areas, warms them, and decreases pain

Melatonin—powerful hormone that has multiple purposes in the body, one of which is to help regulate the sleep cycle; it may also have cancer-preventative properties

Micronutrients—vitamins and minerals

Mitochondria—power stations in every cell where energy is produced

Norepinephrine—one of the stimulating chemicals in the body

Omega 9s—examples are macadamia nut oil, extra-virgin olive oil

Omega-6s—fats found in vegetable oils. Can be pro-inflammatory especially when not balanced with omega-3's.

Omega-3 fats—ALA (alpha-linolenic acid), found in flaxseed; DHA (docosahexaenoic acid) and EPA (eicosapentaenoic acid), found in fish like wild salmon; are anti-inflammatory and keep cell membranes fluid

Oxidize—damage from free radicals

Oxytocin—a chemical often called the "bonding" hormone that is released during stress, nursing, and sex. It can elicit the urge to connect to others

Parasympathetic nervous system—the part of the autonomic nervous system responsible for "rest and digest;" functions in opposition to the sympathetic nervous system

PFCs—used in products to resist oil, stains, heat, water, and grease; studies have shown that some PFCs can cause tumors, damage organs, and affect the reproductive system

Phenylethylamine—a chemical that's released in the brain when you're in love

Phosphatidylcholine—phospholipid with choline as a component; found in eggs; helps keep fat and cholesterol from accumulating in the liver

Phosphatidylserine (PS)—phospholipid and naturally-occurring nutrient that's found in the cell membranes but is most concentrated in the brain

Phthalates—residues of polycarbonate plastics that are endocrine disrupters; used to soften plastic and vinyls and found in many shampoos, makeup, and lotions

Phytoestrogens—plant estrogens

Phytonutrients—nutrients from plants

Polybrominated diphenyl ethers (PBDEs)—class of chemicals found in such things as flame retardants used in electronics, the back coatings of upholstery and drapes, and inside small appliances and other plastic or foam products

Polysaccharide–long string of glucose molecules

Prana–term used during the practice of yoga to signify vital energy

Pranayama–yoga term for breathing techniques

Progesterone–important hormone secreted by the female reproductive system

Propolis–made by bees by mixing wax with a resinous sap from trees with antioxidative, antiulcer, antitumor, and antimicrobial properties

Qi gong–a family of mind-body exercises that share regulation of the body, regulation of breathing, and regulation of the mind

Saturated fats–good form found in coconut oil, bad form in fast-food, French fries

Seasonal Affective Disorder (SAD)–general name for "winter depression," generally experienced during darker months and believed to be related to light

Serotonin–neurotransmitter associated with relaxation, calm, and contentment

Sesamin–member of the lignan family; found in sesame seeds; inhibits the manufacture of inflammatory compounds in the body

Sesaminol–phenolic antioxidant; formed when sesame seeds are refined into oil

Soluble fiber–breaks down as it passes through the digestive tract, forming a gel that traps some substances related to high cholesterol; also helps control blood sugar by delaying the emptying of the stomach and retarding the entry of sugar into the bloodstream

Subluxation–degenerative condition in which one or more of the spinal vertebrae are out of place

Supplements–general name for vitamins, minerals, herbs, and other healthy compounds that can be purchased over the counter

Siylmarin–active ingredient in milk thistle with a liver-protecting effect; inhibits the entrance of toxins into the liver by somehow altering the outer membrane of the liver cells

Sympathetic nervous system–the part of the autonomic nervous system responsible for "fight or flight;" functions in opposition to the parasympathetic nervous system

Taurine–amino acid and natural diuretic

Testosterone–major male sexual hormone belonging to the steroid family; produced in the testes of males but also produced (in smaller amounts) by females in the ovaries

Theobromine–compound that occurs naturally in many plants such as cocoa, tea, and coffee plants; is known for relaxing the lower esophageal sphincter

Theophylline–along with theobromine, it is a well-known stimulant found in coffee and chocolate

Thermogenesis—the production of heat by burning calories; known as "fat burning"

Thyroid—small butterfly-shaped gland that wraps around the windpipe

Thyroid stimulating hormone (TSH)—a hormone secreted by the anterior pituitary gland that tells the thyroid to produce more thyroid hormones; a TSH blood test is frequently used to detect problems affecting the thyroid gland

Thyroxine (T4)—one of the main hormones released by the thyroid along with triiodothryonine (T3). T4 is a largely inactive hormone that has to be converted in the body to the active T3

Trans fat—hydrogenated or partially hydrogenated oil; considered metabolic poison, increases risk for heart disease and stroke; the exception is CLA, or conjugated linoleic acid, a naturally occurring trans fatty acid that actually has health benefits

Triglycerides—main form of fat found in the body, which are nearly always measured on a standard blood test

Triiodothryonine (T3)—one of the main hormones released by the thyroid along with thyroxine (T4); T3 is the active thyroid hormone

Tyrosine—amino acid that the brain converts to dopamine; found in oysters

Vasodilator—helps relax the muscles of the blood vessels, dilating them and allowing blood, nutrients, and oxygen to flow more freely; capsaicin, an ingredient of hot peppers, is a vasodilator

Xanthines—alkaloids in the same family as caffeine; examples are theophylline and theobromine

Xenoestrogen—environmental estrogen

Acknowledgments

Lots of people tell me "I ought to write a book!" The first thing I think to myself is this: You'd better get yourself a first-rate team.

I've got a doozy.

Mary Duffy did endless and invaluable work, tweaking and editing entries as fast as I could churn them out. I could never have completed this book—at least not on time—without her. My treasured assistants, nutritionists Susan Mudd, M.S., C.N.S. and Suzanne Copp, M.S., contributed—as always—valuable research, suggestions, and a critical eye.

My editor Cara Connors—now the veteran of three Jonny Bowden projects (don't ask)—deserves enormous credit for knowing how to "wrangle" a temperamental and often stubborn author who knows exactly what he wants and is not always "editor-friendly" (that would be me). Cara passes my tests with flying colors. The fact that I willingly (and okay, sometimes not-so-willingly) take suggestions and changes from her speaks volumes.

I have the best agent in the world, and that hasn't changed from the last five projects. Coleen O'Shea is the Rolls Royce of literary agents—smart, funny, supportive, and sharp as a tack. They don't come better and I'm lucky to have her.

My publisher—Fair Winds Press—has an all-star cast of people to whom I'm grateful. Ken Fund for his vision, Will Kiester for his perseverance and off-beat humor, and Jill Alexander, Tiffany Hill, Karen Levy, John Gettings, Daria Perreault, and Kate Jylkka for their terrific contributions to making these books look so beautiful.

Everyone needs a coach sometimes. Whenever I do, I have the benefit of one of the best in the business—Laurie Gerber of the Handel Group. Thanks!

Also on my team, editors who continue to give me great and interesting assignments, publish my columns and articles, and generally keep putting me "out there": Tanya Mancini and Jennifer Fields at AOL, Kayla Doner at MedZine and Remedy, Nicole Wise and Sarah Hiner at Bottom Line, Melanie Segala at Total Health Breakthroughs, Suzanne Richardson at Early To Rise, Nicole Brechka at Better Nutrition, Colette Heimowitz, M.S. at Atkins Nutritionals and of course, the wonderful Adam Campbell and Jeff O'Connell, my colleagues at *Men's Health*, who help make that magazine one of the best around and one I am proud to be a part of. And a special thanks to the wonderful Tara Parker Pope of the *New York Times*, who will understand why.

My professional colleagues are always so generous with their information and opinions and are never further than a phone call away—thank you for always making yourselves so graciously available to me: Elson Haas, M.D., Ann Louise Gittleman, Ph.D., C.N.S., Liz Neporent, M.S., Oz Garcia, Charles Poliquin, M.S., Mark Houston, M.D., M.S., Robert Crayhon, M.S., Mary Dan Eades, M.D., Michael Eades, M.D., Glen Depke, N.D.F.A.C.N., JJ Virgin, Ph.D., C.N.S., Linda Lizotte, R.D., Shari Lieberman, Ph.D., C.N.S., Pepper Schwartz, Ph.D., Matthew Mannino, D.C., Bernie Rosen, Ph.D., Suzanne Norman, Sonja Pettersen, N.M.D., Mark Blumenthal, and the many others I didn't call on this time but will next time for sure!

The amazing folks at Eat Drink or Die www.eatdrinkordie.com: Britt Lovett, Talia, Michael the Ping Pong God, Scott, and Jennifer.

Kay, Judy, Phyllis, Krista, Linda, Suzie, and all the folks at Clayton College for Natural Health who are doing wonderful things by empowering people to take charge of their health.

Howard, Robin, Fred, Artie, and Gary for putting a smile on my face virtually every day since 1995.

Jack Canfield, Mark Victor Hansen, T. Harv Eker, Les Brown, Seymour Segnit, Ron Edgar, and Alex Mandossian, all of whom have made a big difference in my life.

Gail Kingsbury and Christine Comaford-Lynch, thank you for your undying and generous support of everything I do.

Mike Adams the original "Health Ranger" of Natural News (www.naturalnews.com), Kevin Gianni, (www.liveawesome.com), and Jimmy Moore (www.livinglavidalowcarb.blogspot.com), all of whom have supported me greatly and all of whom are living their mission of bringing great health information to the masses despite an uphill battle against the Diet Dictocrats and Health Establishment.

An enormous thanks to my webmaster and marketing guru Christopher Loch at (www.whatismysecret.com).

And—as always—a huge thanks to Werner Erhard, whose contribution to my life has been incalculable. And a quiet thanks to the film director Robyn Symon (*Transformation: The Life and Legacy of Werner Erhard*) for finally redeeming his good name.

My family Jeffrey Bowden, Nancy Bowden, Pace Bowden, and Cadence Bowden, all of whom I love very much, even Pace.

All the four legged members of my family who make my life richer: Emily Christy Bowden and Woodstock Bowden, who come to work with me every day and think it's an adventure (almost as great as getting to go in the big box with wheels that goes to Starbucks), and to the late and beloved Allegra, Tigerlily, and Max.

And to the members of my chosen family who make my life amazing: Susan Wood and Christopher Duncan, Jackie "Sky London" Balough, Peter Breger, Oz Garcia, Gina Lombardi and Kevin Sizemore, Liz Neporent, Oliver Becaup and Jennifer Schneider (and Leslie), Scott Ellis, Billy Stritch, Zack Kleinman, my sisters Randy Graff and Lauree Dash, Kimberly Wright the Sushi Goddess, Glen Depke, Sharon Montgomery, Diana Lederman, and Lee Bessinger, I love you all.

All the members of the Warner Center USTA Men's Doubles Team, plus of course, Ron Ellison, Nikki Robbins, and my amazing tennis guru, Delroy Reid.

Many people ask about the secret to having a long and healthy life and are frequently told (only half kiddingly) *"pick the right parents."* I'd add to that *"pick the right life partner."* If I have one secret to my energy, it's having the best life partner in the world: Anja Christy.

She makes life amazing.

Every day in every possible way.

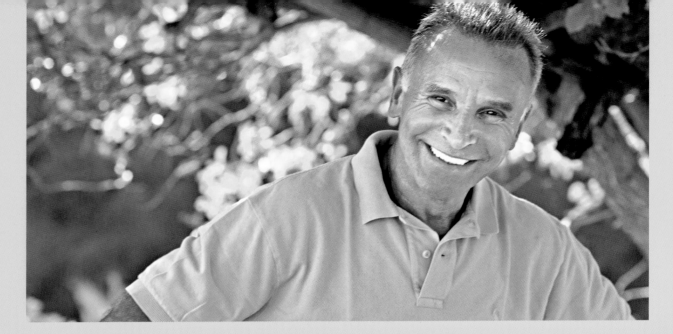

About the Author

Jonny Bowden, Ph.D., C.N.S., a board-certified nutrition specialist with a master's degree in psychology, is a nationally known expert on weight loss, nutrition, and health. A popular speaker and a former personal trainer with six national certifications in exercise, he was the acclaimed "Weight Loss Coach" on iVillage for twelve years, and is now an AOL Coach and a member of the Editorial Advisory Board of *Men's Health*.

His books have been acclaimed by a virtual who's who in the field of nutritional medicine, garnering endorsements by Christiane Northrup, M.D., Mehmet Oz, M.D., Barry Sears, Ph.D. (who calls him "one of the best"), Ann Louise Gittleman, Ph.D. (who calls him "the personal health coach I would want in my corner no matter what"), and many others. His book, *Living the Low Carb Life: Choosing the Diet That's Right for You from Atkins to Zone* has more than 100,000 copies in print. He is also the author of the Amazon best-seller *The Healthiest Foods on Earth: The Suprising Truth About What to Eat*, as well as *The Healthiest Meals on Earth* and *The Most Effective Natural Cures on Earth: The Suprising Truth about What Treatments Work and Why*.

He has been featured in the *New York Times*, the *New York Post*, *Chicago Sun Times*, *Chicago Tribune*, *Time*, *GQ*, *Cosmopolitan*, *Oxygen*, *Remedy*, *Family Circle*, *Self*, *Fitness*, *Allure*, *Essence*, *Men's Health*, *Pilates Style*, *Prevention*, *Woman's World*, *In Style*, *Fitness*, *Natural Health*, and *Shape*, and he has appeared on Fox News, CNN, MSNBC, ABC, NBC, and CBS as an expert on nutrition, weight loss, and health. He is currently a columnist for *Better Nutrition*, a contributing editor for both *Total Health* magazine and *Clean Living* magazine, and on the Editorial Advisory Board of *Men's Health*.

He lives in the Topanga Canyon area of Southern California.

His DVD, *The Truth About Weight Loss*, and his popular motivational CDs, programs, free newsletter, and many of the supplements recommended in this volume can be found at **www.jonnybowden.com**.

Index

communication, 236–240

connection, 273–275

Conrad, Claudius, 171

conversations, 236–238

CoQ10. *See* coenzyme Q10

corn, 60

corn syrup, 44

cortisol, 88, 100, 110, 162, 167, 202

Cow Palace, 262–263

Craig, Gary, 176

Craig, Will, 279

cranberry juice, 71

Crane, Frederick, 124

cravings, 44, 45, 56–57

Crayhon, Robert, 84, 127, 128, 279–280

creativity, 248–250

criticism, 258–259

crunches, *114*, 115–116

cucurbitacins, 68

curcumin, 205

curcurbitacins, 68

D

D'Adamo, Peter, 61

DAF. *See* directed attention fatigue (DAF)

dairy, 60

damaged fats, 40

Damasio, Antonio, 15

dancing, 179–180

David Wolfe's Sunfood Nutrition, 32, 75

dawn simulators, 92–93

de-cluttering, 222–225

deep breathing, 255–256

deltoids, 116

de Mejia, Elvira, 49–50

Dement, William, 81, 85, 87

DePaulis, Tomas, 73

Depke, Glen, 61, 63, 64, 175–177, 279

depressants, 89

depression, 141

Designs for Health, 48, 94

desk lights, 212

desktop, clearing, 222–224

detoxification, 143–159, 278

from air pollution, 152–153

basic program, 146–147

bathing, 149

brushing, 149

cleaning products and, 157–158

fasting, 145–147, 149

of the home, 153–156

of the liver, 158–159

"Master Cleanse", 147–148

milk thistle, 158–159

New Detox Diet, 145–147

from pollutants, 152–156

saunas, 150–152

DHEA, 193

DHT (dihydrotestosterone), 68

diet, 21–75, 279–280. *See also specific diets; specific foods and beverages; specific nutrients;* supplements

diet soda, 56–57

diindolylmethane. *See* DIM (diindolylmethane)

DIM (diindolylmethane), 205

directed attention fatigue (DAF), 250

direction, 241

disasters, fatigue-related, 79

disconnecting, 180–181

distractions, 224

DL-phenylalanine, 134

donations, 265

dopamine, 24, 110, 134, 172

DPBH test, 49

dressing up, 259–260

D-ribose, 127, 130–132

Dr. Tea's Tea Garden and Herbal Emporium, 47

Duke, Kacy, 237

E

Eades, Mary Dan, 26

Eades, Mike, 26, 280

Easy Raw Foods Breakfast, 52

ecotherapy, 169–171

EFT (Emotional Freedom Technique), 175–177, 279

Egan, Josephine M., 57

EGCG (epigallocatechin gallate), 129

L-tyrosine, 134
Lyena yoga, 174
lysine, 69, 127

M

maca, 75
macronutrients, 22, 23, 27, 38
magnesium, 127
Mannino, Matthew, 189, 190, 191
Margolskee, Robert F., 57
martial arts, 264
massage, 177-178
"Master Cleanse", 147-148
maté. *See* yerba maté tea
mattresses, 95
media-free days, 180-181
medial deltoids, 117
meditation, 277. *See also* mindfulness; yoga
medium-glycemic-load foods, 30
melatonin, 82-83, 92, 116, 216
Meltz, Lewis, 151-152
Meltzer, Carole, 252-253
menopause, 200, 201, 202, 203
meridians, 188
metabolic typing, 61
metabolism boosters, 46, 53
metabolites, 204
methanol, 57
micronutrients, 27
milk thistle, 158-159
mind, clearing the, 88
mindfulness, 106, 228, 272-273
minimalism, 223
mitochondria, 124, 126, 127, 133
Mittleman, Stu, 38-39
moderate-intensity cardio workout, 112
moderate-intensity weight training workout, 112
Mona-Vie, 70
mono-tasking, 228-229
Moore, Jimmy, 280
Moreno, Patricia, 101-102, 237, 277
Morinda citrifolia, 70
Morton, R. A., 124

movement, 99-101, 217
Moyad, Mark, 98, 128
multitasking, 228-230, 272
muscle building, 114-117
music, 171-173, 179-180

N

NAD (nicotinamide adenine dinucleotide). *See* ENADA; nicotine adenine dinucleotide (NAD)
Nappen, Lauren, 190
napping, 83-84
National Yogurt Assocation (NYA) "Live and Active Cultures" (LAC) seal, 138
Natural News, 280
nature, 169-171, 216-217, 251
negativity, 234-236, 258-259
Neporent, Liz, 118
neurotransmitters, 166-167, 174. *See also specific neurotransmitters*
New Detox Diet, 145-147
nicotine adenine dinucleotide (NAD), 125
nightcaps, 89
"no-frills-no-excuses-anytime-anywhere" workout, 113
noni juice, 70, 71
norepinephrine, 129
Norman, Suzanne, 278
nothing, doing, 264
Numi Organic Tea, 47
nutmeg, 266-267
nutrition, 21-75, 279-280. *See also specific foods and beverages; specific nutrients;* supplements
nutritional typing, 61-64
nutritional typing eating plans, 63-64
nutritional typing test, 62-63
Nutrition Town Hall, 279-280
nuts, 50-51, 266

O

oatmeal, 69
oats, 60
obesity, vitamin D and, 215
omega-3 fats, 39, 40, 48, 74, 128
omega-6 fats, 40, 74
omega-9 fats, 40

vitamin B_2, 124, 136

vitamin B_3, 124

vitamin B_6, 82, 93, 124, 125, 135-136

vitamin C, 35

vitamin D, 210, 211, 213-215, 217

vitamins. *See* B-complex vitamin; *specific vitamins*; *specific vitamins*

vitamin waters, 54

VOC. *See* volatile organic compounds (VOCs)

volatile organic compounds (VOCs), 154-155

volunteering, 244-246

von Karajan, Herbert, 15

W

Waitzkin, Josh, 229

Walster, Elaine, 246-247

water, 53-55, 91

weight control, 33, 206

weightlifting, 262-263

Weil, Andrew, 163-165

wheat, 60

wheatgrass, 36

Whey Cool, 48

Whey Protein Shake, 48

Wicherts, Ilse, 213

Willett, Walt, 39

Wilshire, Regina, 280

Wilson, Edward O., 251

Wilson's syndrome, 195

Withania somnifera. See ashwagandha

Wolcott, William, 61

Women's Voices for the Earth, 154

workouts. *See also* exercise
   10-minute energy boosting workouts, 110-112
   basic training, *114*, 114-117
   high-intensity workout, 111
   Jonny Bowden's Basic Training for Energy Workout, 118
   low-intensity workout, 110-111
   moderate-intensity cardio workout, 112
   moderate-intensity weight training workout, 112
   muscle building, 114-117
   "no-frills-no-excuses-anytime-anywhere" workout, 113

workplaces, clearing, 222-224

worrying, 88. *See also* anxiety

X

XanGo, 70

xanthines, 49

xenoestrogens, 200, 203, 205, 206

X-iser, 108-109, 277

xylitol, 45

Y

yerba maté tea, 49-50

yoga, 98, 102-104, 173-175, 277-278

Yoga Pulse, 277-278

yogurt, 137-138

Z

Zander, Lauren, 239-240, 279

Zone diet, 26-27